BATES' *Pocket Guide to*

Physical
Examination

AND History Taking

BATES' *Pocket Guide to*
Physical Examination
AND History Taking

NINTH EDITION

Lynn S. Bickley, MD, FACP
Clinical Professor of Internal Medicine
School of Medicine
University of New Mexico
Albuquerque, New Mexico

Peter G. Szilagyi, MD, MPH
Professor of Pediatrics and Executive Vice-Chair
Department of Pediatrics
University of California at Los Angeles (UCLA)
Los Angeles, California

Richard M. Hoffman, MD, MPH, FACP
Professor of Internal Medicine and Epidemiology
Director, Division of General Internal Medicine
University of Iowa Carver College of Medicine
Iowa City, Iowa

Guest Editor
Rainier P. Soriano, MD
Associate Professor of Medical Education, Geriatrics and Palliative Medicine
Brookdale Department of Geriatrics and Palliative Medicine
Associate Dean of Curriculum and Clinical Competence
Icahn School of Medicine at Mount Sinai
New York, New York

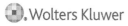 Wolters Kluwer

Philadelphia • Baltimore • New York • London
Buenos Aires • Hong Kong • Sydney • Tokyo

Not authorised for sale in United States, Canada, Australia, New Zealand, Puerto Rico, and U.S. Virgin Islands.

Acquisitions Editor: Crystal Taylor
Development Editor: Andrea Vosburgh
Freelance Development Editor: Kelly Horvath
Senior Editorial Coordinator: Emily Buccieri
Editorial Assistant: Parisa Saranj
Marketing Manager: Phyllis Hitner
Production Project Manager: Catherine Ott
Design Coordinator: Stephen Druding
Art Director, Illustration: Jennifer Clements
Illustrator: Body Scientific International
Photographer: Thibodeau Media Group
Manufacturing Coordinator: Margie Orzech
Prepress Vendor: Aptara, Inc.

Ninth edition

Library of Congress Cataloging-in-Publication Data

Names: Bickley, Lynn S., author. | Szilagyi, Peter G., author. | Hoffman, Richard M., author. | Soriano, Rainier P., editor. | Bickley, Lynn S. Bates' guide to physical examination and history-taking. 13th ed.
Title: Bates' pocket guide to physical examination and history taking / Lynn S. Bickley, Peter G. Szilagyi, Richard M. Hoffman ; guest editor, Rainier P. Soriano.
Other titles: Pocket guide to physical examination and history taking
Description: Ninth edition. | Philadelphia, PA : Wolters Kluwer, 2021. | Abridgement of Bates' guide to physical examination and history-taking. / Lynn S. Bickley, Peter G. Szilagyi, Richard M. Hoffman. Thirteenth edition. [2021]. | Includes bibliographical references and index.
Identifiers: LCCN 2020032374 | ISBN 9781975109875 (paperback)
Subjects: MESH: Physical Examination–methods | Medical History Taking–methods | Handbook
Classification: LCC RC78.7.D53 | NLM WB 39 | DDC 616.07/54–dc23
LC record available at https://lccn.loc.gov/2020032374

This book is dedicated to you,

the ever-constant student, teacher,

and practitioner of this continuously

evolving art and science of medicine.

Faculty Reviewers and Additional Contributors

GEORGE A. ALBA, MD
Instructor, Pulmonary and Critical
Care Medicine
Department of Medicine
Massachusetts General Hospital
Harvard Medical School
Boston, Massachusetts

CATHERINE A. BIGELOW, MD
Maternal-Fetal Medicine Subspecialist
Minnesota Perinatal Physicians
Allina Health
Minneapolis, Minnesota

Y. JULIA CHEN, MD
Clinical Fellow
Department of Pediatric Surgery
Johns Hopkins University School of
Medicine
Baltimore, Maryland

SUZANNE B. COOPEY, MD
Assistant Professor, Harvard University
Faculty of Medicine
Division of Surgical Oncology
Massachusetts General Hospital
Boston, Massachusetts

CHRISTOPHER T. DOUGHTY, MD
Instructor, Neurology
Department of Neurology, Division of
Neuromuscular Disorders
Harvard Medical School/Brigham and
Women's Hospital
Boston, Massachusetts

RALPH P. FADER, MD
Child and Adolescent Psychiatry Fellow
Department of Psychiatry
New York-Presbyterian
New York, New York

RAISA GAO, MD, FACOG
Assistant Professor
Department of Obstetrics, Gynecology,
and Reproductive Science
Icahn School of Medicine at Mount Sinai
New York, New York

SARAH GUSTAFSON, MD
Assistant Clinical Professor, Pediatrics
Division of Pediatric Hospital
Medicine, Harbor-UCLA
David Geffen School of Medicine at
UCLA
Los Angeles, California

ALEXANDER R. LLOYD, MD
Resident Physician
Department of Physical Medicine and
Rehabilitation
University of Pittsburgh Medical Center
Pittsburgh, Pennsylvania

CHRISTOPHER C. LO, MD
Instructor
Stein and Doheny Eye Institutes,
Department of Orbital and Oculofacial
Plastic Surgery
University of California at Los Angeles
Los Angeles, California

S. ANDREW MCCULLOUGH, MD
Assistant Professor, Clinical Medicine
Assistant Director, Graphics Laboratory
Department of Medicine, Division of
Cardiology
Weill Cornell Medicine
New York, New York

MATTHEW E. POLLARD, MD
Fellow, Male Reproductive Medicine
and Surgery
Scott Department of Urology
Baylor College of Medicine
Houston, Texas

KATELYN O. STEPAN, MD
Fellow, Head and Neck Surgical Oncology
and Microvascular Reconstruction
Otolaryngology—Head and Neck
Surgery
Washington University School of
Medicine in St. Louis
St. Louis, Missouri

JOSEPH M. TRUGLIO, MD, MPH
Assistant Professor of Internal Medicine,
Pediatrics and Medical Education
Program Director, Internal Medicine
and Pediatrics Residency
Departments of Internal Medicine and
Pediatrics
Icahn School of Medicine at Mount Sinai
New York, New York

ADDITIONAL CONTRIBUTORS

PAUL J. CUMMINS, PHD
Assistant Professor, Medical Education
Department of Medical Education, The
Bioethics Program
Icahn School of Medicine at Mount
Sinai
New York, New York

ROCCO M. FERRANDINO, MD, MSCR
Resident Physician
Department of Otolaryngology—Head
and Neck Surgery
Icahn School of Medicine at Mount
Sinai
New York, New York

DAVID W. FLEENOR, STM
Director of Education, Center for
Spirituality and Health
Icahn School of Medicine at Mount
Sinai
New York, New York

BEVERLY A. FORSYTH, MD
Associate Professor of Medicine,
Infectious Diseases and Medical
Education
Medical Director of the Morchand
Center for Clinical Competence
Division of Infectious Diseases and
Department of Medical Education
Icahn School of Medicine at Mount
Sinai
New York, New York

NADA GLIGOROV, PHD
Associate Professor, Medical Education
Department of Medical Education, The
Bioethics Program
Icahn School of Medicine at Mount
Sinai
New York, New York

JOANNE R. HOJSAK, MD
Professor, Pediatrics and Medical Education
Director, Pediatric LifeLong Care Team
Pediatric Critical Care/Mount Sinai Kravis Children's Hospital
Icahn School of Medicine at Mount Sinai
New York, New York

SCOTT JELINEK, MD, MED, MPH
Resident Physician
Department of Pediatrics
Icahn School of Medicine at Mount Sinai
New York, New York

GISELLE N. LYNCH, MD
Resident Physician
Department of Ophthalmology
New York Eye and Ear Infirmary of Mount Sinai
New York, New York

ANTHONY J. MELL, MD, MBA
Resident Physician
Boston Combined Residency Program
Boston Children's Hospital and Boston Medical Center
Boston, Massachusetts

ANN-GEL S. PALERMO, DRPH, MPH
Associate Professor
Associate Dean for Diversity and Inclusion in Biomedical Education
Department of Medical Education
Office for Diversity and Inclusion
Icahn School of Medicine at Mount Sinai
New York, New York

KATHERINE A. ROZA, MD
Assistant Professor
Northwell Health House Calls Program
Donald and Barbara Zucker School of Medicine at Hofstra/Northwell
New Hyde Park, New York

ANNETTY P. SOTO, DMD
Clinical Assistant Professor and Team Leader
Division of General Dentistry
Department of Restorative Dental Sciences
University of Florida College of Dentistry
Gainesville, Florida

MITCHELL B. WICE, MD
Integrated Geriatric and Palliative Care Fellow
Brookdale Department of Geriatrics and Palliative Medicine
Icahn School of Medicine at Mount Sinai
New York, New York

STUDENT CONTRIBUTORS

EMILY N. TIXIER, BA
Medical Student
Icahn School of Medicine at Mount Sinai
New York, New York

ISAAC WASSERMAN, MPH
Medical Student
Icahn School of Medicine at Mount Sinai
New York, New York

Preface

Bates' Pocket Guide to Physical Examination and History Taking, ninth edition, is a concise, portable text, with new chapters that expand its scope to include all aspects of clinical skills training and education. This guide:

- Introduces the patient encounter and its critical elements.
- Provides frameworks of advanced communication and interpersonal skills.
- Describes how to interview the patient and take the health history.
- Details and illustrates the steps of each of the regional physical examinations.
- Emphasizes common, normal, and abnormal physical findings.
- Presents a stepwise approach to the process of clinical reasoning.
- Includes visual aids and comparative tables to guide recognition of common and selected findings.

A highlight of this *Pocket Guide,* ninth edition, is the inclusion of clinical diagnostic algorithms for common signs and symptoms at the end of each regional examination chapter. These algorithms are provided as tools to facilitate thinking through tiers of considerations in clinical decision making. These are not presented as definitive but rather as examples of the types of decision-making clinicians might want to consider. Remember that each patient presenting with a particular set of symptoms has unique characteristics. The algorithms presented in this book are intended for use as diagnostic learning guides and not as the sole drivers of diagnostic and management protocols for individual patients.

The *Pocket Guide* is not meant to serve as a primary text for learning the elements of the clinician–patient encounter and its associated skills of history taking or physical examination. Its detail is too brief. It is intended instead as an aid for recall of the regional examinations and examinations for special populations and as a convenient, brief, and portable reference. There are several ways to use the *Pocket Guide:*

- Review and remember the various elements to consider in the clinician–patient encounter.
- Review and remember the content of a health history.
- Review and practice the techniques of examination.

- Look up special maneuvers or techniques related to the physical examination as the need arises.
- Review common variations of normal and selected abnormalities. Observations are keener and more precise when the examiner knows what to look, listen, and feel for.
- Look up additional information about possible findings, including abnormalities and standards of normal.
- Review clinical recommendations related to screening, health maintenance, and disease prevention.

Contents

Faculty Reviewers and Additional Contributors   vi
Preface   ix

CHAPTER **1**
Approach to the Clinical Encounter   1

CHAPTER **2**
Interviewing, Communication, and Interpersonal Skills   19

CHAPTER **3**
Health History   33

CHAPTER **4**
Physical Examination   53

CHAPTER **5**
Clinical Reasoning, Assessment, and Plan   65

CHAPTER **6**
Health Maintenance and Screening   79

CHAPTER **7**
Evaluating Clinical Evidence   102

CHAPTER **8**
General Survey, Vital Signs, and Pain   112

CHAPTER **9**
Cognition, Behavior, and Mental Status   128

CHAPTER **10**
Skin, Hair, and Nails   148

CHAPTER **11**
Head and Neck   176

CHAPTER **12**
Eyes   183

CHAPTER **13**
Ears and Nose   199

CHAPTER **14**
Throat and Oral Cavity   211

CHAPTER **15**
Thorax and Lungs   221

CHAPTER **16**
Cardiovascular System   243

CHAPTER **17**
Peripheral Vascular System   269

CHAPTER **18**
Breasts and Axillae   285

CHAPTER **19**
Abdomen   299

CHAPTER **20**
Male Genitalia   323

CHAPTER **21**
Female Genitalia   336

CHAPTER **22**
Anus, Rectum, and Prostate   354

CHAPTER **23**
Musculoskeletal System   363

CHAPTER **24**
Nervous System   409

CHAPTER **25**
Children: Infancy through Adolescence   453

CHAPTER **26**
Pregnant Woman   503

CHAPTER **27**
Older Adult   533

INDEX   **563**

Approach to the Clinical Encounter

APPROACH TO THE CLINICAL ENCOUNTER

The approach to a clinical encounter is *both* clinician centered and patient centered (Fig. 1-1).

- *Clinician-centered* approach is more symptom focused and concentrates on the pathologic disease.
- *Patient-centered* approach follows the patient's lead to understand their thoughts, ideas, concerns, and requests and evokes the personal context of the patient's symptoms and disease.

The balance between these two essential components results in an effective clinical interview in a patient encounter.

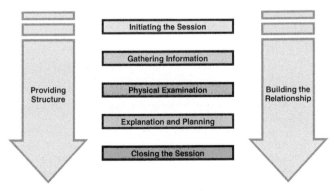

FIGURE 1-1. Enhanced Calgary–Cambridge guides. (Reproduced from Kurtz S, et al. Marrying content and process in clinical method teaching: enhancing the Calgary-Cambridge guides. *Acad Med*. 2003;78(8):802–809.)

General Structure and Sequence of the Clinical Encounter

In general, the clinical encounter moves through several stages (Box 1-1). Throughout this sequence, you must always stay attuned to the patient's feelings, help the patient express them, respond to their content, and validate their significance.

BOX 1-1. Stages of the Clinical Encounter

Stage 1: Initiating the Encounter
- Set the stage/preparation
- Greet the patient and establish initial rapport

Stage 2: Gathering Information
- Initiate information gathering
- Explore patient's perspective of illness
- Explore biomedical perspective of disease including relevant background and context

Stage 3: Performing the Physical Examination

Stage 4: Explaining and Planning
- Provide correct amount and type of information
- Negotiate plan of action
- Pursue shared decision making

Stage 5: Closing the Encounter

Stage 1: Initiating the Encounter

- **Set the stage and prepare for the interview.** Check your appearance. Make sure the patient is comfortable and the environment is conducive to the personal information soon to be shared.
  - *Adjust the environment.* Always consider the patient's privacy. Pull shut any bedside curtains. Suggest moving to an empty room rather than having a conversation that can be overheard. Choose a distance that facilitates conversation and allows good eye contact.
  - *Review the clinical record.* Before seeing the patient, review the electronic health record (EHR). It often provides valuable information about past diagnoses and treatments; however, data may be incomplete or even disagree with what you learn from the patient, so be open to developing new approaches or ideas.
  - *Set your agenda.* Clarify your goals for the interview. A clinician must balance *provider-centered goals* with *patient-centered goals*. The clinician's task is to balance these multiple agendas.

- **Greet the patient.** *Greet the patient* by name and introduce yourself, giving your name. If possible, shake hands. If this is the first contact, explain your role, including your status as a student and how you will be involved in the patient's care. As much as possible, let patients dictate how they would like to be addressed.
  - *Clinicians should ask all patients their preferred name and gender pronouns.* Avoid first names unless you have specific permission from the patient.
  - When asking patients about their pronouns, it can be helpful to share your own pronouns with patients, asking: "Which gender pronouns do you use?" For example, "I use... he and him/she and hers/they and theirs."
- **Establish initial rapport** (Box 1-2). Several measures to establish initial rapport include:
  - *Maintain confidentiality.* Let the patient decide if visitors or family members should remain in the room and ask for the patient's permission before conducting the interview in front of them.
  - *Attend to the patient's comfort.* Ask how he or she is feeling and if you are coming at a convenient time. Look for signs of discomfort, such as frequent changes of position or facial expressions that show pain or anxiety. Arranging the bed may make the patient more comfortable.
  - *Arrange the environment.* Choose a distance that facilitates conversation and good eye contact. Try to sit at eye level with the patient. Move any physical barriers between you and the patient, such as desks or bedside tables, or the computer screen, out of the way.
  - *Provide undivided attention.* Spend enough time on small talk to put the patient at ease. If necessary, jot down short phrases, specific dates, or words rather than trying to put them into a final format. Maintain good eye contact, especially when using the electronic health record. Whenever the patient is talking about sensitive or disturbing material, put down your pen or pause from typing at the keyboard.

BOX 1-2. Establishing Initial Rapport with Patients in Various Age Groups

Specific Population	General Initial Approach
Newborns and infants	▪ While the newborn (birth–30 days) or infant (1 month–1 year) may not be able to talk with you; they will still react to the emotional and physical cues that you convey, so keep your voice calm. ▪ Encourage caregivers to hold the baby wherever he/she is most comfortable for as much of the encounter as possible.

continued

	■ Begin the encounter by focusing on the caregivers and asking about their well-being. This makes it obvious that you are caring as much for them as their child and typically helps place them at ease.
Young and school-aged children	■ Young (1–4 years) and school-aged children (5–10 years) are characterized as having increasing feelings of autonomy, socialization, and curiosity, all things to which you as a clinician will need to be sensitive to. ■ Beginning the encounter from a place of play is a great way to build rapport with the child and the parents. Many of the important milestones to assess in this age group are typical ways of playing (i.e., jumping, drawing, imitating, and throwing a ball). ■ Introduce yourself to the patient first and then to the family. ■ When possible pull the school-aged child into the interview by asking age-appropriate questions. You should ask caregivers to confirm or elaborate as needed.
Adolescents	■ Adolescents generally want to be treated as adults and to be given respect and choices. ■ Frequently the most challenging part of this encounter for clinicians is balancing the needs of the family and the autonomy of the adolescent. ■ It is important that you direct questions to and obtain responses from your adolescent patient while at the same time ensuring that family members and caregivers feel comfortable and that their concerns are heard. ■ Provide ample opportunity for the adolescent to share questions or concerns with you through the use of broad open-ended questions. ■ A significant part of these clinical encounters is the increasing amount of time you will spend with your adolescent patient alone without any family members present. During this time, it is critical that you acknowledge the confidentiality and trust inherent to that space.
Older adults	■ Elicit from older patients their preferred way of being addressed. Calling an older adult patient *"dear," "sweetie,"* or overly familiar names can be perceived as depersonalizing and demeaning. ■ Take the time to adjust the clinical environment. Provide a well-lit, moderately warm setting with minimal background noise, chairs with arms, and access to the examining table. ■ Ensure safety in the examination room for the older adult patient to safely navigate especially if ambulating with an assistive device such as a cane or a walker. ■ Allow time for open-ended questions and reminiscing. ■ Include family and caregivers when indicated, especially if the patient has cognitive impairment.

Patients with Physical and Sensory Disabilities. Use *"people-first" language* especially when referring to patients with disabilities unless the patient asks to be referred to in another manner. You should always speak directly with a patient and not to any companion that the patient with physical and/or sensory disability may have. Box 1-3 provides guidelines on establishing initial rapport with patients with disabilities.

BOX 1-3. **Establishing Initial Rapport with Patients with Physical and Sensory Disabilities**	
Patients who are blind or have low vision	■ Always verbally identify yourself when you approach and introduce other people in the room.
	■ Let the patient know when you are leaving.
	■ Ask before you help how they would like to be assisted. Ask the person before you touch him/her.
	■ Be prepared to provide written materials in an auditory, tactile, or electronic format of the patient's preference (audio file, Braille, large print).
	■ Verbally explain what is about to happen before beginning the encounter and ask the patients if they have any questions.
	■ Tell the patient where personal effects (clothes and other belongings) are in the room and do not move them without telling the patient.
	■ Staff should be welcoming and describe the physical environment (doors, steps, ramps, bathroom location, etc.).
	■ Never distract or touch a service animal without asking the owner.
Patients who are hard of hearing	■ Ask how best to communicate.
	■ Be prepared to give written materials as long as they are not the primary form of communication.
	■ Inform patients that sign language interpreting and real-time captioning services are available.
	■ If requested, promptly provide these services for effective communication.
	■ Do not talk to the patient from a distance or from another room.
	■ Look directly at patients when speaking so they can see your mouth.
	■ Speak normally and clearly. Do not shout, exaggerate mouth movements, or speak rapidly.
	■ Minimize background noise and glare.

continued

Patients who are deaf	■ Ask how best to communicate. ■ Inform patients that sign language interpreting and real-time captioning services are available. ■ If requested, promptly provide these services for effective communication. ■ Family members should not be used to interpret. ■ Address the patient, not the interpreter. ■ Be prepared to give written materials as long as they are not the primary form of communication.
Patients who use wheelchairs	■ Make sure there is a path of access to the room. ■ Respect personal space, including wheelchair and assistive devices. ■ Do not propel the wheelchair unless asked. ■ Provide accessible equipment as needed. ■ Provide assistance as needed, such as by clearing obstacles from the path of travel or helping patients transfer to equipment if accessible equipment is unavailable. ■ Do not separate patients from their wheelchairs.

Source: World Institute on Disability. *Access to Medical Care: Adults with Physical Disabilities.* Available at https://wid.org/2016/01/08/access-to-medical-care-dvd-training/.

Lesbian, Gay, Bisexual, and Transgender (LGBT) Adult Patients

■ In 2013, in a sample of more than 34,000 adults, 1.6% identified as gay or lesbian, 0.7% identified as bisexual, and 1.1% responded either other or did not know. Most respondents were between the ages of 18 and 64 years; more than 726,000 households are same-sex couples; 34% had same-sex spouses.

■ LGBT patients have higher rates of depression, suicide, anxiety, drug use, sexual victimization, and risk of infection with HIV and STIs.

■ One-third (33%) of transgender people who saw a healthcare provider in the past year reported having at least one negative experience related to being transgender, such as "being refused treatment, verbally harassed, or physically or sexually assaulted, or having to teach the provider about transgender people in order to get appropriate care, with higher rates for people of color and people with disabilities."

■ The Institute of Medicine has stated that barriers to accessing quality health care for LGBT adults are "a lack of providers who are knowledgeable about LGBT health needs as well as a fear of discrimination in health care settings."

Learning to make LGBT patients feel comfortable and trust you enough to reveal such personal information will take time (Box 1-4). Practicing and apologizing for mistakes as you learn will help you develop these skills.

BOX 1-4. Establishing Initial Rapport with LGBT Patients

Best Practice	Example
When addressing new patients, avoid pronouns or gender terms like "sir" or "ma'am."	■ "How may I help you today?"
When talking to colleagues about new patients, avoid pronouns and gender terms. Or, use gender-neutral words such as "they." Never refer to someone as "it."	■ "Your patient is here in the waiting room." ■ "They are here for their 3 o'clock appointment."
Politely and privately ask if you are unsure about a patient's preferred name or pronouns.	■ "What name and pronouns would you like us to use?" ■ "I would like to be respectful–how would you like to be addressed?"
Ask respectfully about names if they do not match in your records.	■ "Could your chart be under another name?" ■ "What is the name on your insurance?"
Avoid assuming the gender of patient's partners.	■ "Are you in a relationship?"
Use the terms people use to describe themselves.	■ If someone calls himself "gay," do not use the term "homosexual." ■ If a woman refers to her "wife," then say, "your wife" when referring to her; do not say "your friend."
Only ask for information that is required.	■ Ask yourself: What do I know? What do I need to know? How can I ask in a sensitive way?
Did you make a mistake? Apologize.	■ "I apologize for using the wrong pronoun. I did not mean to disrespect you."

Reprinted with permission from Providing Inclusive Services and Care for LGBT People. National LGBT Health Education Center. Available at https://www.lgbthealtheducation.org/wp-content/uploads/Providing-Inclusive-Services-and-Care-for-LGBT-People.pdf

Stage 2: Gathering Information

■ **Initiate information gathering** by:

■ *Establishing an agenda.* It is important to identify both your own and the patient's issues at the beginning of the encounter. Often, you may need to focus the interview by asking the patient which problem is most pressing. For example, "Do you have some special concerns today? Which one are you most concerned about?" Some patients may not have a specific complaint or problem. *It is still important to start with the patient's story.*

■ *Inviting the patient to tell story.* Encourage patients to tell their own stories, using their own words. Begin with *open-ended questions* that allow full freedom of response: "Tell me more about…" Avoid questions that restrict the patient to a minimally informative "yes" or "no" answer. *Listen to the patient's answers without interrupting.*

■ *Following the patient's leads.* Use verbal and nonverbal cues that prompt patients to recount their stories spontaneously. Use *continuers,* especially at the outset, such as nodding your head and using phrases such as "Uh huh," "Go on," and "I see."

■ **Explore the patient's perspective of illness.** *Disease* is the explanation that the *clinician* uses to organize symptoms that lead to a clinical diagnosis. *Illness* is a construct that explains how the patient experiences the disease, including its effects on relationships, function, and sense of well-being. The interview needs to include both of these views of reality. Learning how patients perceive illness means asking patient-centered questions in the four domains listed below, which follow the mnemonic "FIFE" (Box 1-5).

BOX 1-5. Exploring the Patient's Perspective (F-I-F-E)

	Description
Feelings	Explore patient's feelings, including fears or concerns, about the problem
Ideas	Explore patient's ideas about the nature and the cause of the problem
Function	Explore the effect of the problem on the patient's life and function
Expectations	Explore patient's expectations of the disease, of the clinician, or of health care, often based on prior personal or family experiences

■ **Identify and respond to the patient's emotional cues.** Patients offer various clues to their concerns that may be direct or indirect, verbal or nonverbal; they may express them as ideas or emotions. Acknowledging and responding to these clues help build rapport, expand the clinician's understanding of the illness, and improve patient satisfaction. Clues to the patient's perspective on illness are provided in Box 1-6.

BOX 1-6. Respond to Emotional Cues Using NURSE Statements

NURSE	Example Statements
Name the emotion	*"That sounds like a scary experience"*
Understand or legitimize emotion	*"It's understandable that you feel that way"*
Respect	*"You've done better than most people would with this"*
Support	*"I will continue to work with you on this"*
Explore	*"How else were you feeling about it?"*

- **Explore the biomedical perspective and relevant background information/context.** Each symptom has attributes that must be clarified, including context, associations, and chronology, especially for pain.
  - It is critical to understand fully every symptom's essential characteristics. *Always elicit the attributes of a symptom.* Helpful mnemonic: OLD CARTS, or **O**nset, **L**ocation, **D**uration, **C**haracter, **A**ggravating/**A**lleviating Factors, **R**adiation, and **T**iming; and OPQRST, or **O**nset, **P**alliating/**P**rovoking Factors, **Q**uality, **R**adiation, **S**ite, and **T**iming.
  - The past medical history, family history, personal and social history, and review of systems give shape and depth to the patient's story. The personal and social history is an opportunity for you to see the patient as a person and gain deeper understanding of the patient's outlook and background which strengthens your therapeutic alliance. This segment will be described in detail in Chapter 3, Health History.

Stage 3: Performing the Physical Examination. It is critical that you maintain your patient's comfort throughout, avoid embarrassment, and demonstrate facility with the skills required of the examination to enhance their satisfaction with the clinical encounter. This will be discussed further in Chapter 4, Physical Examination.

Stage 4: Explaining and Planning. This stage includes the generation and explanation of the patient's chief concern from the clinician's (disease) and patient's (illness) perspectives. The goal is to provide information that relates to the patient's perspective of the problem and achieve a shared understanding.

- **Provide correct amount and type of information.** A useful technique to assess the patient's understanding is to "*teach back*," whereby you invite the patient to tell you, in his or her own words, the plan of care (p. 22). Keep in mind "teach back" is not a test of the patient's knowledge. It is a test of how well you explained things in a manner your patient understands.
- **Share the treatment plan.** *Shared decision making* involves a three-step process: introducing choices and describing options, using patient decision support tools when available; exploring patient preferences; and moving to a decision, checking that the patient is ready to make a decision and offering more time if needed.

Stage 5: Closing the Session

- **Close the interview and visit.** Make sure the patient fully understands the plans you have developed together. Review future evaluation, treatments, and follow-up. Give the patient a chance to ask any final questions.
- **Take time for self-reflection.** Because we bring our own values, assumptions, and biases to every encounter, we must look inward to clarify how our expectations and reactions may affect what we hear and how we behave. Self-reflection brings a deepening personal awareness to our work with patients and is one of the most rewarding aspects of providing patient care.

DISPARITIES IN HEALTH CARE

Social Determinants of Health

Social determinants of health are the social, economic, and political conditions that influence the health of individuals and populations. Clinicians and other health care professionals need to improve patient health and reduce inequities at many levels.

- Economic stability (employment, food security, housing stability, level of poverty)
- Education (early childhood education and development, enrollment in higher education, high school graduation, language and literacy)
- Social and community context (civic participation, discrimination, incarceration, social cohesion)
- Health and health care (access to health care, access to primary care, health literacy)
- Neighborhood and built environment (access to foods that support healthy eating patterns, level of crime and violence, environmental conditions, quality of housing)

Racism and Bias

- *Implicit bias* is a set of unconscious beliefs or associations that lead to a negative evaluation of a person on the basis of their perceived group identity.
- *Explicit bias* is the conscious or deliberate decisions or preferences founded on beliefs, stereotypes, or associations on the basis of a perceived group identity.

The aggregation of these biases can lead to a structural system of privilege (*institutional bias*) that misallocates care, particularly for marginalized groups. There are several clinical skills that can mitigate the impact of bias in clinical encounters (Box 1-7).

BOX 1-7. Skills and Practices to Mitigate Bias in Your Clinical Encounters

Reflect on patterns of emotion and behavior.	Pay attention to how you feel and how you behave around patients of different identities. The patterns you begin to recognize may reflect biases that can impact your interactions with patients, as well as your clinical reasoning. Becoming aware of these biases is the first step in reducing their impact on patient care.
Pause before starting an encounter and prepare for potential triggers of bias.	Once you are aware of your potential biases, pay attention to situations that may trigger them. Simply being aware of a bias might help minimize its effect. You may take deliberate actions to reduce the impact of your biases.
Generate alternative hypotheses for biases anchored in behavior.	Many biases are anchored in clinician assumptions about patient behavior (nonadherence, substance use, etc.). Make it a habit to consider what structural forces (socioeconomic status, race/racism, homophobia, etc.) impact patient behaviors, and how these alternative hypotheses can challenge assumptions you make about patients.
Practice universal communication and interpersonal skills.	Often clinicians will not recognize when a bias is at play in a clinical encounter. Universal communication and interpersonal skills can serve to reduce the impact of unconscious biases on the way you interact with patients.
Explore your patients' identities.	Many biases are anchored in clinician assumptions around patient identities. By simply asking patients to clarify what their identities mean to them, clinicians can dismantle their assumptions and better understand their patients.
Explore your patients' experiences of bias.	Clinical encounters are influenced by patients' prior experiences of implicit and explicit bias in health care. Exploring these experiences can help you partner with your patients and better understand their approach to health care.

Cultural Humility. *Cultural humility* is defined as a "process that requires humility as individuals continually engage in self-reflection and self-critique as lifelong learners and reflective practitioners" in an effort to address power imbalances and to advocate for others.

You should engage in self-reflection, critical thinking, and cultural humility as you experience diversity in your clinical training (Box 1-8).

BOX 1-8.   5Rs of Cultural Humility

	Aim	Ask
Reflection	Clinicians will approach every encounter with humility and understanding that there is always something to learn from everyone.	What did I learn from each person in that encounter?
Respect	Clinicians will treat every person with the utmost respect and strive to preserve dignity at all times.	Did I treat everyone involved in that encounter respectfully?
Regard	Clinicians will hold every person in their highest regard, be aware of, and not allow unconscious biases to interfere in any interactions.	Did unconscious biases drive this interaction?
Relevance	Clinicians will expect cultural humility to be relevant and apply this practice to every encounter.	How was cultural humility relevant in this encounter?
Resiliency	Clinicians will embody the practice of cultural humility to enhance personal resiliency and global compassion.	How was my personal resiliency affected by this interaction?

Source: Reprinted with permission from Society of Hospital Medicine. The 5Rs of cultural humility. Available from https://www.hospitalmedicine.org/practice-management/the-5-rs-of-cultural-humility/. Accessed May 30, 2019.

OTHER MAJOR CONSIDERATIONS

Spirituality

Spirituality encompasses religion, but is broader, focusing on larger universal themes such as meaning and purpose, transcendence and connection with others. It is the aspect of humanity that refers to the way individuals seek and express meaning and purpose and the way they experience their connectedness to the moment, to self, to others, to nature, and to the significant and sacred (Spiritual History and FICA, pp. 41–42).

Medical Ethics

Medical ethics, a subdiscipline of applied ethics, which is itself a subdiscipline of philosophy, is the system of norms that has evolved to guide the practice and support clinical decision making.

Respect for autonomy, in addition to the older principles of beneficence, nonmaleficence, and justice, was established as the common core of health care ethics and has been incorporated into most professional codes for health care providers (Box 1-9).

BOX 1-9. Core Values of Medical Ethics

Core Value	Description
Beneficence	■ The dictum that clinicians are to act for the patients' good by preventing or treating disease.
Confidentiality	■ The duty to prevent the disclosure of patients' personal information to parties who are not authorized to learn that information.
Decisional capacity	■ The ability to make an autonomous choice that clinicians should respect.
Informed consent	■ The principle that clinicians must elicit patients' voluntary and informed authorization to test or treat them for illness or injury. ■ Because patients cannot consent to treatment without knowing what they are being treated for, this principle also encompasses the responsibility to inform patients of diagnoses, prognoses, and treatment alternatives.
Justice	■ The value that all patients with similar medical needs should receive similar medical treatment and should be treated fairly by clinicians.
Nonmaleficence ("first, do no harm")	■ The directive that health care professionals should avoid causing harm to patients and minimize the negative effects of treatments.
Respect for autonomy	■ The commitment to accept the choices patients with decisional capacity make about which treatments to undergo, including to reject treatment. The addition of this value to medical ethics changed the clinician–patient relationship from paternalistic one to collaborative.
Truth telling	■ The value that clinicians should disclose information beyond what is required by informed consent that may be relevant to patients (e.g., the number of similar procedures a physician has performed).

Decisional Capacity

If indicated, you may need to determine whether a patient has *decisional capacity* (Box 1-10). *Capacity* is a clinical designation and can be assessed by clinicians, whereas *competence* is a judicial determination and can only be decided by a court. For patients with impaired capacity, a *surrogate informant* or *decision maker* may assist with the history. Check whether the patient has a *durable power of attorney for health care* or a *healthcare proxy*.

BOX 1-10. Elements of Decision-Making Capacity

Patients must have the ability to:

- Understand the relevant information about proposed diagnostic tests or treatment,
- Appreciate their situation (including their underlying values and current clinical situation),
- Use reason to make a decision, and
- Communicate their choice.

Source: Sessums LL, et al. Does this patient have medical decision-making capacity? *JAMA*. 2011;306:420.

APPROACH TO A CLINICAL ETHICAL DILEMMA

When you need to explicitly consider the ethical aspects of the clinical situation, heuristics can provide guidance for how to reason through an ethical dilemma (Box 1-11). This practical method is not guaranteed to be optimal or perfect but instead sufficient for reaching an immediate goal.

BOX 1-11. How to Resolve a Clinical Ethical Dilemma

1. Clearly state the ethical question
2. Collect relevant information
   - Medical facts
   - Patient preferences and interests (e.g., culture, religion, social support, financial concerns, quality of life)
     - Does the patient have capacity?
     - Does the patient have advance directives or a surrogate?
   - Other parties' preferences
3. Identify ethical principles and guidelines
   - Are there legal guidelines that apply to the case?
   - Are there institutional guidelines that apply to the case?
   - What ethical values are relevant to the case?

4. Delineate and relate options to values and principles
   - Identify course of action by prioritizing each of the ethical values.
   - If principle X is primary, then course of action Y is justified, etc.
5. Evaluate the different options
   - Formulate justification for best course of action by identifying the dominant principle based on legal, institutional, and ethical guidelines.
6. Make an action plan

DOCUMENTING THE CLINICAL ENCOUNTER

Quality Clinical Record

The *clinical record* serves a dual purpose—it reflects your analysis of the patient's health status, and it documents the unique features of the patient's history, examination, laboratory and test results, assessment, and plan in a formal written format. A clear, well-organized clinical record is one of the most important adjuncts to patient care. Think especially about the *order and readability* of the record and the *amount of detail* needed. Use the checklist in Box 1-12 to make sure your record is informative and easy to follow.

BOX 1-12. Checklist to Ensure a Quality Clinical Record

- **Is the order clear?**
  Order is imperative. Make sure that readers can easily find specific points of information. Keep the *subjective* items of the history, for example, in the history; do not let them stray into the physical examination. Did you:
  - Make the headings clear?
  - Accent your organization with indentations and spacing?
  - Arrange the *History of Present Illness* in chronologic order, starting with the current episode, then filling in relevant background information?

- **Do the data included contribute directly to the assessment?**
  Spell out the supporting evidence, both positive and negative, for each problem or diagnosis. Make sure there is sufficient detail to support your differential diagnosis and plan.

continued

- **Are pertinent negatives specifically described?**
  Often portions of the history or examination suggest that an abnormality might exist or develop in that area. For example, for the patient with notable bruises, record the "pertinent negatives," such as the absence of injury or violence, familial bleeding disorders, or medications or nutritional deficits that might lead to bruising. For the patient who is depressed but not suicidal, recording both facts is important. In the patient with a transient mood swing, on the other hand, a comment on suicide is unnecessary.

- **Are there overgeneralizations or omissions of important data?**
  Remember that data not recorded are data lost. No matter how vividly you can recall clinical details today, you will probably not remember them in a few months. The phrase "neurologic exam negative," even in your own handwriting, may leave you wondering in a few months' time, "Did I really check the reflexes?"

- **Is there too much detail?**
  Is there excess information or redundancy? Is important information buried in a mass of detail, to be discovered by only the most persistent reader? Make your descriptions concise. "Cervix pink and smooth" indicates you saw no redness, ulcers, nodules, masses, cysts, or other suspicious lesions, but this description is shorter and more easily read. You can omit unimportant structures even though you examined them, such as normal eyebrows and eyelashes.

  Omit most of your negative findings unless they relate directly to the patient's complaints or specific exclusions in your differential diagnosis. *Instead, concentrate on major negative findings* such as "no heart murmurs."

- **Is the written style succinct? Are phrases, short words, and abbreviations used appropriately? Is data unnecessarily repeated?**
  Omit repetitive introductory phrases such as "The patient reports no …" because readers assume the patient is the source of the history unless otherwise specified.

  - Using words or brief phrases instead of whole sentences is common, but abbreviations and symbols should be used only if they are readily understood. Use shorter words when possible such as "felt" for "palpated" or "heard" for "auscultated." Omit unnecessary words, such as those in parentheses in the examples below. For example, "Cervix is pink (in color).""Lungs are resonant (to percussion)."
  - Describe what you observed, not what you did. "Optic discs seen" is less informative than "disc margins sharp."

- **Are precise measurements included where appropriate?**
  To ensure accurate evaluations and future comparisons, make measurements in centimeters, not in fruits, nuts, or vegetables.

  - "1 × 1 cm lymph node" versus a "pea-sized lymph node…"
  - Or "2 × 2 cm mass on the left lobe of the prostate" versus a "walnut-sized prostate mass."

- **Is the tone of the write-up neutral and professional?**
  It is important to be objective. Hostile or disapproving comments have no place in the patient's record. Never use inflammatory or demeaning words or punctuation.

  Comments such as "Patient DRUNK and LATE TO CLINIC AGAIN!!" are unprofessional and set a bad example for other clinicians reading the chart. They also might prove difficult to defend in a medico-legal setting.

INTERPRETATION AIDS

Box 1-13 represents the types of common abbreviations that may be used in the clinical record. Note that it is not intended to be a complete list of acceptable abbreviations. If you are in doubt about the correct abbreviation, write or type it out.

BOX 1-13. Common Abbreviations for the Clinical Record

Units of Measure		Medical Abbreviations	
C	Celsius	Ø	Without or no
cm	Centimeter	+ or pos	Positive
F	Fahrenheit	– or neg	Negative
hr	Hour	Abd	Abdomen
kg	Kilogram	AIDS	Acquired immune deficiency syndrome
lbs	Pounds		
mcg	Microgram	AP	Anteroposterior
mg	Milligram	CABG	Coronary artery bypass grafting
min	Minute		
oz	Ounces	CBC	Complete blood count
Vital Signs		CHF	Congestive heart failure
BP	Blood pressure	COPD	Chronic obstructive pulmonary disease
HR	Heart rate		
RR	Respirations	CPR	Cardiopulmonary resuscitation
T	Temperature		
Routes of Drug Administration		CT	Computed tomography
IM	Intramuscularly	CVA	Cerebrovascular accident
IV	Intravenously	CVP	Central venous pressure
PO	Orally	CXR	Chest x-ray

continued

DM	Diabetes mellitus	MRI	Magnetic resonance imaging
DTR	Deep tendon reflexes		
ECG or EKG	Electrocardiogram	MVA	Motor vehicle accident
ED	Emergency department	Neuro	Neurologic
EMT	Emergency medical technician	NIDDM	Noninsulin-dependent diabetes mellitus
ENT	Ears, nose, and throat	NKA	No known allergies
EOM	Extraocular muscles	NKDA	No known drug allergy
EtOH	Alcohol	nl	Normal/Normal limits
Ext	Extremities	PA	Posteroanterior
f	Female	PERRLA	Pupils equal, round, and reactive to light and accommodation
FH or FHx	Family history		
GI	Gastrointestinal		
GU	Genitourinary	PMH or PMHx	Past medical history
h/o	History of		
HEENT	Head, eyes, ears, nose, and throat	PT	Prothrombin time
		PTT	Partial thromboplastin time
HIV	Human immunodeficiency virus	R	Right
		RBC	Red blood cells
HRT	Hormone replacement therapy	ROM	Range of motion
		SH or SHx	Social history
HTN	Hypertension Hx History	SOB	Shortness of breath
JVD	Jugular venous distention	TIA	Transient ischemic attack
L	Left	U/A	Urinalysis
LMP	Last menstrual period	URI	Upper respiratory tract infection
LP	Lumbar puncture		
m	Male	WBC	White blood cells
Meds	Medications	wnl	Within normal limits
MI	Myocardial infarction	yo	Year old

Source: Federation of State Medical Boards of the United States, Inc., The National Board of Medical Examiners® (NBME®). 2018. *Step 2 CS content description and information*. Available at https://www.usmle.org/pdfs/step-2-cs/cs-info-manual.pdf. Updated November 2018. Accessed May 30, 2019.

Interviewing, Communication, and Interpersonal Skills

The *interviewing process* is more than just a series of questions; it requires a highly refined sensitivity to the patient's feelings and behavioral cues. This process generates a patient's story that draws on various relational skills to respond effectively to patient cues, feelings, and concerns.

FUNDAMENTALS OF SKILLED INTERVIEWING

Skilled interviewing requires the use of global communication and interpersonal techniques that can be used across all stages of the clinical encounter (Box 2-1).

BOX 2-1. Skilled Interviewing Techniques

Skilled Interviewing Technique	Description
Active or attentive listening	Listen closely to what the patient is communicating, being aware of the patient's emotional state, and using verbal and nonverbal skills to encourage the patient to continue and expand both concerns and fears.
Guided questioning ■ Moving from open-ended to focused questions	*Proceed from the general to the specific.* Directed questions should not be leading questions that call for a "yes" or "no" answer: not "Did your stools look like tar?" but "Please describe your stools."

continued

■ Using questioning that elicits a graded response	Ask questions that require a graded response rather than a single answer. "What physical activity do you do that makes you short of breath?" is better than "Do you get short of breath climbing stairs?"
■ Asking a series of questions, one at a time	Be sure to ask one question at a time. Try "Do you have any of the following problems?" Be sure to pause and establish eye contact as you list each problem.
■ Offering multiple choices for answers	Offer multiple-choice answers. Sometimes patients may seem unable to describe symptoms.
■ Clarifying what the patient means	Request clarification for patients using words that are ambiguous, as in "Tell me exactly what you meant by 'the flu.'"
■ Encouraging with continuers	Use *continuers*, such as postures, actions, or words that encourage the patient to say more but are not overly specific. Nod your head or remain silent. Lean forward, make eye contact, and use phrases like "Mm-hmm," "Go on," or "I'm listening."
■ Using echoing/ repetition	Repetition and echoing of the patient's words encourage the patient to express both factual details and feelings.
Empathic responses	Patients may express—with or without words—feelings they have not consciously acknowledged. Empathic responses are vital to patient rapport and convey that you experience some of the patient's suffering. *To express empathy, you must first recognize the patient's feelings.* Elicit these feelings rather than assume how the patient feels.
	Respond with understanding and acceptance. Responses may be as simple as "I understand," "That sounds upsetting," or "You seem sad." Empathy also may be nonverbal—for example, placing your hand on the patient's arm if the patient is crying.
Summarization	Give a capsule summary that lets the patient know that you have been listening carefully. It also clarifies what you know and don't know. Summarization allows you to organize your clinical reasoning and to convey your thinking to the patient, which makes the relationship more collaborative.
Transitions	Tell patients when you are changing topics during the interview. This gives patients a greater sense of control.

Partnering	Express your desire to work with patients in an ongoing way. Reassure patients that regardless of what happens with their health, as their provider, you are committed to a continuing partnership. Even in your role as a student, such support makes a big difference.
Validation	Provide verbal support that legitimizes or validates the patient's experience to help the patient feel accepted.
Reassurance	Avoid premature or false reassurance. Such reassurance may block further disclosures, especially if the patient feels that exposing anxiety is a weakness. *The first step to effective reassurance is identifying and accepting the patient's feelings without offering reassurance at that moment.*

Empower the Patient

The clinician–patient relationship is inherently unequal. Patients have many reasons to feel vulnerable: pain, worry, feeling overwhelmed with the healthcare system, lack of familiarity with the clinical evaluation process. Differences of gender, ethnicity, race, or class may also create power differentials. Ultimately, patients must be empowered to take care of themselves and follow through on your advice (Box 2-2).

BOX 2-2. Empowering the Patient: Techniques for Sharing Power

- Evoke the patient's perspective.
- Convey interest in the person, not just the problem.
- Follow the patient's lead.
- Elicit and validate emotional content.
- Share information with the patient, especially at transition points during the visit.
- Make your clinical reasoning transparent to the patient.
- Reveal the limits of your knowledge.

Use Understandable Language

It is critical to use short sentences and words and only communicate essential information. Simple words avoid the use of medical jargon, abbreviations, or any complex words or phrases. You can use these two approaches.

- **"Ask Me Three" approach.** This approach is intended to help patients become more active members of their healthcare team. It encourages patients to ask—and clinicians to answer—three main questions during each clinical encounter.

1. What is my main problem?
2. What do I need to do?
3. Why is it important for me to do this?

Modify this approach to **"Tell Them Three"** which can also help clinicians keep their message focused and simple.

- **Teach-Back Method.** Another useful technique to assess the patient's understanding is to "*teach back*," whereby you invite the patient to tell you, in his or her own words, the plan of care (Box 2-3). Keep in mind "teach back" is not a test of the patient's knowledge. It is a test of how well you explained things in a manner your patient understands.

BOX 2-3. Teach-Back Method

- Plan your approach. Think about how you will ask your patient to teach back the information. An example would be: "We covered a lot today and I want to make sure that I explained things clearly. So, let's review what we discussed."
- "Chunk and check." Chunk out information into small segments and have your patient teach it back.
- Clarify and check again. If teach back uncovers a misunderstanding, explain things again using a different approach.
- Start slowly and use consistently.
- Practice. It will take a little time, but once it is part of your routine, teach back can be done without awkwardness and does not lengthen a visit.
- Use the *show-me* method especially when prescribing new medicines or changing a dose.
- Use handouts along with teach back. Point out important information by reviewing written materials to reinforce your patients' understanding.

Source: Agency for Healthcare Research and Quality. 2015. *Use the teach-back method: Tool #5.* Rockville, MD. Available at http://www.ahrq.gov/professionals/quality-patient-safety/quality-resources/tools/literacy-toolkit/healthlittoolkit2-tool5.html. Last reviewed February 2015. Accessed May 30, 2019.

Use Nonstigmatizing Language

The language we use to reference people should reflect their full identities and acknowledge their capacity to change and grow. Unintentionally, stigmatizing language can distance and traumatize patients, create barriers to patients seeking help or accessing treatment, and perpetuate negative stereotypes (Box 2-4).

BOX 2-4. Examples of Stigmatizing and Corresponding Nonstigmatizing Language

What you should AVOID saying...	What you should say...
Ex-offender, thug, criminal, ex-felon, ex-con, convict, inmate, offender, felon, prisoner	A person who was/is incarcerated, formerly incarcerated person
Parolee, probationer	A person on parole, a person on probation
Drug abuser, addict, junkie	A person who uses/injects drugs, a person with an addiction
Schizophrenic, depressive	A person who has been diagnosed with schizophrenia or depression
AIDS or HIV patient, suffering from HIV, AIDS victim	A person living with HIV, a person living with AIDS
Prostitute, hooker, streetwalker	Sex worker, a person who is involved in transactional or survival sex
Rape victim	Sexual assault survivor, a rape survivor
The handicapped, the disabled	People with disabilities
Normal, healthy, whole or typical people	People without disabilities
Dwarf, a midget	Person of short stature, little person
Confined to a wheelchair; wheelchair bound	A person who uses a wheelchair or a mobility chair

Source: Texas Council for Developmental Disabilities. *People first language.* Available at http://www.tcdd.texas.gov/resources/people-first-language/. Accessed May 30, 2019.

Use Appropriate Nonverbal Communication

Pay close attention to eye contact, facial expression, posture, head position, and movement such as shaking or nodding, interpersonal distance, and placement of the arms or legs, such as crossed, neutral, or open. Physical contact can convey empathy or help the patient gain control of feelings. You also can mirror the patient's *paralanguage,* or qualities of speech such as pacing, tone, and volume, to increase rapport. Be sensitive to cultural variations in uses and meanings of nonverbal behaviors.

OTHER CONSIDERATIONS

Broaching Sensitive Topics

Guidelines for how to broach sensitive topics with your patients are provided in Box 2-5.

BOX 2-5. Guidelines for Broaching Sensitive Topics

- Be nonjudgmental. Your role is to learn from the patient and help the patient achieve better health.
- Explain why you need to know certain information. This makes patients less apprehensive. For example, say to patients, "Because sexual practices put people at risk for certain diseases, I ask all of my patients the following questions."
- Find opening questions for sensitive topics and learn the specific kinds of information needed for your shared assessment and plan.
- Consciously acknowledge whatever discomfort you are feeling. Denying your discomfort may lead you to avoid the topic altogether.

Obtaining Informed Consent

Informed consent is a communication process in which a clinician educates a patient about the risks, benefits, and alternatives of a given procedure or intervention.

Required elements for informed consent discussion:

- Nature of the procedure or treatment
- Risks and benefits of the procedure or treatment
- Reasonable alternatives
- Risks and benefits of alternatives
- Assessment of the patient's understanding of the first four elements

Working with a Medical Interpreter

The ideal interpreter is a "cultural navigator" who is neutral and trained in both languages and cultures (Box 2-6). Both face-to-face and telephone interpreting have important roles in healthcare settings, but they do not replace each other, and telephonic interpreters do not replace on-site interpretation. Telephonic interpreters are helpful for basic services, especially for rarely encountered languages and issues involving anonymity. Face-to-face interpreters rather than telephonic interpreters are best suited for:

- Serious diagnoses or other bad news
- When the patient is hard-of-hearing

- Family meetings or group discussions
- Interaction requiring visual elements
- Complicated or personal medical procedures or news

BOX 2-6. Guidelines for Working with an Interpreter: "INTERPRET"

I	**Introductions:** Make sure to introduce all the individuals in the room. During the introduction, include information as to the roles individuals will play.	
N	**Note Goals:** Note the goals of the interview. What is the diagnosis? What will the treatment entail? Will there be any follow-up?	
T	**Transparency:** Let the patient know that everything said will be interpreted throughout the session.	
E	**Ethics:** Use qualified interpreters (not family members or children) when conducting an interview. Qualified interpreters allow the patient to maintain autonomy and make informed decisions about his or her care.	
R	**Respect beliefs:** Patients with limited English proficiency (LEP) may have cultural beliefs that need to be taken into account as well.	
P	**Patient focus:** The patient should remain the focus of the encounter. Providers should interact with the patient and not the interpreter. Make sure to ask and address any questions the patient may have before ending the encounter. If you don't have trained interpreters on staff, the patient may not be able to call in with questions.	
R	**Retain control:** It is vital as the clinician that you remain in control of the interaction and not let the patient or the interpreter take over the conversation.	
E	**Explain:** Use simple language and short sentences when working with an interpreter. This will ensure that comparable words can be found in the second language and that all the information can be conveyed clearly.	
T	**Thanks:** Thank the interpreter and the patient for their time. On the electronic health record (EHR), note that the patient needs an interpreter and who served as an interpreter this time.	

Source: Administration for Children and Families, U.S. Department of Health and Human Services. *INTERPRET tool: working with interpreters in cultural settings.* Available at https://www.acf.hhs.gov/sites/default/files/otip/hhs_clas_interpret_tool.pdf. Accessed May 30, 2019.

Obtaining Advance Directives

In general, it is important to encourage any adult, but especially older adults or chronically ill, to have an *advance directive* and establish a *healthcare proxy* or *healthcare power of attorney* who can act as the patient's health decision maker. For patients who are terminally ill or frail and toward the end of life (prognosis is within a year), completion of a *Physician Orders for Life Sustaining Treatment (POLST)* form (also called *Medical Orders for Life-Sustaining Treatment [MOLST]*) is recommended. It is an actionable medical order form that tells others the patient's medical orders for life-sustaining treatment.

Disclosing Serious News

The SPIKES protocol for disclosing serious news is recommended due to the complexity of these interactions and the possibility of miscommunication (Box 2-7).

BOX 2-7. SPIKES: Six-Step Protocol for Delivering Bad News

	Steps	Information
S	**S**etting up the interview	■ Arrange for some privacy. ■ Involve significant others. ■ Sit down. ■ Make a connection with the patient. ■ Manage time constraints and interruptions.
P	Assessing the patient's **P**erception	■ The clinician uses open-ended questions to create a reasonably accurate picture of how the patient perceives the medical situation.
I	Obtaining the patient's **I**nvitation.	■ Find out how much the patient wants to know. ■ In any conversation about bad news the real issue is not "do you want to know?" but "at what level do you want to know?"
K	Giving **K**nowledge and information to the patient	■ Present information based on the assessed level of patient's understanding, compliance, and wishes for disclosure. ■ Start with a "warning shot." ■ Pause after sharing the primary information before proceeding further. ■ Avoid jargon.

E	Addressing the patient's **E**motions with **E**mpathic responses	▪ Expect the patient's first response to be an emotion. ▪ Be prepared to acknowledge the emotion explicitly.
S	**S**trategy and **S**ummary	▪ Ensure that the patient understands the information that has been provided first before discussing the next steps.

Source: Baile WF, et al. SPIKES-A six-step protocol for delivering bad news: application to the patient with cancer. *Oncologist.* 2000;5(4):302–311. VitalTalk. Serious News. Available at https://www.vitaltalk.org/guides/serious-news/. Accessed May 30, 2019.

Another framework in clarifying a patient's understanding and perspective of their illness is using the **Ask-Tell-Ask** framework. This patient-centered technique begins the patient conversation with asking their current understanding of the situation (*Ask*) before giving any new information (*Tell*). This information sharing is then followed by checking (*Ask*) for understanding of what has been told.

Building Interprofessional Communication

Without a doubt, working as a team using effective communication is key in providing efficient, quality care that leads to excellence in patient outcomes. An environment of mutual respect is essential because it helps facilitate shared goals, collaborative decisions and plans, and shared responsibilities. One of the frameworks to improve interprofessional communication and teamwork is the SBAR, **S**ituation-**B**ackground-**A**ssessment-**R**ecommendation (Box 2-8).

BOX 2-8. SBAR: A Tool to Facilitate Interprofessional Communication

SBAR	Examples
Situation	"I am . . . I am calling because . . . ""I have a patient who is . . ."
Background	"The patient was admitted on . . . because of . . ."
Assessment	"I think this patient is likely having a . . ."
Recommendation	"Let us transfer . . . ""Let us monitor and then . . ."

Source: Agency for Health Research and Quality (AHRQ). *TeamSTEPPS.* Available at http://teamstepps.ahrq.gov/. Accessed May 27, 2019.

CHALLENGING ENCOUNTERS

Box 2-9 provides examples of challenging patient behaviors or situations and suggested approaches for handling them.

BOX 2-9. Challenging Patient Encounters

Challenging Encounter	Suggested Approach
Patient who is silent	■ Silence has many meanings. Watch closely for nonverbal cues such as difficulty controlling emotions. ■ You may need to shift your inquiry to symptoms of depression or begin an exploratory mental status examination. ■ Silence may be the patient's response to how you are asking questions. Are you asking too many direct questions? Have you offended the patient?
Patient who is verbose	■ For the first 5 or 10 minutes, listen closely. Does the patient seem obsessively detailed or unduly anxious? Is there a flight of ideas or disorganized thought process? ■ Try to focus on what seems most important to the patient. "You've described many concerns. Let's focus on the hip pain first. Can you tell me what it feels like?" Or you can ask, "What is your primary concern today?"
Patient with confusing narrative	■ The patient may give a history that is vague and difficult to understand, and patients may describe symptoms in bizarre terms. ■ Some patients have *multiple symptoms* or a somatization disorder. Focus on the context of the symptoms and guide the interview into a psychosocial assessment. ■ When you suspect a psychiatric or neurologic disorder, shift to a mental status examination, focusing on level of consciousness, orientation, and memory.
Patient with altered state or cognition	■ Determine whether the patient has *decision-making capacity,* or the ability to understand information related to health, to make clinical choices based on reason and a consistent set of values, and to declare preferences about treatments. ■ If a patient lacks capacity to make a healthcare decision, then identify the health care proxy or the agent with power of attorney for health care.

Patient with emotional lability	▪ Usually crying is therapeutic, as is quiet acceptance of the patient's distress. ▪ Make a facilitating or supportive remark like "I'm glad that you were able to express your feelings."
Patient who is angry or aggressive	▪ Many patients have reasons to be angry and they may direct this anger toward you. Accept angry feelings from patients and allow them to express such emotions without getting angry in return. ▪ Validate their feelings without agreeing with their reasons. ▪ Some angry patients become hostile and disruptive. Before approaching them, alert security. Stay calm, appear accepting, and avoid being challenging. ▪ Keep your posture relaxed and nonthreatening. Once you have established rapport, gently suggest moving to a different location.
Patient who is flirtatious	▪ If you become aware of sexual feelings, accept them as a normal human response, and bring them to the conscious level so they will not affect your behavior. ▪ Denying these feelings makes it more likely that you will act inappropriately. ▪ *Any* sexual contact or romantic relationship with patients is *unethical*; keep your relationship with the patient within professional bounds and seek help if you need it.
Patient who is discriminatory/ racist	▪ Discriminatory or racist patient behavior should be named and processed appropriately. ▪ First, you should assess the illness acuity of the patient. Options include continuing care for your patient, reaching out to another team member for assistance, or removing yourself from the situation entirely. ▪ Next, you can seek to cultivate a therapeutic alliance with your patient. Acknowledging these factors does not make the behavior acceptable or easier to manage. ▪ Finally, it is the role of your supervising clinician to establish a supportive learning environment for you on the clinical team.
Patient who is nonadherent	▪ The term *adherence* is preferred over *compliance* because when a patient does not cooperate with suggested therapy, it is not fair to assume that the patient is always at fault. ▪ Strategies for better adherence include the use of informational handouts; cues and reminders using e-mails or form letters; positive feedback to the patient; steps to minimize discomfort and inconvenience such as simplifying dosing schedule; disease monitoring to alter management; and obtaining counseling, if appropriate.

continued

Patient with hearing loss	■ Find out the patient's preferred method of communicating. Patients may use American Sign Language (ASL), a unique language with its own syntax, or various other communication forms combining signs and speech. ■ Determine whether the patient identifies with the deaf or hearing culture. ■ Handwritten questions and answers may be the best solution. ■ When patients have partial hearing impairment or can read lips, face them directly, in good light. If the patient has a unilateral hearing loss, sit on the hearing side. If the patient has a hearing aid, make sure it is working. ■ Eliminate background noise such as a television.
Patient with low or impaired vision	■ Shake hands to establish contact and explain who you are and why you are there. ■ If the room is unfamiliar, orient the patient to the surroundings.
Patient with limited intelligence	■ Patients of moderately limited intelligence usually can give adequate histories. Pay special attention to the patient's schooling and ability to function independently. How far has the patient gone in school? If he or she didn't finish, why not? ■ Assess simple calculations, vocabulary, memory, and abstract thinking. ■ For patients with severe mental retardation, obtain the history from the family or caregivers. ■ Avoid "talking down" or using condescending behavior. The sexual history is equally important and often overlooked.
Patient burdened by personal problems	■ Patients may ask you for advice about personal problems outside the range of health. Letting the patient talk through the problem is usually more valuable and therapeutic than any answer you could give.
Patient with low literacy or low health literacy	■ Assess the ability to read. Some patients may try to hide their reading problems. Ask the patient to read whatever instructions you have written. Simply handing the patient written material upside down to see if the patient turns it around may settle the question. ■ Assess *health literacy*, or the skills to function effectively in the healthcare system: interpreting documents, reading labels and medication instructions, and speaking and listening effectively.

Patient with limited language proficiency	▪ If the patient speaks a different language, make every effort to find a trained interpreter. The ideal interpreter is a neutral, objective person trained in both languages and cultures. ▪ Avoid using family members or friends: confidentiality may be violated. ▪ As you work with the interpreter, *make questions clear, short, and simple.* Speak directly to the patient. ▪ Bilingual written questionnaires are valuable.
Patient with terminal illness or who is dying	▪ Offer openings for patients and family members to talk about their feelings and ask questions. ▪ Dying patients rarely want to talk about their illnesses all the time, nor do they wish to confide in everyone they meet. Give them opportunities to talk and then listen receptively, but be supportive if they prefer to stay at a social level. ▪ Work through your own feelings about death and dying and acquiring necessary skills to ensure excellent communication are essential, as you will come into contact with patients of all ages near the end of their lives.

MAINTAINING PATIENT-CENTEREDNESS IN COMPUTERIZED CLINICAL SETTINGS

Effective EHR use has been shown to facilitate the process of communication, clarification, and discussion as well as some potentially patient-centered communication behaviors, such as screen sharing, signposting, cessation of typing during sensitive discussions (Box 2-10).

BOX 2-10. Strategies to Maintain Patient-Centeredness in Computerized Clinical Settings

- Review the patient's medical record before calling the patient in.
- Start the visit by asking about the patient's concerns and building rapport before turning to computer.
- Move the computer/patient to facilitate communication while using the EHR (i.e., construct a clinician/patient/computer triangle).
- Maintain body orientation toward the patient (especially lower body); maintain eye contact intermittently with the patient despite using the EHR.

continued

- Talk while working on the computer to maintain engagement with the patient and break long silences.
- Explain the purpose for using the computer; verbalize actions on the computer (e.g., describe what you are looking for); read out loud while typing.
- Visually or verbally share EHR information using the screen with the patient.
- Involve the patient in building their chart.
- Separate use of the computer from communication with the patient, especially when building rapport or discussing treatment options; verbalize or use gestures to indicate switches in attention between the patient and the computer.
- Use gaps in the interaction with the patient for computer work (e.g., when the patient is dressing up after a physical examination).
- Document the patient encounter in the patient's electronic health record after the visit.

Sources: Crampton NH, et al. Computers in the clinical encounter: a scoping review and thematic analysis. *J Am Med Inform Assoc.* 2016;23(3):654–665; Biagioli FE, et al. The electronic health record objective structured clinical examination: assessing student competency in patient interactions while using the electronic health record. *Acad Med.* 2017;92(1):87–91.

Health History

The *health history* is a structured framework for organizing patient information into written or verbal form. This format focuses on needed information that facilitates clinical reasoning and clarifies patient concerns, diagnoses, and plans to other healthcare providers involved in the patient's care.

For adults, the comprehensive history includes Identifying Data and Source of the History, Chief Complaint (CC), History of Present Illness (HPI), Past Medical History, Family History, Personal and Social History, and Review of Systems (ROS) (Box 3-1). New patients in the office or hospital merit a comprehensive health history; however, in many situations, a more flexible, focused, or problem-oriented interview is appropriate. The components of the comprehensive health history structure the patient's story and the format of your written record, but the order shown below should not dictate the sequence of the interview. The interview is more fluid and should follow the patient's leads and cues.

BOX 3-1. Components of the Adult Health History

Identifying patient information	■ *Identifying data*—such as patient's name, age, and sex assigned at birth and/or gender identity
Source/reliability	■ *Source of the history*—usually the patient, but can be a family member, caregiver or friend, or the clinical record ■ *Reliability* varies according to the patient's memory, trust, and mood
Chief complaint(s)	■ Primary symptom or concern causing the patient to seek care that may be one or two concerns and rarely more than that
History of present illness	■ Amplifies the *Chief Complaint;* describes the chronology of events as to how each symptom developed ■ Includes patient's thoughts and feelings about the illness ■ Pulls in relevant portions of the *Review of Systems,* called "pertinent positives and negatives" (see pp. 42–44)

continued

Past medical history	■ Describes *adult illnesses* with dates for events in at least four categories: *medical, surgical, obstetric/ gynecologic,* and *psychiatric*
	■ May list *childhood illnesses*
	■ Includes *health maintenance practices* such as immunizations, screening tests, lifestyle issues, and home safety
	■ Includes *medications* and *allergies*
Family history	■ Outlines or diagrams age and health, or age and cause of death, of siblings, parents, and grandparents
	■ Includes presence or absence of specific illnesses in family, such as hypertension, diabetes, or type of cancer
Personal and social history	■ Includes any history of *tobacco, alcohol,* or *recreational drug use*
	■ Describes *sexual history*
	■ Describes *educational level, family of origin, current household, personal interests,* and *lifestyle*
Review of systems	■ Includes presence or absence of common symptoms related to each of the major body systems

Decide if your assessment will be *comprehensive* or *focused.* Be sure to distinguish *subjective* from *objective* data (Box 3-2).

BOX 3-2. Subjective versus Objective Data

Subjective Information	Objective Information
What the patient tells you	What you detect during the examination, laboratory information, and test data
The *symptoms* and history, from Chief Complaint through Review of Systems	All physical examination findings, or *signs*

COMPREHENSIVE ADULT HEALTH HISTORY

As you elicit the adult health history, be sure to note the following: date and time of history; identifying data, which include age and gender, and reliability, which reflects the quality of information the patient provides.

Chief Complaint(s)

The *CC* or *presenting complaint* is the term used to describe the primary problem or condition prompting the clinician encounter. The CC is the starting point that triggers information gathering from the clinician's perspective.

Make every attempt to document the patient's own words, especially if it is descriptive, unusual, or unique. "My stomach hurts and I feel awful"; or "I have come for my regular checkup."

History of Present Illness

This section is a complete, clear, and chronologic account of the problems prompting the patient to seek care. It should include the problem's onset, the setting in which it has developed, its manifestations, and any treatments. The HPI in its most basic form is the story of the patient's problem. It is where you characterize the CC fully by describing its attributes listed in Boxes 3-3 and 3-4 and *pertinent positives* and *negatives* from relevant areas of the ROS that help clarify the *differential diagnosis*.

BOX 3-3. Attributes of a Symptom

Attribute	Description
Location	Where in/on the body the problem, symptom, or pain occur or move to other areas
Quality	An adjective describing the type of problem, symptom, or pain
Quantity or severity	Patient's nonverbal actions or verbal description of the extent of the problem, symptom, or pain (on a scale of 1 to 10), compared to previous experiences
Timing including:	Describes when the symptom or pain started
Onset	Setting in which it occurs, what actions or circumstances cause the problem, symptom, or pain to occur, worsen, or improve
Duration	How long the problem, symptom, or pain has been present or how long the problem, symptom, or pain lasts
Frequency	How often the problem, symptom, or pain occurs
Modifying factors	Actions or activities taken to improve the problem, symptom, or pain and its outcome
Associated manifestations	Other signs or symptoms that occur when the problem, symptom, or pain occurs

---

BOX 3-4. Helpful Mnemonics for Characterizing the Chief Complaint

OPQRST	OLD CARTS
■ **O**nset	■ **O**nset
■ **P**recipitating and **P**alliating factors	■ **L**ocation
■ **Q**uality	■ **D**uration
■ **R**egion or **R**adiation	■ **C**haracter
■ **S**everity	■ **A**ggravating or **A**lleviating factors
■ **T**iming or **T**emporal characteristics	■ **R**adiation
	■ **T**iming
	■ **S**etting

Past Medical History

The past medical history includes all medical problems whether they are currently active or remote. It should include *childhood illnesses* and *adult illnesses* and their four types of health information *medical, surgical, psychiatric, obstetric/gynecologic.* Also ask about the patient's immunizations and age-appropriate preventive measures.

Childhood Illnesses: Ask patients about illnesses such as measles, rubella, mumps, whooping cough, chicken pox, rheumatic fever, scarlet fever, and polio. Also included are any chronic childhood illnesses such as asthma or diabetes mellitus.

Adult Illnesses: Ask the patient to provide information in each of the four areas:

■ *Medical:* Illnesses such as diabetes, high blood pressure, heart attack, hepatitis, asthma, human immunodeficiency virus (HIV); seizures, arthritis, tuberculosis, cancer; including time frame, and hospitalizations

■ *Surgical:* Dates and types of operations or procedures; if the patient is unable to recall the name of the operation or procedure, ask for the reason why it was performed (indication)

■ *Obstetric/Gynecologic:* Obstetric history, menstrual history, methods of contraception, and sexual function

■ *Psychiatric:* Illnesses such as depression, anxiety, suicidal ideations/ attempts; including time frame, diagnoses, hospitalizations, and treatments

Also discuss *Health Maintenance*, including *immunizations* and *screening tests,* together with the results and the dates they were last performed.

Mental Health History. Ask open-ended questions initially: "Have you ever had any problem with emotional or mental illnesses?" Then move to more specific questions: "Have you ever visited a counselor or psychotherapist?" "Have you taken medication for emotional issues?" "Have you or a family member ever been hospitalized for a mental health problem?"

Be sensitive to reports of mood changes or symptoms such as fatigue, tearfulness, appetite or weight changes, insomnia, and vague somatic complaints. Two validated screening questions are: "Over the past 2 weeks, have you felt down, depressed, or hopeless?" and "Over the past 2 weeks, have you felt little interest or pleasure in doing things?" Ask about thoughts of suicide: "Have you ever thought about hurting yourself or ending your life?" Evaluate severity.

Medications. Medications should be noted, including name, dose, route, and frequency of use. Also list nonprescription or over-the-counter (OTC) medications, vitamins, mineral or herbal supplements, eye drops, ointments, oral contraceptives, and home remedies.

Family History

Outline the age and health, or age and cause of death, of each immediate relative, including grandparents, parents, siblings, children, and grandchildren. Record the following conditions as either *present* or *absent* in the family: hypertension, coronary artery disease, elevated cholesterol levels, stroke, diabetes, thyroid or renal disease, cancer (specify type), arthritis, tuberculosis, asthma or lung disease, headache, seizure disorder, mental illness, suicide, alcohol or drug addiction, and allergies, as well as conditions that the patient reports.

Personal and Social History

Include the patient's *personal and social history,* which captures their personality and interests, their coping style, strengths, and concerns (Box 3-5). This information helps personalize your relationship with the patient and builds rapport. This personal history includes *sexual orientation* and *gender identification (SOGI)*, place of birth, and personal environmental map; *occupation and education*; significant *relationships* including *safety* in those relationships; *home environment* including family and household composition; important *life experiences* such as military service, job history, financial situation, and retirement; *leisure activities; sexuality, spirituality;* and *social support systems.*

BOX 3-5. Social History Domains

- Sexual orientation and gender identity (SOGI)
- Personal geographic map
- Significant relationships
- Local support systems
- Work history/occupation
- Education
- Lifestyle
- Activities of daily living
- Nutrition
- Exercise
- Alcohol use
- Tobacco use
- Illicit drug use
- Safety measures
- Spirituality
- Sexual history

Sexual Orientation and Gender Identity. Discussing SOGI touches a vital and multifaceted core of your patients' lives. Reflect on any biases and providing a supportive nonjudgmental approach is essential for exploring your patients' health and well-being. You should ask open-ended questions and use language that is inclusive, allowing your patient to decide when and what to disclose:

- "How would you describe your sexual orientation?" The range of responses can include heterosexual or straight, lesbian, gay, bisexual, pansexual, queer, and questioning, among others.
- "How would you describe your gender identity?" Responses include male, female, transgender, transmale, transfemale, genderqueer, gender nonbinary, unsure or questioning, or even "prefer not to answer."
- "What is the sex on your original birth certificate?" This question helps elicit further gender history when asked as a follow-up to gender identity and will give the clinician a sense of which organs the patient may have in order to help guide sexually transmitted infection (STI) and cancer screening recommendations.

Familial and Social Relationships. Ask about parents, children, partners, friends, acquaintances, and distant relatives. Seek those that your patient identifies as providing *social support* which refers to the emotionally sustaining qualities of relationships.

Social relationships can also be extremely stressful, overburdened, strained, conflicted, or abusive, which then undermines health (Box 3-6). Begin with normalizing statements such as "Because abuse is common in many of my patients' lives, I've begun to ask about it routinely." Follow-up with "Are you in a relationship where you have been hit or threatened?" Has anyone ever treated you badly or made you do things you don't want to?" or "Is there anyone you are afraid of?" or "Have you ever been hit, kicked, punched, or hurt by someone you know?" Following disclosure, empathic validating and nonjudgmental responses are critical.

BOX 3-6. Clues to Physical and Sexual Abuse

- Injuries that are unexplained, seem inconsistent with the patient's story, are concealed by the patient, or cause embarrassment
- Delay in getting treatment for trauma
- History of repeated injuries or "accidents"
- Presence of alcohol or drug abuse in patient or partner
- Partner tries to dominate the visit, will not leave the room, or seems unusually anxious or solicitous
- Pregnancy at a young age; multiple partners
- Repeated vaginal infections and STIs
- Difficulty walking or sitting due to genital/anal pain
- Vaginal lacerations or bruises
- Fear of the pelvic examination or physical contact
- Fear of leaving the examination room

Alcohol History. It is important to learn about your patient's *patterns* of alcohol consumption, not just their average levels of consumption. "Tell me about your use of alcohol" is an opening query that avoids the easy yes–no response. Positive answers to two additional questions are highly suspicious for problem drinking: "Have you ever had a drinking problem?" and "When was your last drink?" The most widely used screening questions are the *CAGE* questions about **C**utting down, **A**nnoyance when criticized, **G**uilty feelings, and **E**ye-openers. Two or more affirmative answers suggest lifetime alcohol abuse and dependence alcohol use disorders (AUD).

Tobacco Use History. Determine tobacco use, including the type (smoking, chewing). Ask: "Do you smoke?" "Have you ever smoked?" "What do you smoke?" "How many cigarettes per day? For how many years?" "Do you chew tobacco?" Cigarettes are often reported in pack-years calculated by multiplying the number of packs of cigarettes smoked per day by the number of years the person has smoked. If someone has quit, note for how long and note as a former smoker.

Illicit Drug Use History. Ask a highly sensitive and specific single question: "How many times in the past year have you used an illegal drug or used a prescription medication for nonclinical reasons?" If there is a positive response, ask specifically about nonclinical use of illicit and prescription drugs: "In your lifetime have you ever used: marijuana; cocaine; prescription stimulants; methamphetamines; sedatives or sleeping pills; hallucinogens like lysergic acid diethylamide (LSD), ecstasy, mushrooms...; street opioids like heroin or opium; prescription opioids like fentanyl, oxycodone, hydrocodone...; or other substances."

Sexual History. Answering questions about sexual health may be uncomfortable for some patients, particularly if they have experienced judgment or discrimination. An orienting sentence or two is often helpful. "To help me take better care of you, I need to ask you some questions about your sexual health and practices" or "I routinely ask all patients about their sexual function." If you are straightforward, the patient is more likely to follow your lead.

The most common sexual history script is the 5 Ps: *partners, practices, protection from STIs, past history of STIs,* and *prevention of pregnancy* (Box 3-7). Add a sixth "P" for "plus" encompassing an assessment of trauma, violence, sexual satisfaction, sexual health concerns/problems, and support for gender identity and sexual orientation. These questions are designed to help patients reveal their concerns. Note that these questions make no assumptions about marital status, sexual orientation, or attitudes about pregnancy or contraception.

BOX 3-7. Sexual History: The Five Ps+	
General	■ "Do you have any specific concerns or questions we can start with, about your sexual health or sexual practices?"
Partners	■ "When was the last time you had intimate physical contact with someone?" "Did that contact include sexual intercourse?" ■ "What are the genders of your sexual partners?" ■ "How many sexual partners have you had in the last 6 months? In the last 5 years? In your lifetime?" ■ "Have you had any new partners in the past 6 months?"
Practices	■ "How do you have sex? or "What kinds of sex are you having? (for example, oral sex, vaginal sex, anal sex, sharing sex toys)" ■ "What parts of your body do you use for sex?" or "What body parts go where when you are sexually active?" (penis, mouth, anus, vagina, hands, toys, and other objects)

Protection from STIs	▪ "What do you do to protect yourself from HIV and STDs?"
	▪ "Can you tell me when you use condoms? With which partners?" "There are a lot of reasons why people don't use condoms. Can you tell me why you are not using them for sex?"
	▪ "Do you have any concerns about HIV infection or AIDS?"
Past history of STIs	▪ "Have you ever had a sexually transmitted disease?" If yes: "What kind have you had?" "When did you have it?" "How were you treated/what medications did you take?"
	▪ "Have you ever been tested for any (other) STDs? If yes, when and what were the test results?
Pregnancy plans	▪ "Do you have any plans or desires to have (more) children?"
	▪ "Are you concerned about getting pregnant or getting your partner pregnant?" "Are you doing anything to prevent yourself or your partner from getting pregnant?" "Do you want information on birth control?" "Do you have any questions or concerns about pregnancy prevention?"
Plus	▪ The "plus" should encompass an assessment of trauma, violence, sexual satisfaction, sexual health concerns/problems, and support for sexual orientation and gender identity (SOGI).

Sources: U.S. Department of Health and Human Services: Centers for Disease Control and Prevention. *Taking a sexual history: a guide to taking a sexual history.* Last Reviewed August 22, 2018. Available at https://www.cdc.gov/std/treatment/sexualhistory.pdf. Accessed May 27, 2019; National LGBT Health Education Center. *Taking routine histories of sexual health: a system-wide approach for health centers.* Originally published February 15, 2016. Available at https://www.lgbthealtheducation.org/publication/taking-routine-histories-of-sexual-health-a-system-wide-approach-for-health-centers/. Accessed May 27, 2019.

Spiritual History. The spiritual history helps to better understand patients' spiritual and/or religious needs and resources. It may be part of a new patient visit, annual examination, or a follow-up visit. Keep it patient centered and listen actively. The most widely used is the FICA Spiritual Tool (Box 3-8).

BOX 3-8. FICA Spiritual Tool

Faith or beliefs	▪ *What is your faith or belief?*
	▪ *Do you consider yourself spiritual or religious?*
	▪ *What gives your life meaning?*

continued

Importance and Influence	■ Is it important in your life? ■ What importance does your spirituality have in life? ■ Has your spirituality influenced how you take care of yourself, your health? ■ How have your beliefs influenced your behavior during this illness? ■ Does your spirituality influence you in your healthcare decision making? ■ What role do your beliefs play in regaining your health?
Community	■ Are you part of a spiritual or religious community? Is this a support to you and how? ■ Is there a group of people you really love or who are important to you?
Address	■ How would you like me, your healthcare provider, to address these issues in your health care?

Source: Borneman T, Ferrell B, Puchalski CM. Evaluation of the FICA Tool for spiritual assessment. *J Pain Symptom Manage*. 2010;40(2):163–173; Puchalski C, Romer AL. Taking a spiritual history allows clinicians to understand patients more fully. *J Palliat Med* 2000;3(1):129–137. Reprinted with permission from Christina Puchalski, MD.

Review of Systems (ROS)

These "yes/no" questions go from "head to toe" and conclude the interview. The *ROS* questions may uncover problems that the patient overlooked. Remember to move major health events to the History of Present Illness or Past Medical History in your write-up.

General. Usual weight, recent weight change, clothing that fits more tightly or loosely than before; weakness, fatigue, fever.

Skin. Rashes, lumps, sores, itching, dryness, color change; changes in hair or nails; changes in size or color of moles.

Head, Eyes, Ears, Nose, Throat (HEENT). *Head:* Headache, head injury, dizziness, light-headedness. *Eyes:* Vision, glasses or contact lenses, last examination, pain, redness, excessive tearing, double or blurred vision, spots, specks, flashing lights, glaucoma, cataracts. *Ears:* Hearing, tinnitus, vertigo, earache, infection, discharge. If hearing is decreased, use or nonuse of hearing aid. *Nose and sinuses:* Frequent colds, nasal stuffiness, discharge or itching, hay fever, nosebleeds, sinus trouble. *Throat (or mouth and pharynx):* Condition of teeth and gums; bleeding gums; dentures, if any, and how they fit; last dental examination; sore tongue; dry mouth; frequent sore throats; hoarseness.

Neck. Lumps, "swollen glands," goiter, pain, stiffness.

Breasts. Lumps, pain or discomfort, nipple discharge.

Respiratory. Cough, sputum (color, quantity), hemoptysis, dyspnea, wheezing, pleurisy, last chest x-ray. You may wish to include asthma, bronchitis, emphysema, pneumonia, and tuberculosis.

Cardiovascular. "Heart trouble," hypertension, rheumatic fever, heart murmurs, chest pain or discomfort, palpitations, dyspnea, orthopnea, paroxysmal nocturnal dyspnea, edema.

Gastrointestinal. Trouble swallowing, heartburn, appetite, nausea. Bowel movements, color and size of stools, change in bowel habits, rectal bleeding or black or tarry stools, hemorrhoids, constipation, diarrhea. Abdominal pain, food intolerance, excessive belching or passing of gas. Jaundice, liver or gallbladder trouble, hepatitis.

Peripheral Vascular. Intermittent claudication; leg cramps; varicose veins; past clots in veins; swelling in calves, legs, or feet; color change in fingertips or toes during cold weather; swelling with redness or tenderness.

Urinary. Frequency of urination, polyuria, nocturia, urgency, burning or pain on urination, hematuria, urinary infections, kidney stones, incontinence; in males, reduced caliber or force of urinary stream, hesitancy, dribbling.

Genital. *Male:* Hernias, discharge from or sores on penis, testicular pain or masses, history of STIs and treatments, sexual function. *Female:* menstrual regularity, frequency, and duration; amount of bleeding, bleeding between periods or after intercourse, last menstrual period; dysmenorrhea, premenstrual tension. Age at menopause, menopausal symptoms, postmenopausal bleeding. Vaginal discharge, itching, sores, lumps, STIs and treatments. Number of pregnancies, number and type of deliveries, number of abortions (spontaneous and induced), complications of pregnancy, birth control methods. Sexual interest, function, satisfaction, problems (including dyspareunia).

Musculoskeletal. Muscle or joint pain, stiffness, arthritis, gout, backache. If present, describe location of affected joints or muscles, any swelling, redness, pain, tenderness, stiffness, weakness, or limitation of motion or activity; include timing of symptoms (e.g., morning or evening), duration, and any history of trauma. Neck or low back pain. Joint pain with systemic features such as fever, chills, rash, anorexia, weight loss, or weakness.

Psychiatric. Nervousness; tension; mood, including depression, memory change, suicide attempts, if relevant.

Neurologic. Changes in mood, attention, or speech; changes in orientation, memory, insight, or judgment; headache, dizziness, vertigo; fainting, blackouts, seizures, weakness, paralysis, numbness or loss of sensation, tingling or "pins and needles," tremors or other involuntary movements, seizures.

Hematologic. Anemia, easy bruising or bleeding, transfusion reactions.

Endocrine. "Thyroid problem," heat or cold intolerance, excessive sweating, excessive thirst or hunger, polyuria, change in glove or shoe size.

Modification of the Clinical Interview for Various Clinical Settings

Box 3-9 provides guidelines for modifying the clinical interview when warranted.

BOX 3-9. Modifying the Clinical Interview for Various Clinical Settings	
Clinical Setting	**Modification**
Ambulatory care clinic	▪ Patients are mostly mobile, independent with Chief Complaints which tend to be of low acuity. ▪ Since patients are seen on a regular basis in the ambulatory setting, focus your information gathering not only on the Chief Complaint (if there is one) but also on chronic health issues and any changes that may have occurred since their last visit. ▪ Also ask about routine health maintenance.
Emergency care	▪ Ask about symptoms related to possible causes of the patient's problem to help quickly rule out life-threatening illnesses. ▪ If patient is incapable of providing information due to confusion or change in mental status, obtain the health history from family members, caregivers, other clinicians, emergency medical providers, or their patient's clinical records if available.
Intensive care unit	▪ Most of these patients have limited abilities to communicate due to their serious illness, altered mental states, being medically sedated, on ventilatory support or from a combination of these. ▪ Your clinical information will need to come from a family member, other clinicians, or prior documentations in the clinical record. ▪ If the patient is able to communicate, information gathering should also include how they wish they would like to direct their care.

Nursing home	▪ Always attempt to obtain the health history from the resident first.
	▪ If you suspect that the patient may have cognitive dysfunction, you may need to confirm certain information with family or the clinical staff.
Home	▪ Patients are often chronically ill and with functional impairments that make it difficult to leave home without supportive devices or another person's help (*homebound or home-limited status*).
	▪ Try to focus on function. A patient's ability to function within his or her home setting has a profound impact on his or her overall health status.
	▪ Evaluate for environmental hazards and level of cleanliness or upkeep, presence of available food and medications.

DOCUMENTING THE HEALTH HISTORY

Be sure to include the following: date and time of history and identifying data, which include age, gender, and reliability. The patient's full name is frequently abbreviated to initials. Key areas in the health history documentation are highlighted here.

Documenting the Chief Complaint

Make every attempt to quote the patient's own words especially if it is descriptive, unusual, or unique. For example, you may document, "My stomach hurts and I feel awful." or "My urine is darkly colored and smells funny." or "I feel like an elephant is sitting on my chest." For those with multiple complaints, one may predominate. If there are multiple presenting problems of equal importance, then the CC documentation will list the multiple problems, and you should then describe and fully elaborate each one in the HPI. If patients have no specific complaints, report their reason for the visit, such as "I have come for my regular checkup."

Documenting the History of Present Illness

Structuring how to document the HPI in the clinical record is one of the most challenging tasks for any beginning student. A framework that could guide you in structuring this section of the documentation is outlined in Box 3-10.

> ### BOX 3-10. Suggested Structure in Documenting the HPI (One Chief Complaint)
>
> - Start with an opening statement
> - Further characterize the Chief Complaint with attention to chronology of events
> - Then describe accompanying symptoms and their pertinence
> - Include absent symptoms and their pertinence
> - Add information from other parts of the health history that are relevant

Opening Statement. Opening statements for the health history provide a foundation for the reader to begin thinking of possible causes for the patient's condition. This first statement should be stated in the patient's clinical context, i.e., critical historical elements that are most related to the CC that hints at possible causes of the patient's condition. For example: *JM is a 48-year-old man with poorly controlled diabetes mellitus presenting with 3 days of fever.*

Elaboration of Chief Complaint with Attention to Chronology. In the HPI, the CC should be well characterized by its attending attributes (Box 3-11). Based on the patient's responses to your questions, pay particular attention to the clarity of the story. This section should be a chronologic account of events as well, so pay attention to the timing of symptoms.

> ### BOX 3-11. Documentation of Attributes of the Chief Complaint
>
> | Attribute | Examples |
> | --- | --- |
> | **Location** | Area of body, bilateral, unilateral, left, right, anterior, posterior, upper, lower, diffuse or localized, fixed or migratory, radiating to other areas |
> | **Quality** | Dull, sharp, throbbing, constant, intermittent, itching, stabbing, acute, chronic, improving or worsening, red or swollen, cramping, shooting, scratchy |
> | **Quantity or severity** | 8/10 on the pain scale, moderately dizzy, approximately half a cup of bloody urine |

Timing	
■ Onset	■ This morning, last night, 6 days ago
■ Duration	■ Since last night, for the past week, until today, it lasted for 2 hours
■ Frequency	■ Every six hours, daily, comes and goes
Setting in which it occurs	Worse when standing, improved with sitting, aggravated by eating, fell going down the stairs, during a football game
Modifying factors	Clinically, relief more likely from ibuprofen, less likely from acetaminophen; it felt better/worse when I ....
Associated manifestations	Generalized symptoms (constitutional), frequency and urgency with urination, headache with blurred vision, back pain leads to numbness and tingling down the leg.

One method to maintain clarity of the patient's story is to anchor each event to a timeline or chronology. Keep the time anchors consistent to make it easier for your readers to follow.

Accompanying Symptoms and Absent Pertinent Symptoms. In this section, you should describe:

- *Pertinent positives*—any symptoms brought up during the encounter that may be related to the CC
- *Pertinent negatives*—the absence of any symptoms related to your differential diagnosis

The pertinent positives and especially the negatives reflect the clinician's perspective as to possible causes of the patient's condition as well as eliminate less likely possibilities based on the patient's story.

Additional Pertinent Information. Here you should note any additional facts pertinent to the CC, regardless of where they are typically documented. For example, if your patient has a fever and cough you believe is pneumonia, you may want to include the patient's smoking history in the HPI. These additional pertinent facts would typically be documented elsewhere in the health history, but are included in the HPI because they impact the evolving list of possible causes of the CC.

Box 3-12 provides additional suggestions on how to structure the HPI. These templates emphasize clarity of the story in the HPI as well as provide clues to the reader to possible causes of the patient's problems.

> ### BOX 3-12. Additional Suggested Templates for Documenting the HPI
>
> **History of Present Illness Template (Chief Complaint which you believe is a symptom of an exacerbation of the patient's chronic illness):**
>
> - Opening statement: Chief Complaint in light of the patient's clinical context
> - Description of condition and symptom control of the chronic illness:
>   - Diagnosis or symptom
>   - When diagnosed
>   - Complications
>   - Treatments
>   - Recent symptom control prior to this exacerbation
> - Elaborate description of the Chief Complaint
> - Accompanying symptomatology
> - Absent pertinent symptomatology
> - Pertinent past medical history, family history, or social history
> - Concluding statement: How the patient got to the care site
>
> **History of Present Illness Template (No Chief Complaint)**
>
> - Opening statement: Simple statement of the patient's medical problems
> - Status report of the patient's chronic conditions/illnesses
>   - Pertinent symptoms—present and absent
>   - Current treatment and response
>   - Prior relevant labs/studies
> - Concluding statement: How the patient got to the care site

Documenting the Past Medical History

List *childhood illnesses*, then list *adult illnesses* in each of four areas (Box 3-13):

- *Medical* (e.g., diabetes, hypertension, hepatitis, asthma, HIV), with dates of onset; also, information about hospitalizations with dates
- *Surgical* (dates, indications, and types of operations)
- *Obstetric/gynecologic* (obstetric history, menstrual history, birth control, and sexual function)
- *Psychiatric* (illness and time frame, diagnoses, hospitalizations, and treatments)

Recall that your goal is to produce a clear, concise, but comprehensive report that documents key findings and communicates your assessment in a succinct format to clinicians, consultants, and other members of the healthcare team. Note the standard format of the clinical record from *Initial Information* including *Source and Reliability* to *Review of Systems.*

BOX 3-13. Sample Health History Note

8/25/20 11:00 AM

MN, 54 years old, female

Source and Reliability
Self-referred; reliable.

Chief Complaint
"My head has been aching for the past 3 months."

History of Present Illness:
MN is a 54-year-old female with a remote history of intermittent headaches who states that her "head has been aching for the past 3 months." She was in her usual state of health until 3 months prior to consultation when she started experiencing episodes of headache. These episodes occur on both sides of the front of her head without any radiation elsewhere. They are described as throbbing, and mild to moderately severe in intensity (rated as 3 to 6 out of 10 in the 10-point pain scale). The headaches usually last 4 to 6 hours, started as one to two episodes a month but now average once a week. The episodes are usually related to stress. The headaches are relieved with sleep and placing a damp cool towel over her forehead. There is little relief from acetaminophen.

MN has missed work on several occasions because of associated nausea and occasional vomiting during the episodes. There are no associated visual changes, motor-sensory deficits, loss of consciousness, or paresthesia. She had headaches with nausea and vomiting beginning at age 15 years. These recurred throughout her mid-20s, then decreased to one every 2 or 3 months, and almost disappeared. She thinks her headaches may be like those in the past but wants to be sure because her mother had a headache just before she died of a stroke. She is concerned because her headaches interfere with her work and make her irritable with her family. She reports increased pressure at work from a demanding supervisor as well as being worried about her daughter. She eats three meals a day and drinks three cups of coffee a day and tea at night. Due to the

continued

increasing frequency of the headaches, she decided to come to the clinic today.

Allergies: Ampicillin causes rash. No environmental or food allergies.

Medications:

- Acetaminophen, one to two tablets every 4 to 6 hours as needed.

Past Medical History:

Childhood Illnesses: Measles, chicken pox. No scarlet fever or rheumatic fever.

Adult Illnesses: Medical: Pyelonephritis, 2016, with fever and right flank pain; treated with ampicillin; developed generalized rash with itching several days later; no recurrence of infection. Last dental visit 2 years ago. *Surgical:* Tonsillectomy, age 6; appendectomy, age 13. Sutures for laceration, 2012, after stepping on piece of glass. *Ob/Gyn:* G3P3 (3–0–0–3), with normal vaginal deliveries. Three living children. Menarche age 12. Last menses 6 months ago. *Psychiatric:* None.

Health Maintenance: Immunizations: Age-appropriate immunizations up to date as per immunization registry. *Screening tests:* Last Pap smear, 2018, normal. Mammograms, 2019, normal.

Family History:

Father died at age 43 years in a train accident. Mother died at age 67 years from stroke; had varicose veins, headaches.

One brother, age 61 years, with hypertension, otherwise well; one brother, age 58 years, well except for mild arthritis; one sister, died in infancy of unknown cause.

Husband died at age 54 of heart attack.

Daughter, age 33 years, with migraine headaches, otherwise well; son, age 31 years, with headaches; son, age 27 years, well.

No family history of diabetes, heart or kidney disease, cancer, epilepsy, or mental illness.

Personal and Social History:

Born and raised in Las Cruces, was assigned female sex at birth, and currently identifies as female, finished high school, married at age 19 years. Worked as a salesclerk for 2 years, then moved with her husband to Española, had three children. Returned to work as a salesclerk 15 years ago to improve family finances. Children all married. Four years ago, her husband died suddenly of a heart attack, leaving little savings. MN has moved to a small apartment to be near daughter, Isabel. Isabel's husband, John, has an alcohol problem. MN's apartment is now a haven for Isabel and her two children, Kevin, age 6 years, and Lucia, age 3 years. MN feels responsible for helping them; she feels tense and nervous but denies feeling depressed. She has friends, but rarely discusses family problems: "I'd rather keep them to myself. I don't like gossip." During the "FICA" assessment she reports being raised as a Catholic, but that she stopped attending church after the death of her husband. Although she states her faith is still important to her now describes having no faith community or spiritual support system. She feels this has contributed to her sense of anxiety and agrees to meet with a chaplain. She is typically up at 7:00 AM, works 9:00 AM to 5:30 PM, and eats dinner alone.

Exercise and diet. Gets little exercise. Diet high in carbohydrates.

Safety measures. Uses seat belt regularly. Uses sunblock. Medications kept in an unlocked medicine cabinet. Cleaning solutions in unlocked cabinet below sink. Handgun stored in unlocked dresser in bedroom.

Tobacco. About 1 pack of cigarettes per day since age 18 (36 pack-years).

Alcohol/drugs. Wine on rare occasions. No illicit drugs.

Sexual history. Little interest in sex, and not sexually active. Her deceased husband was her only sexual partner. Never had STIs before. Could not recall if she has had testing done for STIs before. No concerns about HIV infection.

Review of Systems

General: Has gained 10 lb in the past 4 years.

Skin: No rashes or other changes.

Head, Eyes, Ears, Nose, Throat (HEENT): See *Present Illness*. *Head:* No history of head injury. *Eyes:* Reading glasses for 5 years, last checked 1 year ago. No symptoms. *Ears:* Hearing good. No tinnitus, vertigo, infections. *Nose, sinuses:* No hay fever, sinus trouble. *Throat* (or mouth and pharynx): No tooth pain or gum bleeding.

Neck: No lumps, goiter, pain. No swollen glands.

Breasts: No lumps, pain, discharge.

Respiratory: No cough, wheezing, shortness of breath.

Cardiovascular: No dyspnea, orthopnea, chest pain, palpitations.

Gastrointestinal: Appetite good; no nausea, vomiting, indigestion. Bowel movement about once daily, though sometimes has hard stools for 2 to 3 days when especially tense; no diarrhea or bleeding. No pain, jaundice, gallbladder or liver problems.

Urinary: No frequency, dysuria, hematuria, or recent flank pain; occasionally loses urine when coughing.

continued

Genital: No vaginal or pelvic infections. No dyspareunia.
Peripheral vascular: No history of phlebitis or leg pain.
Musculoskeletal: Mild low backaches, often at the end of the workday; no radiation into the legs; used to do back exercises, but not now. No other joint pain.
Psychiatric: No history of depression or treatment for psychiatric disorders.
Neurologic: No fainting, seizures, motor or sensory loss. No memory problems.
Hematologic: No easy bleeding or bruising.
Endocrine: No known heat or cold intolerance. No polyuria, polydipsia.

Physical Examination

COMPREHENSIVE PHYSICAL EXAMINATION

Conduct a *comprehensive physical examination* on most new patients or patients being admitted to the hospital. For more *problem-oriented*, or *focused, assessments*, the presenting complaints will dictate which segments you elect to perform.

- The key to a thorough and accurate physical examination is a systematic sequence of examination. With effort and practice, you will acquire your own routine sequence. This book recommends examining from the patient's *right side*.
- Apply the techniques of inspection, palpation, auscultation, and percussion to each body region, but be sensitive to the whole patient.
- *Minimize the number of times you ask the patient to change position* from supine to sitting or standing to lying supine.
- For an overview of the physical examination, study the sequence that follows. *Note that clinicians vary in where they place different segments, especially for the musculoskeletal and nervous systems.*

Beginning the Examination: Setting the Stage

Take the steps in Box 4-1 to prepare for the physical examination.

> **BOX 4-1. Steps in Preparing for the Physical Examination**
>
> - Reflect on your approach to the patient.
> - Adjust the lighting and the environment.
> - Check your equipment.
> - Make the patient comfortable.
> - Observe standard and universal precautions.
> - Choose the sequence, scope, and positioning of examination.

Think through your approach, your professional demeanor, and how to make the patient comfortable and relaxed. Always wash your hands in the patient's presence before beginning the examination.

Reflect on Your Approach to the Patient. Identify yourself as a student. Try to appear calm, organized, and competent, even if you feel differently. If you forget to do part of the examination, simply examine that area out of sequence, but smoothly. This is not uncommon, especially at first!

Adjust the Lighting and Environment. Adjust the bed to a convenient height (be sure to lower it when finished). Ask the patient to move toward you if this makes it easier to do your physical examination. Good lighting and a quiet environment are important.

Check Your Equipment. Use the checklist in Box 4-2 to check your equipment.

BOX 4-2. Tools of the Trade: Instruments and Supplies for the Physical Examination

- Stethoscope
- Sphygmomanometer
- Ophthalmoscope
- Visual acuity card or chart
- Otoscope. If you are examining children, the otoscope should allow pneumatic otoscopy.
- Tuning forks—128-Hz and 256-Hz Thermometer
- Neurologic reflex or percussion hammer
- Vaginal speculum
- Sampling equipment for cytologic and bacteriologic studies
- Light source
- A timepiece with second hand (timer)
- Cotton swabs, safety pins, or other disposable objects for testing light touch sensation and two-point discrimination
- Tongue depressor
- Ruler or a flexible tape measure, preferably marked in centimeters
- Disposable face mask
- Disposable gown
- Gloves and lubricant for oral, vaginal, and rectal examinations
- Hand sanitizer
- Paper and pen or pencil
- Handheld ultrasound
- Dermoscope
- Access to the electronic health record via desktop or laptop computer

Make the Patient Comfortable. Show concern for privacy and modesty.

- Close nearby doors and draw curtains before beginning.
- Acquire the art of *draping the patient* with the gown or draw sheet as you learn each examination segment in future chapters. The goal is to visualize one area of the body at a time maximizing the patient's comfort but without compromising your diagnostic goals as a clinician.
- As you proceed, keep the patient informed, especially when you anticipate embarrassment or discomfort, as when checking for the femoral pulse. Also try to gauge how much the patient wants to know.
- Make sure your instructions to the patient at each step are courteous and clear.
- Watch the patient's facial expression and even ask "Is it okay?" as you move through the examination.

Concluding the Examination. When you have finished, tell the patient your general impressions and what to expect next. Lower the bed to avoid risk of falls and raise the bedrails if needed. As you leave, clean your equipment, dispose of waste materials, and wash your hands.

Observing Standard and MRSA Precautions. Observe standard and universal precautions. Use rigorous handwashing before and after all patient contact and, whenever indicated, personal protective equipment (gloves; gowns; and mouth, nose, and eye protection); safe injection practices; safe handling of contaminated equipment or surfaces; respiratory hygiene and cough etiquette; patient isolation criteria; and precautions relating to equipment, toys, solid surfaces, and laundry handling.

Observing Universal Precautions. Universal precautions are a set of precautions designed to prevent transmission of HIV, HBV, and other blood-borne pathogens when providing first aid or health care. The following fluids are considered potentially infectious: all blood and other body fluids containing visible blood, semen, and vaginal secretions; and cerebrospinal, synovial, pleural, peritoneal, pericardial, and amniotic fluids. Protective barriers include gloves, gowns, aprons, masks, face shields, and protective eyewear. All healthcare workers should observe the important precautions for safe injections and prevention of injury from needlesticks, scalpels, and other sharp instruments and devices (Box 4-3). Report to your health service immediately, if such injuries occur.

BOX 4-3. Transmission-Based Precautions in Patient Care Facilities

Type of Precaution	Description	Type of Personal Protective Equipment Required			
		Gloves	Gown	Mask	Respirator Mask
Contact precautions	Conditions that can be contracted through touching or contact such as MRSA and *Clostridium difficile*	✓	✓		
Droplet precautions	Conditions that could be spread through contact with secretions from the mouth, nose, and lungs especially when a patient coughs or sneezes; usually, the droplets can only travel ~3 ft. (e.g., influenza, whooping cough), but COVID-19 droplets can travel up to 6 ft	✓	✓	✓	
Airborne precautions	Conditions that could spread through the air over long distances such as tuberculosis and chickenpox Patients also placed in a *negative pressure room* designed to prevent the air from flowing into the hallways	✓	✓		✓
Reverse isolation	To protect the patient from any germs the staff or visitors are carrying; those with a decreased immune system, usually from chemotherapy, may be placed in reverse isolation	✓	✓	✓	

Source: CDC. *Guideline for isolation precautions: preventing transmission of infectious agents in healthcare settings.* 2007. Available at https://www.cdc.gov/infectioncontrol/pdf/guidelines/isolation-guidelines-H.pdf. Updated November 14, 2018. Accessed May 26, 2019.

Choose the Sequence, Scope, and Positioning of the Examination.
The sequence of the examination should:

- Maximize the patient's comfort.
- Avoid unnecessary changes in position.
- Enhance the clinician's efficiency.

Choose whether to do a *comprehensive* or *focused examination*. In general, move from "head to toe." An important goal as a student is to develop your own sequence with these principles in mind.

Practice examining the patient from the patient's right side. Note that the right side is more reliable to estimate jugular venous pressure from the right, the palpating hand rests more comfortably on the apical impulse, the right kidney is more frequently palpable than the left, and examining tables are frequently positioned to accommodate a right-handed approach.

To examine the *supine patient* who is unable to sit up, you can examine the head, neck, and anterior chest. Then roll the patient onto each side to listen to the lungs, examine the back, and inspect the skin. Roll the patient back and finish the rest of the examination with the patient again supine.

Suggested "Head-to-Toe" Physical Examination

Use the checklist in Box 4-4 to do the head-to-toe examination.

BOX 4-4. Physical Examination: Suggested Sequence and Positioning

- General survey
- Vital signs
- Skin: upper torso, anterior and posterior
- Head and neck, including thyroid and lymph nodes
- *Optional:* Nervous system (mental status, cranial nerves, upper extremity motor strength, bulk, tone, cerebellar function)
- Thorax and lungs
- Breasts
- Musculoskeletal as indicated: upper extremities

- *Optional:* thorax and lungs—anterior
- Breasts and axillae
- Abdomen
- Peripheral vascular
- *Optional:* skin—lower torso and extremities
- Nervous system: lower extremity motor strength, bulk, tone, sensation; reflexes; plantar reflex
- Musculoskeletal, as indicated
- *Optional:* skin, anterior and posterior

---

continued

- Cardiovascular, including jugular venous pressure (JVP), carotid upstrokes and bruits, point of maximal impulse (PMI), S_1, S_2, murmurs, extra sounds
- Cardiovascular, for S_3 and murmur of mitral stenosis
- Cardiovascular, for murmur of aortic insufficiency

- *Optional:* nervous system, including gait
- *Optional:* musculoskeletal, comprehensive
- *Women:* pelvic and rectal examination
- *Men:* prostate and rectal examination

Key to the Symbols for the Patient's Position

♀	Sitting	ᴏ—	Lying supine
⌇	Lying supine, with head of bed raised 30°	⸋	Standing
⌇	Same, turned partly to left side	ᴧ	Lying supine, with hips flexed, abducted, and externally rotated, and knees flexed (lithotomy position)
⸋	Sitting, leaning forward	ᴏⱼ—	Lying on the left side (left lateral decubitus)

Each symbol pertains until a new one appears. Two symbols separated by a slash indicate either or both positions.

General Survey. Observe general state of health, height, build, and sexual development. Note posture, motor activity, and gait; dress, grooming, and personal hygiene; and any odors of the body or breath. Watch facial expressions and note manner, affect, and reactions to persons and things in the environment. Listen to the patient's manner of speaking and note the state of awareness or level of consciousness.

⸋ Vital Signs. Ask the patient to sit on the edge of the bed or examining table, unless this position is contraindicated. Stand in front of the patient, moving to either side as needed. Measure the blood pressure. Count pulse and respiratory rate. If indicated, measure body temperature.

Skin. Observe the face. Identify any lesions, noting their location, distribution, arrangement, type, and color. Inspect and palpate the hair and nails. Study the patient's hands. Continue to assess the skin as you examine the other body regions.

HEENT. *Head:* Examine the hair, scalp, skull, and face. *Eyes:* Check visual acuity and screen the visual fields. Note position and alignment of the eyes. Observe the eyelids. Inspect the sclera and conjunctiva of each eye. With oblique lighting, inspect each cornea, iris, and lens. Assess extraocular movements. Darken the room to promote pupillary dilation and visibility of the fundi. Compare the pupils and test their reactions to light. With an ophthalmoscope, inspect the ocular fundi. *Ears:* Inspect the auricles, canals, and drums. Check auditory acuity. If acuity is diminished, check lateralization (Weber test) and compare air and bone conduction (Rinne test). *Nose and sinuses:* Examine the external nose; using a light and nasal speculum, inspect nasal mucosa, septum, and turbinates. Palpate for tenderness of the frontal and maxillary sinuses. *Throat (or mouth and pharynx):* Inspect the lips, oral mucosa, gums, teeth, tongue, palate, tonsils, and pharynx. You may wish to assess the cranial nerves at this point in the examination.

Neck. Move behind the sitting patient to feel the thyroid gland and to examine the back, posterior thorax, and lungs. Inspect and palpate the cervical lymph nodes. Note any masses or unusual pulsations in the neck. Feel for any deviation of the trachea. Observe sound and effort of the patient's breathing. Inspect and palpate the thyroid gland.

Back. Inspect and palpate the spine and muscles.

Posterior Thorax and Lungs. Inspect and palpate the spine and muscles of the *upper* back. Inspect, palpate, and percuss the chest. Identify the level of diaphragmatic dullness on each side. Listen to the breath sounds; identify any adventitious (or added) sounds, and, if indicated, listen to transmitted voice sounds (see p. 228).

Breasts, Axillae, and Epitrochlear Nodes. The patient is still sitting. Move to the front again. In a woman, inspect the breasts with patient's arms relaxed, then elevated, and then with her hands pressed on her hips. In either sex, inspect the axillae and feel for the axillary nodes; feel for the epitrochlear nodes. Palpate the breasts, while continuing your inspection.

Note on the Musculoskeletal System. By this time, you have made preliminary observations of the musculoskeletal system. You have inspected the hands and surveyed the upper back. If indicated, *with the patient still sitting,* examine the hands, arms, shoulders, neck, and temporomandibular joints. Inspect and palpate the joints and check their range of motion. You may choose to examine upper extremity muscle bulk, tone, strength, and reflexes at this time, or wait until later as part of the nervous system exam.

Anterior Thorax and Lungs. Ask the patient to lie down. Stand at the *right side* of the patient's bed. Inspect, palpate, and percuss the chest. Listen to the breath sounds, any adventitious sounds, and, if indicated, transmitted voice sounds.

Cardiovascular System. Elevate the head of bed to about 30 degrees, adjusting as necessary to see the jugular venous pulsations. Observe the jugular venous pulsations and measure the jugular venous pressure in relation to the sternal angle. Inspect and palpate the carotid pulsations. Listen for carotid bruits.

Ask the patient to roll partly onto the left side while you listen at the apex. Then have the patient roll back to supine while you listen the rest of the heart. Ask the patient to sit, lean forward, and exhale while you listen for the murmur if you suspect an aortic regurgitation. Inspect and palpate the precordium. Note the location of the apical impulse. Attempt to note its diameter, amplitude, and duration. Listen at the apex and the lower sternal border with the bell of a stethoscope. Listen at each auscultatory area with the diaphragm. Listen for S_1 and S_2 and for physiologic splitting of S_2. Listen for any abnormal heart sounds or murmurs.

Abdomen. Lower the head of the bed to the flat position. Inspect, auscultate, and percuss. Palpate lightly, then deeply. Assess the liver and spleen by percussion and then palpation. Try to palpate the kidneys; palpate the aorta and its pulsations. If you suspect kidney infection, percuss posteriorly over the costovertebral angles (CVAs).

Peripheral Vascular System. With the patient supine, palpate the femoral pulses and, if indicated, popliteal pulses. Palpate the inguinal lymph nodes. Inspect for edema, discoloration, or ulcers in the lower extremities. Palpate for pitting edema. With the patient standing, inspect for varicose veins.

Lower Extremities. With the patient in supine, examine the legs, assessing the peripheral vascular, musculoskeletal, and nervous systems. Each of these systems can be further assessed when the patient stands.

Nervous System. The patient is sitting or supine. The examination of the nervous system can also be divided into the upper extremity examination (when the patient is still sitting) and the lower extremity examination (when the patient is supine) after examination of the peripheral nervous system.

Mental Status. If indicated and not done during the interview, assess orientation, mood, thought process, thought content, abnormal perceptions, insight and judgment, memory and attention, information and vocabulary, calculating abilities, abstract thinking, and constructional ability.

Cranial Nerves. If not already examined, check sense of smell, funduscopic examination, strength of the temporal and masseter muscles, facial movements, gag reflex, strength of the trapezius and sternocleidomastoid muscles, and protrusion of tongue.

Motor System. Assess muscle bulk, tone, and strength of major muscle groups.

Sensory System. Assess pain, temperature, light touch, vibrations, and discrimination. Compare right and left sides and distal with proximal areas on the limbs.

Reflexes. Include biceps, triceps, brachioradialis, patellar, Achilles deep tendon reflexes; also, plantar reflexes or Babinski reflex (see pp. 425–427).

Coordination, Station and Gait. Perform rapid alternating movements (RAMs), point-to-point movements such as finger to nose (F → N) and heel to shin (H → S); gait. Perform a Romberg test for station. Observe patient's gait and ability to walk heel to toe, on toes, and on heels.

Additional Examinations. The *rectal* and *genital* examinations are often performed at the end of the physical examination.

◔/♂ *Genital Examination in Men.* Examine the penis and scrotal contents. Check for hernias.

♂ *Rectal Examination in Men.* The patient is lying on left side for the rectal examination. Inspect the sacrococcygeal and perianal areas. Palpate the anal canal, rectum, and prostate. (If the patient cannot stand, examine the genitalia before doing the rectal examination.)

♀ *Genital and Rectal Examination in Women.* The patient is in the lithotomy position. Sit during the examination with the speculum, then stand during bimanual examination of uterus, adnexa, and rectum (Box 4-5). Examine the external genitalia, vagina, and cervix. Obtain a Pap smear. Palpate the uterus and adnexa. Do a bimanual and rectal examination.

BOX 4-5. Modifications of Physical Examination for Specific Patient Situations	
Specific Patient Situation	**Modification**
Patient on bed rest	■ Patients on bed rest are often required to refrain from weightbearing or certain activities as a precaution after an injury or after a procedure. ■ Often this restriction only allows the examination of the patient's head, neck, and chest anteriorly with the patient lying supine. ■ Examine the posterior region of the body (e.g., auscultation of the posterior chest) if it is safe for the patient to roll over on the bed.

continued

Patient using a wheelchair	▪ Certain maneuvers of the head and neck, cardiovascular, and pulmonary examination can be performed with the patient sitting in the wheelchair and leaning forward if necessary.
	▪ Certain maneuvers, like the abdominal examination, require the patient to transfer from their wheelchair to the examination table or bed.
Patient who is postprocedure	▪ Before examining the patient, confirm any restrictions of movement.
	▪ Pay particular attention to the condition of the surgical site and its dressing, return of bowel function and, depending on the procedure, peripheral vascular or neurologic examinations.
	▪ Also assess drains, lines, and tubes such as chest tubes, indwelling catheters, or intravenous lines.
Patient who is obese	▪ When examining patients, note the patient's fat distribution.
	▪ When examining the skin, you should examine within body folds. Since these areas are usually moist, warm, and often missed in daily hygiene, they are prone to skin breakdown and development of infections.
	▪ Also inspect the lower extremities for any signs of skin breakdown, swelling, or vascular changes.
Patient in pain	▪ The first step in examining a patient in pain is observation. Look for signs of distress like an increased respiratory rate, sweating, tearing, and facial expressions such as grimacing or biting.
	▪ Pain commonly elevates blood pressure and heart rate.
	▪ An attempt to control the pain prior to examination may be warranted.

DOCUMENTING THE PHYSICAL EXAMINATION

Recall that your goal is to produce a clear, concise, but comprehensive report that documents key findings and communicates your assessment in a succinct format to clinicians, consultants, and other members of the healthcare team (Box 4-6). Note the standard format of the clinical record from *General Survey* to *Neurological Examination*.

BOX 4-6. Sample Physical Examination Note

General Survey: MN is a short, overweight, middle-aged woman, who is animated and responds quickly to questions. Her hair is well groomed. Her color is good, and she lies flat without discomfort.

Vital Signs: Ht (without shoes) 157 cm (5'2"). Wt (dressed) 65 kg (143 lb). BMI 26. BP 164/98 right arm, supine; 160/96 left arm, supine; 152/88 right arm, supine with wide cuff. Heart rate (HR) 88 and regular. Respiratory rate (RR) 18. Temperature (oral) 98.6 °F.

Skin: Palms cold and moist, but color good. Scattered cherry angiomas over upper trunk. Nails without clubbing, cyanosis.

Head, Eyes, Ears, Nose, Throat (HEENT): Head: Hair of average texture. Scalp without lesions, normocephalic/atraumatic (NC/AT). *Eyes:* Vision 20/30 in each eye. Visual fields full by confrontation. Conjunctiva pink; sclera white. Pupils 4 mm constricting to 2 mm, round, regular, equally reactive to light. Extraocular movements intact. Disc margins sharp, without hemorrhages, exudates. No arteriolar narrowing or A-V nicking. *Ears:* Cerumen partially obscures right tympanic membrane (TM); left canal clear, TM with good cone of light. Acuity good to whispered voice. Weber midline. AC > BC. *Nose:* Mucosa pink, septum midline. No sinus tenderness. *Mouth:* Oral mucosa pink. Dentition good. Tongue midline. Tonsils absent. Pharynx without exudates.

Neck: Neck supple. Trachea midline. Thyroid isthmus barely palpable, lobes not felt.

Lymph Nodes: No cervical, axillary, or epitrochlear nodes.

Thorax and Lungs: Thorax symmetric with good excursion. Lungs resonant on percussion. Breath sounds vesicular with no added sounds. Diaphragms descend 4 cm bilaterally.

Cardiovascular: Jugular venous pressure 1 cm above the sternal angle, with head of examining table raised to 30°. Carotid upstrokes brisk, without bruits. Apical impulse discrete and tapping, barely palpable in the 5th left interspace, 8 cm lateral to the midsternal line. Good S_1, S_2; no S_3 or S_4. A II/VI medium-pitched midsystolic murmur at the 2nd right interspace; does not radiate to the neck. No diastolic murmurs.

Breasts: Pendulous, symmetric. No masses; nipples without discharge.

Abdomen: Protuberant. Well-healed scar, right lower quadrant. Bowel sounds active. No tenderness or masses. Liver span 7 cm in right midclavicular line; edge smooth, palpable 1 cm below right costal margin (RCM). Spleen not felt. No costovertebral angle tenderness (CVAT).

continued

Genitalia: External genitalia without lesions. Mild cystocele at introitus on straining. Vaginal mucosa pink. Cervix pink, parous, and without discharge. Uterus anterior, midline, smooth, not enlarged. Adnexa not palpated due to obesity and poor relaxation. No cervical or adnexal tenderness. Pap smear taken. Rectovaginal wall intact.

Rectal: No external hemorrhoids, with tight sphincter tone, rectal vault without masses. Stool brown, negative for occult blood.

Extremities: Warm and without edema. Calves supple, nontender.

Peripheral Vascular: Trace edema at both ankles. No varicosities in lower extremities. No stasis pigmentation or ulcers. Pulses (2+ = brisk, or normal):

	Radial	Femoral	Popliteal	Dorsalis Pedis	Posterior Tibial
RT	2+	2+	2+	2+	2+
LT	2+	2+	2+	2+	2+

Musculoskeletal: No joint deformities or swelling on inspection and palpation. Good range of motion in hands, wrists, elbows, shoulders, spine, hips, knees, ankles.

Neurologic: Mental Status: Alert and cooperative. Thought processes are coherent and insight is good. Oriented to person, place, and time. *Cranial Nerves:* II to XII intact. *Motor:* Good muscle bulk and tone. *Strength:* 5/5 bilaterally in deltoids, biceps, triceps, hand grips, iliopsoas, hamstrings, quadriceps, tibialis anterior, and gastrocnemius. *Cerebellar:* rapid alternating movement (RAMs) and point-to-point movements intact. *Gait:* stable, fluid. *Sensory:* Pinprick, light touch, position sense, vibration, and stereognosis intact. *Station:* Romberg negative. *Reflexes:*

Clinical Reasoning, Assessment, and Plan

The basic process of *clinical reasoning* starts with the information you have gathered from your patient including historical information, findings from your physical examination, and any preliminary diagnostic and laboratory testing (Box 5-1).

The next step is to organize and interpret these sets of information with the goal of creating a concise and appropriate *problem representation* (documented in the clinical record as the *Summary Statement*).

From this problem representation, generate, prioritize, and test a list of possible diagnoses until you have selected a *working diagnosis*—one that fits your patient's problem best. Your working diagnosis will then be the basis for determining your patient's *plan*.

BOX 5-1. Basic Structure of the Clinical Reasoning Process

- Gather initial patient information (health history and physical examination).
- Organize and interpret information to synthesize the problem (problem representation).
- Generate hypotheses (*differential diagnosis*) for the patient's problem.
- Test hypotheses until you have working diagnosis.
- Plan the diagnostic and treatment strategy.

Gather Initial Patient Information

This step includes gathering the patient's *symptoms,* the *signs* you observed during the physical examination, and any laboratory and other reports available to you. It is critical to be methodical and organized, such that all abnormal and unexpected findings are identified.

Organize and Interpret Clinical Information

Once you have a list of abnormal findings, begin to organize them in order to narrow the list of possible their causes. A helpful approach is to *tease out separate clusters of observations and analyze one cluster at a time.*

- *Anatomic Location.* Clustering your findings *anatomically* could point to a potential source of the problem. Sometimes you may have to settle for a body region or system.
- *Age:* Younger patients are more likely to have a single disease compared to older patients.
- *Timing of symptoms.*
- *Involvement of different body systems.* If symptoms and signs occur in a single system, one disease may explain them. Problems in different, apparently unrelated, systems often require more than one explanation.
- *Multisystem conditions:* With experience, you will become increasingly adept at recognizing *multisystem conditions* and building plausible explanations that link manifestations that are seemingly unrelated. Related risk factors should be explored promptly.

Synthesize Clinical Information and Develop the Problem Representation

As you gather and organize clinical data during the patient encounter, you simultaneously *synthesize* this information to form a *problem representation*—your evolving sense of the clinical picture (Box 5-2). It usually contains the patient's initial information (chief complaint, epidemiology, and risk factors), key features in the history and physical examination, and results of diagnostic testing. In your clinical documentation, the problem representation is called the *Summary Statement.*

BOX 5-2. Example: Development of a Problem Representation

A 57-year-old male comes to the emergency room with a chief complaint of pain in his chest for the past 2 hours. He says that he was shoveling snow from his driveway when he suddenly developed a moderately severe pain in the center of his chest right behind the sternum. The pain lasted for approximately 1 to 2 minutes and did not move anywhere else. He said that the pain was accompanied by shortness of breath. He has smoked a pack of cigarettes per day for the last 35 years and has a history of congestive heart failure. His physical examination is notable for new S_3 gallop, crackles in both lung bases, and swelling of both legs.

Your resulting problem representation for the case could be:
*A 57-year-old man with congestive heart failure and a 35 pack-year
smoking history presents with acute, severe, exertional, retrosternal pain
and associated shortness of breath. His examination is notable for a
new S₃ gallop, bibasilar crackles, and bilateral lower extremity edema.*

Generate Hypotheses by Searching for the Probable Cause of the Findings

For each identified problem or cluster of problems, you will generate
a clinical hypothesis. Draw on the full range of your knowledge and
experience and read widely. It is at this point that reading about diseases
and abnormalities is most useful. The approaches in Boxes 5-3 and 5-4
may help.

BOX 5-3. Approaches to Searching for Probable Causes of the Findings

- Generate an exhaustive list.
- Select the most specific and critical findings to support your hypothesis.
- Match these findings against all conditions that can produce them.
- Eliminate diagnostic possibilities that fail to explain the findings.
- Weigh competing possibilities and select the most likely diagnosis.
- Give special attention to potentially life-threatening conditions.

BOX 5-4. Memory Aids for Generating Differential Diagnosis

Tom G. Prince, MD, Psychiatrist, General Hospital

Toxin/Trauma including medications	**C**ardiovascular
Oncologic	**E**ndocrine
Musculoskeletal/Rheumatologic	**M**etabolic/Genetic
Gastrointestinal	**D**ermatologic
Pulmonary	**P**sychiatric
Renal	**G**enitourinary/Gynecologic
Infectious	**H**ematologic
Neurologic	

continued

VINDICATE

Vascular	**C**ongenital
Infectious	**A**utoimmune/**A**llergic
Neoplastic	**T**rauma/**T**oxic
Drug related	**E**ndocrine/**M**etabolic
Inflammatory/**I**diopathic/**I**atrogenic	

Illness scripts trigger a memory response from previously learned information that often includes a disease's pathophysiology, epidemiology, time course, salient symptoms and signs, diagnostics, and treatment (Box 5-5). Try to see if the patient's problem can match one of these patterns.

BOX 5-5. Sample Illness Script for Acute Coronary Syndrome

	Acute Coronary Syndrome
Epidemiology/ Pathophysiology	Older age, risk factors include diabetes, hypertension, dyslipidemia, family history, tobacco use
Time course	Acute onset, not necessarily preceded by exertional angina
Clinical presentation	Chest pain, with crescendo to maximal pain; often dull and substernal, radiating to arms/shoulders; diaphoresis; dyspnea; nausea/vomiting, diaphoresis; tachycardia on examination
Diagnostic studies	Elevated cardiac biomarkers; ST elevation/depression, T-wave changes on ECG; regional wall motion abnormality on echocardiogram

Test Your Hypotheses

After you have made a hypothesis about the patient's problem, you are ready to *test your hypothesis*. You are likely to need further history, additional maneuvers on physical examination, or laboratory studies to confirm or rule out your tentative diagnosis or to clarify which of two or three possible diagnoses are most likely.

Establish a Working Diagnosis

Establish a working definition of the problem at the highest level of explic-itness and certainty that the data allow. You may be limited to a symptom. At other times, you can define a problem more specifically based on its anatomy, disease process, or cause. Be aware of common cognitive errors as shown in Box 5-6.

BOX 5-6. Common Types of Clinical Cognitive Errors	
Cognitive Error	**Description**
Anchoring bias	Tendency to perceptually lock onto salient features in the patient's initial presentation too early in the diagnostic process and failure to adjust in light of later information
Availability heuristic	Assumption that a diagnosis is more likely, or more frequently occurring, if it more readily comes to mind
Confirmation bias	Seeking supportive evidence for a diagnosis at the exclusion of more persuasive information refuting it
Diagnostic momentum	Prioritizing a diagnosis made by prior clinicians, discounting evidence of alternative explanations
Framing effect	Interpretation of information is influenced heavily by the way information about the problem is presented (*framed*)
Representation error	Failure to take prevalence into account when estimating the probability of a diagnosis
Visceral bias	Visceral arousal (negative and positive feelings toward patients) leads to poor diagnostic decisions

Sources: Croskerry P. The importance of cognitive errors in diagnosis and strategies to minimize them. *Acad Med.* 2003;78(8):775–780; Weinstein A, et al. Diagnosing and remediating clinical reasoning difficulties: a faculty development workshop. *MedEdPORTAL.* 2017;13:10650.

Plan the Diagnostic and Treatment Strategy

Planning the diagnostic and treatment strategy flows logically from the working diagnosis you have identified and discussed with the patient. These steps are often wide ranging and incorporate the diagnostic and therapeutic interventions that you recommend, patient education, changes in medications, needed tests, referrals to other clinicians, and return visits for counseling and support.

Use Shared Decision Making to Develop a Plan. It is critical to both obtain patient agreement and encourage patient participation in decision making whenever possible. These discussions should use evidence-based medicine, clinician judgment, and the patient's values. These practices promote optimal therapy, adherence to treatment, and patient satisfaction, especially since there is often no single "right" plan, but a range of variations and options.

DOCUMENTING THE SUMMARY STATEMENT, ASSESSMENT, AND PLAN

The *Summary Statement, Assessment*, and *Plan* represent the most robust reflection of your clinical reasoning and data synthesis skills. You proceed to go from the description and observation of subjective and objective data to their analysis and interpretation. You select and cluster relevant pieces of information, analyze their significance, and try to explain them logically using principles of biopsychosocial and biomedical science.

Documenting the Summary Statement

The problem representation is a synthesis and distillation of the salient information which "makes a case" for your working diagnosis. This is written in your patient's health record as the *Summary Statement* and often starts the *Assessment* section of the clinical record. The goal is for the summary statement to elicit the working diagnosis in the mind of the reader by aligning with the illness script.

For example: *A 57-year-old man with congestive heart failure and a 35 pack-year smoking history presents with acute, severe, exertional, retrosternal pain and associated shortness of breath. His examination is notable for a new S₃ gallop, bibasilar crackles, and bilateral lower extremity edema.*

A well-developed summary statement often contains important qualifying adjectives called *semantic qualifiers* (Box 5-7). Semantic qualifiers are qualitative terms that are binary in nature (opposing descriptors) that can be used to compare and contrast diagnostic considerations and are associated with strong clinical reasoning.

BOX 5-7. Examples of Semantic Qualifiers	
■ acute—chronic	■ mild—severe
■ at rest—with activity (*exertional*)	■ old—new
■ constant—intermittent	■ sharp—dull
■ diffuse—localized	■ unilateral—bilateral
	■ young—old

Documenting the Assessment and Plan

In general, an assessment and plan can be *diagnostic, therapeutic,* or *both.* Your *assessment* will include a brief description of the potential causes (your *differential diagnosis*), and your *plan* will describe your steps in reaching a diagnosis and/or addressing the problem (Box 5-8). Start by making a list of all of the patient's problems addressed during the clinical encounter. This list should include known diagnoses, symptoms, abnormalities, and psychosocial concerns. It is related to the initial list of abnormalities you have made at the start of the clinical reasoning process; however, it reflects how those observations are analyzed and synthesized. As such the problem list:

- Is a synthesis of all abnormal and unexpected findings during an encounter
- Includes known diagnoses and new/undiagnosed symptoms/signs
- Includes significant social factors that impact health such as food or housing insecurity
- Is prioritized, with the patient's chief complaint on top

Another increasingly prominent item on problem lists is *Health Maintenance.* Routinely listing Health Maintenance helps you track several important health concerns more effectively: immunizations, screening tests such as mammograms or colonoscopies, instructions regarding nutrition or self-examinations, recommendations about exercise or use of seat belts, and responses to important life events.

BOX 5-8. Sample of Summary Statement, Assessment, and Plan

In a well-constructed record, the *Assessment* and *Plan* section stems from the list of problems addressed in the clinical encounter. Each problem is listed in order of priority and expanded with an explanation of supporting findings and a differential diagnosis, followed by a plan for addressing that problem.

Summary Statement: MN is a 54-year-old female with a history of migraines since childhood presenting with chronic intermittent, progressive pulsatile headaches which are similar to prior attacks and precipitated by current life stressors. The headaches are accompanied by nausea and vomiting. On examination, she has elevated blood pressure but otherwise a normal cardiovascular and nonfocal neurologic examination.

continued

Assessment and Plan:

1. Headaches:

   The differential diagnosis includes:
   - Migraine headache—This is most likely as the patient has a history of migraine headaches and describes her current headaches as similar in quality. The pulsatile quality, duration between 4 and 72 hours, associated nausea and vomiting, and disability intensity all support this diagnosis, as does the normal neurological examination.
   - Tension headaches—This is also a possibility as the headaches are bilateral, which is less common in migraine headaches. Headaches are associated with stress and relieved by sleep and cold compresses. There is no papilledema, and there are no motor or sensory deficits on the neurologic examination.
   - Other dangerous conditions are less likely. There is no fever, stiff neck, or focal findings to suggest meningitis, and the lifelong recurrent pattern makes subarachnoid hemorrhage unlikely (usually described as "the worst headache of my life"). A normal neurologic and funduscopic examination make a space-occupying lesion such as tumor less likely as well.

   Plan:
   - Discuss features of migraine versus tension headaches with the patient. Also discuss warning signs that would prompt urgent reevaluation.
   - Discuss biofeedback and stress management.
   - Advise patient to avoid caffeine, including coffee, colas, and other carbonated beverages.
   - Start nonsteroidal anti-inflammatory drugs (NSAIDs) for headache, as needed.
   - If needed next visit, begin prophylactic medication if headaches are occurring more than 2 days a week or 8 days a month.

2. Elevated blood pressure: Elevated systolic and diastolic blood pressure are noted. The patient denies chest pain and shortness of breath and is not symptomatic at the time of the interview, making hypertensive urgency unlikely.

   Plan:
   - Discuss standards for assessing blood pressure.
   - Check a hemoglobin A1c to assess for diabetes, which would impact the target blood pressure.
   - Recheck blood pressure in 2 weeks.
   - Discuss weight reduction and exercise programs (see #4).
   - Reduce salt intake.

3. Cystocele with occasional stress incontinence: Cystocele on pelvic examination, probably related to bladder relaxation. Patient is perimenopausal. Incontinence reported with coughing, suggesting alteration in bladder neck anatomy. No dysuria, fever, flank pain. Not taking any contributing medications. Usually involves small amounts of urine, no dribbling, so doubt urge or overflow incontinence.

   Plan:
   - Explain cause of stress incontinence.
   - Review urinalysis.
   - Recommend Kegel exercises.
   - Consider topical estrogen cream to vagina during next visit if no improvement.

4. Overweight: Patient 5'2", weighs 143 lb. BMI is ~26.

   Plan:
   - Explore diet history, ask patient to keep food intake diary.
   - Explore motivation to lose weight, set target for weight loss by next visit.
   - Schedule visit with dietitian.
   - Discuss exercise program, specifically, walking 30 minutes most days a week.

5. Stress and housing insecurity: Son-in-law with alcohol problem; daughter and grandchildren seeking refuge in patient's apartment, leading to tensions in these relationships. Patient also has financial constraints and describes spiritual duress with lack of social and spiritual support. Stress currently situational. No current evidence of depression (PHQ2 = 0).

   Plan:
   - Explore patient's views on strategies to cope with stress.
   - Explore sources of support, including Al-Anon for daughter and financial counseling for patient. Refer to social work and discuss in interdisciplinary team meeting.
   - Refer to chaplain to discuss spiritual support systems.
   - Continue to monitor for possible signs of depression.

6. Occasional musculoskeletal low back pain: Usually with prolonged standing. No history of trauma or motor vehicle accident. Pain does not radiate; no tenderness or motor-sensory deficits on examination. Doubt disc or nerve root compression, trochanteric bursitis, sacroiliitis.

   Plan:
   - Review benefits of weight loss and exercises to strengthen low back muscles.

continued

7. Tobacco misuse: 1 pack per day for 36 years. No signs of oral cancer on examination today. Seems precontemplative for smoking cessation in setting of multiple life stressors and progressive headaches.
   Plan:
   - Check peak flow or FEV_1/FVC on office spirometry to assess for obstructive lung disease.
   - Discuss low-dose CT for lung cancer screening.
   - Precontemplative at this point, but offered ongoing support moving forward should she change her mind and provided information resources regarding nicotine replacement therapy and oral medications to review. Can readdress after improvement of life stressors and relief from headaches.

8. Murmur: A II/IV midsystolic murmur was appreciated on examination. Given its location in the aortic position and the patient's age, this most likely represents aortic sclerosis or stenosis. The patient has no shortness of breath, chest pain or syncope to suggest severe aortic stenosis. Will monitor symptoms examination and consider a transthoracic echocardiogram if the murmur changes in intensity or if she develops any symptoms.

9. Health maintenance: Last Pap smear, 2018; Mammogram, 2019; has never had a colonoscopy.
   Plan:
   - Referred for colonoscopy, prescribed prep medications and discussed use. Provided hand out with instructions and discussed using teach-back technique.
   - Referred to dentist for oral cancer screening in light of smoking.
   - Advise patient to move medications and caustic cleaning agents to locked cabinet above shoulder height. Urge patient to store handgun in a secured locked location, unloaded with trigger lock, and to store ammunition in a separate locked location.

PATIENT PROBLEM LIST

After you complete the clinical record for the current patient encounter, generate a *Patient Problem List* that summarizes the patient's problems to be included on the patient's summary page in the electronic health record (EHR), as shown in Box 5-9. List the most active and serious problems first and record their date of onset.

BOX 5-9. Sample Patient Problem List

Date	Problem No.	Problem
8/25/21	1	Headaches probably migraine
	2	Elevated blood pressure
	3	Cystocele with occasional stress incontinence
	4	Overweight
	5	Social stress with housing insecurity
	6	Low back pain
	7	Tobacco use since age 18 years
	8	Murmur
	9	Allergy to ampicillin
	10	Health maintenance

On follow-up visits, the *Patient Problem List* provides a quick summary of the patient's clinical history and a reminder to review the status of problems the patient may not mention. It also allows other members of the healthcare team to learn about the patient's health status at a glance.

PROGRESS NOTE

The format of the progress note should be clear, sufficiently detailed, and easy to follow. It should reflect your clinical reasoning and delineate your assessment and plan. A widely adopted framework is the Subjective, Objective, Assessment, and Plan (SOAP) format, which provides a cognitive framework for evaluation of information and reasoning activities (Box 5-10).

BOX 5-10. SOAP Structural Framework for Progress Notes

Header	Description
Subjective	Documentation of data that comes from patients' experiences. These are the *"subjective"* experiences of patients (history of illness, symptoms experienced, pain and anxiety, and other features as elicited by the clinician or other healthcare providers

continued

Objective	Documentation of *"objective"* data as assessed by the clinician (physical examination findings, diagnostic testing, and radiologic examinations) that govern the processing of subjective reports of illness into medical diagnoses.
Assessment	The Assessment section documents the synthesis of "subjective" and "objective" evidence to arrive at a diagnosis. The Assessment section details the differential diagnosis and may include some risk/benefit trade-offs in decision making.
Plan	The Plan section details the needs for additional testing and consultation with other clinicians to address the patients' illnesses, in addition to the steps being taken to treat the patient.

Adapted with permission from Lenert LA. Toward medical documentation that enhances situational awareness learning. *AMIA Annu Symp Proc*. 2017;2016:763–771.

ORALLY COMMUNICATING THE CLINICAL ENCOUNTER

The *oral presentation* is a structured, accurate, and tailored account of the patient and the patient's clinical story (Box 5-11). It serves as the primary means of communication between clinicians and the rest of the patient's clinical teams and is an expression of your clinical reasoning.

The oral presentation condences the information you have obtained for the patient's clinical record and includes only what is most relevant to your differential diagnosis for or management of the patient's chief complaint. A suggested framework of a comprehensive oral presentation of a new patient is shown. The types of information and level of detail you provide in the oral presentation, however, will vary depending on the context.

BOX 5-11. Guideline for Oral Patient Presentation– New Patient

Make a convincing case for the important problems, the differential, and the plan. Make it structured, organized, and targeted, as it should take only 3–5 minutes.

Opening Statement
- Briefly state the chief complaint and why the patient was admitted.
- Include pointed and relevant historical information.

Source
- If indicated, briefly note if/why the patient cannot give a reliable history.
- Note any information sources besides the patient.
- If there is no comment on the source, it will be assumed that all information came from a reliable patient.

Present Illness
- Your differential diagnosis should guide what you include.
- Consider starting with: "... *usual state of health until* ... "
- Be chronologically organized and clear without analyzing.
- Remember the attributes of the chief complaint.
- Include elements of the past history (with supporting studies and therapeutic interventions), medications, family history, social history (including psychosocial factors) that specifically contribute to the Present Illness.
- Include pertinent positives and negatives to help the listener understand your differential diagnosis.
- Only include an ER course if it significantly affects/alters triage or immediate treatment decisions prior to coming to your care.

Other History
- Include important Past Medical History (with supporting history/data).
- Exclude minor diagnoses without impact on current care.
- Include important meds with doses of relevant ones. Omit unimportant medications.
- Include allergies.
- Include focused Family History/Social History/Review of Systems. Do not repeat previously stated information.

Physical Examination
- Always include general appearance and specific vitals.
- Include pertinent elements of examination and any abnormal findings.
- Note the remainder as "unremarkable."

Labs/Data
- Include pertinent or otherwise significant labs/studies
- Start with basic blood tests first.
- It is appropriate to mention other tests as being "normal."

continued

Synthesis
- Consider beginning with: *"And in summary ... "*
- Assess and synthesize, avoid summarizing and regurgitating information.
- Demonstrate your thinking about the patient-specific differential diagnosis.
- If multiple issues are present, weave together or discuss lesser issues in problem list.

Enumerated Problem List
- Start with most important problem first.
- Use most specific label for the problem you can.
- Avoid labeling a problem solely by its organ system.
- Include your understanding of the cause of the problem.
- Include a diagnostic and/or therapeutic specific plan for addressing it.

Source: Modified from Green EH, et al. Developing and implementing universal guidelines for oral patient presentation skills. *Teach Learn Med*. 2005;17(3):263–267. Reprinted by permission of Taylor & Francis Ltd, http://www.tandfonline.com.

Health Maintenance and Screening

CONCEPT OF PREVENTIVE CARE

- *Primary prevention* refers to interventions designed to prevent disease that include immunizations, chemoprevention, surgical procedures, and behavioral counseling.
- *Secondary prevention* refers to interventions (screening tests) designed to find disease or disease processes at an early stage when the patient has not yet manifested any signs or symptoms (*asymptomatic*) of the condition. The rationale for secondary prevention is that treating an early-stage disease is often more effective than treating disease at a later more advanced stage.

GUIDELINE RECOMMENDATIONS

Following is one of the many approaches for rating the strength of recommendations (Box 6-1).

BOX 6-1. U.S. Preventive Service Task Force (USPSTF) Ratings: Grade Definitions and Implications for Practice

Grade	Definition	Suggestions for Practice
A	The USPSTF recommends the service. There is high certainty that the net benefit is substantial.	Offer or provide this service.
B	The USPSTF recommends the service. There is high certainty that the net benefit is moderate or there is moderate certainty that the net benefit is moderate to substantial.	Offer or provide this service.

continued

C	The USPSTF recommends selectively offering or providing this service to individual patients based on professional judgment and patient preferences. There is at least moderate certainty that the net benefit is small.	Offer or provide this service for selected patients depending on individual circumstances.
D	The USPSTF recommends against the service. There is moderate or high certainty that the service has no net benefit or that the harms outweigh the benefits.	Discourage the use of this service.
I	The USPSTF concludes that the current evidence is insufficient to assess the balance of benefits and harms of the service. Evidence is lacking, of poor quality, or conflicting, and the balance of benefits and harms cannot be determined.	If the service is offered, patients should understand the uncertainty about the balance of benefits and harms.

The USPSTF defines *certainty* as the "likelihood that the USPSTF assessment of the net benefit of a preventive service is correct." The *net benefit* is defined as benefit minus harm of the preventive service as implemented in a general, primary care population.

SCREENING

Screening involves testing to identify asymptomatic patients with early-stage disease or precursors to disease who could benefit from early treatment (Box 6-2). Most screening programs target common diseases that have substantial morbidity and mortality, such as cancers, diabetes, chronic viral infections, substance abuse, and cardiovascular disease.

BOX 6-2. Selected USPSTF Screening Recommendations for Adults

Screening	USPSTF Grade (Year)	USPSTF Description
Abdominal aortic aneurysm (AAA)	B (2019)	The USPSTF recommends one-time screening for AAA with ultrasonography in men aged 65 to 75 years who have ever smoked.

Alcohol use	B (2018)	The USPSTF recommends screening for unhealthy alcohol use in primary care settings in adults 18 years or older, including pregnant women, and providing persons engaged in risky or hazardous drinking with brief behavioral counseling interventions to reduce unhealthy alcohol use.
HIV infection	A (2019)	The USPSTF recommends that clinicians screen for HIV infection in adolescents and adults aged 15 to 65 years. Younger adolescents and older adults who are at increased risk should also be screened.
Intimate partner violence (IPV)	B (2018)	The USPSTF recommends that clinicians screen for IPV in women of reproductive age and provide or refer women who screen positive to ongoing support services.
Sexually transmitted infections (STIs) including chlamydia, gonorrhea, and syphilis	B (2014)	The USPSTF recommends intensive behavioral counseling for all sexually active adolescents and for adults who are at increased risk for STIs.
Tobacco use	A (2015)	The USPSTF recommends that clinicians ask all adults about tobacco use, advise them to stop using tobacco, and provide behavioral interventions and U.S. FDA–approved pharmacotherapy for cessation to adults who use tobacco
Weight (unhealthy) and diabetes mellitus	B (2015)	The USPSTF recommends screening for abnormal blood glucose as part of cardiovascular risk assessment in adults aged 40 to 70 years who are overweight or obese.

Screening Guidelines for Adults

- Unhealthy weight and diabetes mellitus
- Substance use disorders, including misuse of prescription and illicit drugs
- Screening for intimate partner violence, elder abuse, and abuse of vulnerable adults

Screening for Unhealthy Weight and Diabetes Mellitus

- Nearly 38% of US adults are obese, including about 8% who are severely obese.
- Overweight and obesity are associated with a 20% increased risk for all-cause mortality.
- Diabetes is a major risk factor for cardiovascular disease and was either a cause or contributor to more than 330,000 deaths in 2015.

The body mass index (BMI), often used to screen for being overweight, is calculated using the person's weight divided by the square of their height (Box 6-3). Although BMI does not directly measure body fat, it is correlated with percentage of body fat and body fat mass as determined by more direct measures.

BOX 6-3. Classification of Weight by Body Mass Index (BMI)

BMI (kg/m^2)	Weight Status
<18.5	Underweight
18.5 to <25	Normal or healthy
25.0 to <30	Overweight
30.0 to <35	Obesity Class 1
35 to <40	Obesity Class 2
≥40	Obesity Class 3 ("severe")

The diagnosis of type 2 diabetes can be made based on repeated measurements of hemoglobin A1c levels ≥6.5%, fasting blood glucose ≥126 mg/dL, or an oral glucose tolerance test result ≥200 mg/dL. Because diabetes is an important modifiable risk factor for cardiovascular disease, the USPSTF has issued a grade B recommendation to screen for abnormal blood glucose in overweight or obese adults aged 40 to 70 years.

Screening for Substance Use Disorders, Including Misuse of Prescription and Illicit Drugs

- The 2017 National Survey on Drug Use and Health (NSDUH) report estimated that 30.5 million Americans used an illicit drug during the month before the survey, including:
  - 26 million marijuana users,

■ 3.2 million users of prescription drugs for nonmedical indications, and
■ 2.2 million users of cocaine.
■ An estimated 7.5 million people met DSM-IV criteria for having at least one illicit drug disorder.
■ Drug overdoses accounted for 70,237 deaths in 2017 with more than two-thirds involving opioids.

The National Institute on Drug Abuse (NIDA) recommends first asking a highly sensitive and specific single question: "How many times in the past year have you used an illegal drug or used a prescription medication for nonclinical reasons?"

If the response is positive, ask specifically about nonclinical use of illicit and prescription drugs: "In your lifetime have you ever used: marijuana; cocaine; prescription stimulants; methamphetamines; sedatives or sleeping pills; hallucinogens like lysergic acid diethylamide (LSD), ecstasy, mushrooms...; street opioids like heroin or opium; prescription opioids like fentanyl, oxycodone, hydrocodone...; or other substances." For those answering yes, a series of further questions is recommended.

The USPSTF, however, concluded in 2008 that evidence was insufficient to recommend screening for illicit drug use. The USPSTF guideline is currently being reviewed and updated.

Screening for Intimate Partner Violence, Elder Abuse, and Abuse of Vulnerable Adults

■ The Centers for Disease Control and Prevention (CDC) reports that more than one in three US women and about one in three US men experience intimate partner violence (IPV) during their lifetime.
■ Overall, 21% of women experienced severe physical violence during their lifetime compared to 15% of men.
■ More than half of all female homicides (55.3%) with known circumstances were IPV related.

The USPSTF defines *IPV* as "physical violence, sexual violence, psychological aggression (including coercive tactics, such as limiting access to financial resources), or stalking by a romantic or sexual partner, including spouses, boyfriends, girlfriends, dates, and casual 'hookups.'"

Screening for IPV can begin with general "normalizing" questions: "Because abuse is common in many lives of my patients, I've begun to ask about it routinely." "Are there times in your relationships that you feel unsafe or afraid?" "Have you ever been hit, kicked, punched, or hurt by someone you know?"

The USPSTF has issued a grade B recommendation to screen for IPV among women of reproductive age and refer those screening positive to support services. It recommends several screening instruments, including the Humiliation, Afraid, Rape, Kick (HARK); Hurt, Insult, Threaten, Scream (HITS); Extended-HITS (E-HITS); Partner Violence Screen (PVS); and Woman Abuse Screening Tool (WAST) with ranges in sensitivity from 64% to 87%, while specificity ranged from 80% to 95%. Effective interventions following screen-detected IPV include ongoing delivery of support services, including counseling and home visits.

The term *elder abuse* refers to "acts whereby a trusted person (e.g., a caregiver) causes or creates risk of harm to an older adult. *Vulnerable adult* is generally defined as "a person who is or may be mistreated and who, because of age, disability, or both, is unable to protect him or herself." A 2008 national survey of adults ages 60 and older found that 1 in 10 reported abuse or potential neglect in the past year. The USPSTF found insufficient evidence (I statement) to determine whether to recommend screening for abuse and neglect in all older or vulnerable adults.

Behavioral Counseling

A useful model characterizing patients who should be adopting healthy behaviors or stopping unhealthy behaviors is the Prochaska and DiClemente's *Transtheoretical* or *Stages of Behavioral Change Model,* conceptualized as a process that unfolds over time and involves progression through a series of five stages: *precontemplation, contemplation, preparation, action, and maintenance* (Box 6-4).

BOX 6-4. Transtheoretical Model for Behavioral Change

Stage	Description	Statement
Precontemplation	Patients have no intention to change behavior in the foreseeable future. They are often unaware of their problems.	*"I do not think that I need to change any behaviors."*
Contemplation	Patients are aware that a problem exists and are seriously thinking about overcoming it. No commitment has been made to take action.	*"I'm concerned about my behavior, but not ready to make any changes now."*

Preparation	Patients have expressed intention to take action soon and are reporting small behavioral changes.	*"I'm ready to change my behavior now."*
Action	Patients modify their behavior to overcome their problems.	*"I'm changing my behavior now."*
Maintenance	Patients continue their action for behavioral change and work to prevent relapse.	*"I've changed my behavior."*
Relapse[a]	Cessation of behavioral changes and patients revert to old behavior.	*"I've returned to my old behavior."*

[a]Not a stage in itself but rather the "return from action or maintenance to an earlier stage."

Motivational Interviewing. *Motivational interviewing* is a set of well-documented techniques that encourages you to help your patients, especially those in the precontemplative or contemplative stages, to discover their interest in considering and making a change in their behaviors, such as change in diet, exercise habits, cessation of smoking or drinking, adherence to medication regimens, or self-management strategies (Boxes 6.5 and 6.6).

BOX 6-5. Guiding Style of Motivational Interviewing

- "Ask" open-ended questions—invite the patient to consider how and why they might change.
- "Listen" to understand your patient's experience—"capture" their account with brief summaries or reflective listening statements such as "quitting smoking feels beyond you at the moment"; these express empathy, encourage the patient to elaborate, and are often the best way to respond to resistance.
- "Inform"—by asking permission to provide information, and then asking what the implications might be for the patient.

Source: Reproduced from Rollnick S, et al. Motivational interviewing. *BMJ.* 2010;340:1243, with permission from BMJ Publishing Group Ltd.

BOX 6-6. Selected USPSTF Behavioral Counseling Guidelines for Adults

Behavioral Counseling	USPSTF Grade	USPSTF Description
Healthful diet and physical activity		
Population: Adults who are overweight or obese and have additional cardiovascular disease (CVD) risk factors	B (2014)	The USPSTF recommends offering or referring adults who are overweight or obese and have additional CVD risk factors to intensive behavioral counseling interventions to promote a healthful diet and physical activity for CVD prevention.
Population: Adults without obesity who do not have known cardiovascular disease risk factors	C (2017)	The USPSTF recommends that primary care professionals individualize the decision to offer or refer adults without obesity who do not have hypertension, dyslipidemia, abnormal blood glucose levels, or diabetes to behavioral counseling to promote a healthful diet and physical activity.
Weight loss		
Population: Adults with a body mass index (BMI) of 30 or higher (obese)	B (2018)	The USPSTF recommends that clinicians offer or refer adults with a BMI of 30 or higher (obese) to intensive, multicomponent behavioral interventions.

Behavioral Counseling Guidelines for Adults

- Weight loss
- Healthful diet and physical activity

Behavioral Counseling for Weight Loss. The USPSTF supported (B recommendation) intensive, multicomponent behavioral interventions to prevent CVD in adults with a BMI ≥30 and adults with a BMI 25 to <30 with CVD risk factors (hypertension, dyslipidemia, abnormal blood glucose levels). The USPSTF found that effective intensive behavioral interventions (self-monitoring of weight, tools to support and maintain weight loss such as pedometers, food scales, or exercise videos, and motivational counseling sessions), which combined dietary changes with increased physical activity, could result in a 5% or greater weight loss (Box 6.7).

A 5% to 10% weight loss is realistic and proven to reduce risk of diabetes and other obesity-associated health problems. A safe goal for weight loss is 0.5 to 2 lb per week.

BOX 6-7. Steps to Promote Optimal Weight

1. Measure BMI and waist circumference.
   - Adults with a BMI ≥25 kg/m², men with waist circumferences >40", and women with waist circumferences >35" are at increased risk for heart disease and obesity-related diseases.
   - Measuring the waist-to-hip ratio (waist circumference divided by hip circumference) may be a better risk predictor for individuals older than 75 years. Ratios >0.95 in men and >0.85 in women are considered elevated.
2. Determine additional risk factors for cardiovascular diseases, including smoking, high blood pressure, high cholesterol, physical inactivity, and family history.
3. Assess dietary intake.
4. Assess the patient's motivation to change.
5. Provide counseling about nutrition and exercise.

Behavioral Counseling for Healthful Diet and Physical Activity. To help reduce the risk for CVD, clinicians should offer behavioral counseling to promote a healthful diet and physical activity to adults who are overweight or obese and who have at least one other known risk factor for CVD. However, clinicians should individualize the decision to offer behavioral counseling to nonobese patients without specific risk factors for CVD.

Healthful Diet. A *heart-healthy diet* is rich in vegetables, fruits, fiber, and whole grains and is low in salt, red and processed meats, and saturated fats (Box 6-8). Key recommendations include:

- Limit sodium intake to <2,300 mg/day since excess sodium intake can lead to hypertension, a major risk factor for cardiovascular disease.
- Limit added sugars and saturated fats each to ≤10% of total calories.
- Alcohol, if consumed, should be consumed in moderation.

BOX 6-8. Nutrition Counseling: Sources of Nutrients

Nutrient	Food Source
Calcium	Dairy foods such as milk, natural cheeses, and yogurt
	Calcium-fortified cereals, fruit juice, soy milk, and tofu
	Dark green leafy vegetables like collard, turnip, and mustard greens; bok choy
	Sardines

continued

Iron	Lean meat, dark turkey meat, liver
	Clams, mussels, oysters, sardines, anchovies
	Iron-fortified cereals
	Enriched and whole grain bread
	Spinach, peas, lentils, turnip greens, and artichokes
	Dried prunes and raisins
Folate	Cooked dried beans and peas
	Oranges, orange juice
	Liver
	Spinach, mustard greens
	Black-eyed peas, lentils, okra, chickpeas, peanuts
	Folate-fortified cereals
Vitamin D	Vitamin D–fortified milk, orange juice, and cereals
	Cod liver oil; swordfish, salmon, herring, mackerel, tuna, trout
	Egg yolk
	Mushrooms

Adapted from U.S. Department of Agriculture and U.S. Department of Health and Human Services. *Dietary Guidelines for Americans, 2010.* Washington, DC: U.S. Government Printing Office; 2010; *Choose MyPlate.gov.* Available at http://www.choosemyplate.gov/index.html. Accessed June 8, 2019; Office of Dietary Supplements, National Institutes of Health. *Dietary supplement fact sheets: calcium; vitamin D.* Available at http://ods.od.nih.gov/factsheets/list-all/. Accessed June 8, 2019.

The USDA has issued the "10 Tips: Choose MyPlate" to provide additional dietary guidance (Fig. 6-1 and Box 6-9).

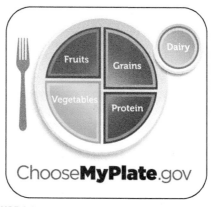

FIGURE 6-1. Rate your plate. (Source: From choosemyplate.gov.)

BOX 6-9. 10 Tips: Choose MyPlate

1. Find your healthy eating style
2. Make half your plate fruits and vegetables
3. Focus on whole fruits
4. Vary your veggies
5. Make half your grains whole grains
6. Move to low-fat or fat-free milk or yogurt
7. Vary your protein routine
8. Drink and eat beverages and foods with less sodium, saturated fat, and added sugars
9. Drink water instead of sugary drinks
10. Everything you eat and drink matters

Source: USDA Center for Nutrition Policy & Promotion. *Choose MyPlate.* Available at https://www.choosemyplate.gov/. Accessed May 30, 2019.

Physical Activity. Physical activity benefits include reducing risks for early death, cardiovascular disease, hypertension, type 2 diabetes, breast and colon cancer, obesity, osteoporosis, falls, and depression (Box 6-10). It also helps improve cognition and functional capacity in older adults. Inactive adults should start with lower-intensity activities and gradually increase how often and how long they perform these activities—*"start low and go slow."* Clinicians should assess patients with chronic pulmonary, cardiac, or musculoskeletal conditions to determine the appropriate types and amounts of activity.

BOX 6-10. Physical Activity Guidelines for Americans

■ Adults should do at least 150 to 300 minutes of moderate-intensity aerobic activity or 75 to 150 minutes of vigorous-intensity aerobic activity each week.

■ Adult should also do moderate- or greater-intensity muscle-strengthening activity that involves all major muscle groups on 2 or more days a week.

■ Greater health benefits can be achieved by increasing the frequency, duration, and/or intensity of physical activity.

■ Adults should avoid being sedentary; doing any amount of moderate-to-vigorous intensity physical activity has health benefits.

■ Older adults should also engage in balance training activities.

The USPSTF recommended referring adults with a BMI ≥30 for intensive, multicomponent behavioral interventions (grade B recommendation). However, they recommend individualizing decisions about referrals for adults without cardiovascular risks for behavioral counseling that promotes physical activity, suggesting that counseling is most beneficial for those motivated to change.

Screening and Behavioral Counseling Guidelines for Adults

Clinicians are encouraged to use screening questions and tests for the health behaviors in Box 6-11 to identify at risk patients and then provide effective *behavioral counseling* and *prevention* strategies.

- Unhealthy alcohol use
- Tobacco misuse
- Sexually transmitted infections (STIs): chlamydia, gonorrhea, and syphilis
- HIV/AIDS

BOX 6-11. Selected USPSTF Behavioral Counseling Guidelines for Adults

Screening and Behavioral Counseling	Counseling	
	USPSTF Grade (Year)	USPSTF Recommendation
Alcohol use (unhealthy)	B (2018)	The USPSTF recommends providing persons engaged in risky or hazardous drinking with brief behavioral counseling interventions to reduce unhealthy alcohol use.
Sexual practices to prevent STIs and HIV/AIDS	B (2014)	The USPSTF recommends intensive behavioral counseling for all sexually active adolescents and for adults who are at increased risk for STIs.
Tobacco misuse	A (2015)	The USPSTF recommends that clinicians ask all adults about tobacco use, advise them to stop using tobacco, and provide behavioral interventions and U.S. FDA–approved pharmacotherapy for cessation to adults who use tobacco.

Screening and Behavioral Counseling for Unhealthy Alcohol Use

▪ The 2017 NSDUH estimated that over 140 million Americans aged 12 years and older were current alcohol users based on consumption of alcoholic beverages in the past 30 days.

▪ 16.7 million were classified as heavy drinkers, 66.6 million were classified as binge drinkers.

▪ An estimated 16 million Americans met the *Diagnostic and Statistical Manual of Mental Disorders, 4th edition (DSM-IV)* definition for alcohol use disorder based on meeting criteria for dependence or abuse.

Alcohol: Screening. Because early detection of at-risk behaviors may be challenging, the USPSTF recommends screening for risky or hazardous alcohol use and brief behavioral counseling interventions when indicated for all adults in primary care settings, including pregnant women (grade B).

If your patient reports drinking alcoholic beverages, you can begin to assess for unhealthy alcohol use (Box 6-12) by asking some simple screening questions.

▪ The Single Alcohol Screening Question (sensitivity = 73% to 88%, specificity = 74% to 100%) asks "How many times in the past year have you had 5 or more drinks in a day (men) or 4 or more drinks in a day (women)?"

BOX 6-12. Unhealthy Alcohol Use

Standard Drink Equivalents: 1 standard drink is equivalent to 12 oz of regular beer or wine cooler, 8 ounces of malt liquor, 5 ounces of wine, or 1.5 ounces of 80-proof spirits.
  Definitions of Drinking Levels for Adults—National Institute of Alcohol Abuse and Alcoholism

	Women	Men
Moderate drinking	≤1 drink/day	≤2 drinks/day
Unsafe drinking levels (increased risk for developing an alcohol use disorder)[a]	>3 drinks/day and >7 drinks/wk	>4 drinks/day and >14 drinks/wk
Binge drinking[b]	≥4 drinks on one occasion	≥5 drinks on one occasion

[a]Pregnant women and those with health problems that could be worsened by drinking should not drink any alcohol.
[b]Brings blood alcohol level to 0.08 g% within, usually within 2 hrs.

- The Alcohol Use Disorders Identification Test-Consumption (AUDIT-C) questionnaire asks about how often the person drinks alcohol, how many standard alcohol drinks are consumed on a typical day, and how often the person consumes six or drinks on one occasion.
- The AUDIT-C, which is scored from 0 to 12, has sensitivities ranging from 0.73 to 1.00 using cutoffs of ≥3 (women) or ≥4 (men). The corresponding specificities range from 0.28 to 0.94.
- The widely used CAGE tool, which asks about **C**utting down, **A**nnoyance when criticized, **G**uilty feelings, and **E**ye-openers, is best at detecting alcohol dependence.

Alcohol: Behavioral Counseling. The USPSTF recently issued a B recommendation advising primary care clinicians to provide behavioral counseling interventions to adults with unhealthy alcohol use. The screening tools described previously can be used to identify adults with at-risk or hazardous alcohol use. The USPSTF identified a number of effective behavioral interventions, which varied by elements (feedback, motivational interviewing, drinking diaries, cognitive behavioral therapy, and action plans on alcohol use), delivery method (in-person, web based, one-on-one, group), frequency (most involved ≤4 sessions), and intensity (most involved ≤2 hours of contact time).

Screening, Brief Intervention, and Referral to Treatment (SBIRT) Program. This program is designed to be administered in a series of encounters conducted by practitioners who are not experts in substance abuse to reduce and prevent harms for those with nondependent alcohol use. Brief interventions target people at low risk for unhealthy alcohol use by educating them about the harms of exceeding drinking limits and, if applicable, identifying any links between alcohol use and other health problems. Motivational techniques are used to help those at moderate to high risk for unhealthy alcohol use to reduce their alcohol intake or to seek additional treatment, particularly those with a high-risk screening result.

Screening and Behavioral Counseling for Tobacco Use

- An estimated 47.4 million (19%) of US adults aged 18 years or older were using tobacco products in 2017, including 41.1 smoking combustible tobacco products.
- E-cigarettes or electronic nicotine delivery systems (ENDS) have become the most frequently used tobacco product among youth, many of whom use two or more tobacco products. Use of these devices is called "*vaping.*"

- Cigarette smoking causes more than 480,000 deaths in the United States each year, nearly one fifth of all deaths.
- Nonsmokers exposed to smoke have increased risk of lung cancer, ear and respiratory infections, and asthma.

Tobacco: Screening. The USPSTF has given a grade A recommendation to screening all adults, particularly pregnant women, for tobacco use and providing behavioral interventions and/or pharmacotherapy for tobacco cessation to all who are using tobacco.

Questions you may ask at every visit include *"Have you ever used tobacco (smoke, chew, e-cigarettes) or vapor products?"* For nonsmokers, ask about exposure to secondhand smoke and tobacco use by other persons in the household or workplace.

Tobacco: Behavioral Counseling. The USPSTF recommends (grade A) that clinicians ask all adult patients about tobacco use, advise tobacco cessation for tobacco users, and then offer behavioral support and pharmacotherapy.

Use the "5 As" framework or the stages of change model to assess readiness to quit using tobacco products (Box 6-13).

BOX 6-13. Assessing Readiness to Quit Smoking: Brief Interventions Models

5 As Model	Transtheoretical or Stages of Change Model
▪ **Ask** about tobacco use ▪ **Advise** to quit ▪ **Assess** willingness to make a quit attempt ▪ **Assist** in quit attempt ▪ **Arrange** follow-up	▪ **Precontemplation**—"I don't want to quit." ▪ **Contemplation**—"I am concerned but not ready to quit now." ▪ **Preparation**—"I am ready to quit." ▪ **Action**—"I just quit." ▪ **Maintenance**—"I quit 6 months ago."

The most commonly used pharmacotherapies are nicotine replacement therapy (NRT), including patches, gum, lozenges, and inhalers, as well varenicline, and bupropion SR. Combining multiple types of NRT has additive benefits and combining pharmacotherapy with behavioral counseling is more effective than either modality alone.

Screening and Behavioral Counseling for Sexually Transmitted Infections. Box 6-14 provides facts about STIs including human immunodeficiency virus (HIV) and acquired immune deficiency syndrome (AIDS).

BOX 6-14. Facts About Chlamydia, Gonorrhea, Syphilis, and HIV/AIDS

- Of the nearly 2.4 million reported new STI cases in 2017, about 72% were infections from chlamydia, 24% from gonorrhea, and 4% from syphilis; rates of all three infections have been increasing with almost half in persons between the ages of 15 and 24 years.
- More than 1.1 million Americans age ≥13 years are currently infected with HIV, although up to 18% remain undiagnosed. Most HIV is being transmitted by HIV-positive persons who are unaware of their status or who are not receiving medical care.
- At highest risk are men who have sex with men (82% of new infections among males), African Americans (43% of new infections), and Hispanics/Latinos (26% of new infections); injection-drug users represent 6% of new HIV infections.

STIs (Chlamydia, Gonorrhea, and Syphilis): Screening. The USPSTF has given a grade B recommendation for chlamydia and gonorrhea screening in sexually active women aged 24 years and younger; the evidence is insufficient to make a recommendation for sexually active men. The USPSTF issued a grade A recommendation for screening high-risk nonpregnant adults and adolescents for syphilis infection. Risk factors for syphilis include being a man who has sex with men, being infected with HIV, and having a history of incarceration or commercial sex work. The USPSTF issued a grade A recommendation for screening all pregnant women for syphilis infection.

HIV: Screening. In 2019, the USPSTF gave a grade A recommendation for HIV screening of adolescents and adults from age 15 to 65 years and for screening all pregnant women. Screening is also recommended for younger adolescents and older adults who are at increased risk for infection. The CDC recommends universal HIV testing for adolescents and adults ages 13 to 64 years in healthcare settings and prenatal testing of all pregnant women. At least annual testing is recommended for high-risk groups, defined as men with male sex partners, individuals with multiple sexual partners, past or present injection-drug users, persons who exchange sex for money or drugs, and sex partners of persons who are HIV infected, bisexual, or injection-drug users. Patients beginning treatment for TB and those with any STI or requests for STI testing, should be tested for coinfection with HIV.

STIs Including HIV: Behavioral Counseling. The USPSTF issued a grade B recommendation supporting behavioral counseling for all sexually active adolescents and for adults who are at increased risk for STIs including HIV/AIDS. The USPSTF noted that behavioral counseling can reduce the risk of acquiring an STI, and successful interventions usually "provide basic information about STIs and STI transmission; assess risk for transmission; and provide training in pertinent skills, such as condom use, communication about safe sex, problem solving, and goal setting." Patient counseling should be interactive, nonjudgmental, and combine information about general risk reduction with personalized messages based on the patient's personal risk behaviors.

Standard recommendations for preventing HIV infection include choosing less risky sexual behaviors, getting treated for injection-drug use and using sterile equipment, getting HIV tests with partners, and using condoms correctly. Another strategy for preventing HIV infections is preexposure prophylaxis (PrEP), which involves taking a daily pill containing two antiretroviral drugs (tenofovir and emtricitabine). PrEP is recommended for HIV-negative people who are at risk for HIV through sexual transmission or illicit drug injection. Consistent use has been shown to reduce the risk of HIV infections.

Correct use of male condoms is highly effective in preventing the transmission of HIV, human papillomavirus (HPV), and other STIs. Recommendations include:

- Using a new condom with each sex act
- Applying the condom before any sexual contact occurs
- Adding only water-based lubricants
- Immediately withdrawing if the condom breaks during sexual activity and holding the condom during withdrawal to keep it from slipping off.

Immunization

Immunization denotes the process of inducing or providing immunity by administering an immunobiologic agent. Immunization can be *active* or *passive*. Although often used interchangeably, the terms vaccination and immunization are not synonymous.

The recommendations for *immunization* are in Box 6-15 and throughout this chapter and in the regional examination chapters.

BOX 6-15. Selected ACIP/CDC Immunization Recommendations for Adults

Immunization	ACIP/CDC Recommendation (Routine Vaccination)
Hepatitis A vaccine (HepA)	■ Not at risk but want protection from hepatitis A: two-dose series HepA or ■ Three-dose series HepA-HepB at 0, 6 mo
Hepatitis B vaccine (HepB)	■ Not at risk but want protection from hepatitis B: two- or three-dose series HepB at least 4 weeks apart or ■ Three-dose series Engerix-B or Recombivax HB at 0, 1, 6 mo or ■ Three-dose series HepA-HepB at 0, 1, 6 mo
Human papillomavirus (HPV) vaccine	■ Females through age 26 yrs and males through age 21 yrs: two- or three-dose series HPV vaccine depending on age at initial vaccination; males age 22 through 26 yrs may be vaccinated based on individual clinical decision (HPV vaccination routinely recommended at age 11–12 yrs) ■ Age 15 yrs or older at initial vaccination: three-dose series HPV vaccine at 0, 1–2, 6 mo ■ Consider discussing vaccination with adults ages 27 through 45 years who are not adequately vaccinated and might be at risk for new HPV infection ■ Age 9 through 14 yrs at initial vaccination and received one dose, or two doses less than 5 mo apart: one dose HPV vaccine ■ Age 9 through 14 yrs at initial vaccination and received two doses at least 5 mo apart: HPV vaccination complete, no additional dose needed
Influenza vaccine—inactivated (IIV), recombinant (RIV) or live attenuated (LAIV)	■ Persons age 6 mo or older: one dose IIV, RIV, or LAIV appropriate for age and health status annually
Measles, mumps, rubella (MMR) vaccine	■ No evidence of immunity to measles, mumps, or rubella: one dose MMR

Pneumococcal vaccine—conjugated (PCV13) and polysaccharide (PPSV23)	▪ Age 65 years or older (immunocompetent): one dose PCV13 if previously did not receive PCV13, followed by one dose PPSV23 at least 1 year after PCV13 and at least 5 years after last dose PPSV23 ▪ Previously received PPSV23 but not PCV13 at age 65 years or older: one dose PCV13 at least 1 year after PPSV23 ▪ When both PCV13 and PPSV23 are indicated, administer PCV13 first (PCV13 and PPSV23 should *not* be administered during same visit)
Tetanus/diphtheria (Td) or Tetanus/ diphtheria/pertussis (Tdap) vaccine	▪ Previously did not receive Tdap at or after age 11 years: one dose Tdap, then Td booster every 10 years
Varicella (VAR)	▪ No evidence of immunity to varicella: two-dose series VAR 4–8 wks apart if previously did not receive varicella-containing vaccine (VAR) ▪ If previously received one dose varicella-containing vaccine: one dose VAR at least 4 wks after first dose
Zoster vaccine— recombinant (RZV) or live (ZVL)	▪ Age 50 years or older: two-dose series RZV 2–6 mo apart regardless of previous herpes zoster or previously received ZVL

Hepatitis A Vaccine. Recommend a two-dose series for those at risk for hepatitis A infection including those with chronic liver disease, clotting factor disorders, men who have sex with men, injection or noninjection-drug use, homelessness, travel in countries with high or intermediate endemic hepatitis A, and household members and close personal contacts of new international adoptees from countries with high or intermediate endemic hepatitis A. Those not at risk but wanting protection from hepatitis A infection should also receive the full two-dose series.

Hepatitis B Vaccine. Recommend a two- or three-dose series for those at risk for hepatitis B infection including those with hepatitis C virus infection, chronic liver disease, HIV infection, sexual exposure risk, current or recent injection drug use, percutaneous or mucosal risk for exposure to blood, persons who are incarcerated, and travel in countries with high or intermediate levels of endemic hepatitis B. Those not at risk but wanting protection from hepatitis B infection should also receive the full two- or three-dose series.

Human Papillomavirus Vaccine
- HPV is the most common STI in the United States. Approximately half of new infections occur among persons aged 15 through 24 years.
- HPV is associated with cervical, vulvar, and vaginal cancer in females, penile cancer in males, and anal and oropharyngeal cancer in both women and men.

The CDC recommends vaccinating all adolescents at ages 11 or 12 (though vaccination can begin at age 9) with the 9-valent HPV vaccine. Depending upon age at initial vaccination, either a two-dose (ages 9 through 14) or 3-dose (ages 15 and older) series will be administered within a period of 6 to 12 months. A three-dose series is recommended for those who are immunocompromised or have a history of sexual abuse or assault. Guidelines recommend giving HPV vaccination to adults through age 26; however, the FDA recently approved using the 9-valent vaccine for men and women ages 27 through 45.

Influenza Vaccine
- Influenza season usually begins during the late fall and can last into the spring, peaking between December and February.
- The number of annual deaths related to influenza varies depending on the virus type and subtype, ranging in recent years from 12,000 to nearly 80,000 deaths.

The CDC Advisory Committee on Immunization Practices (ACIP) updates its recommendations for vaccination annually. Two types of vaccines are available. The "flu shot" is an inactivated vaccine-containing killed virus, which comes in a standard dose for those younger than 65 years and a high dose for those ≥65 years. It is recommended for all people aged 6 months and older, especially the groups listed below:

- Adults and children with chronic pulmonary and cardiovascular conditions (except hypertension) and renal, hepatic, neurologic, hematologic, or metabolic disorders (including diabetes mellitus); persons who are immunosuppressed due to any cause; persons who are morbidly obese
- Adults ≥50 years of age
- Women who are or will be pregnant during influenza season
- Residents of nursing homes and long-term care facilities
- American Indians and Alaska natives
- Healthcare personnel
- Household contacts and caregivers of children ≤5 years of age (especially infants ≤age 6 months) and of adults ≥50 years of age with clinical conditions placing them at higher risk for complications of influenza

Pneumococcal Vaccine

- *Streptococcal pneumonia* causes pneumonia, bacteremia, and meningitis.
- In 2015, invasive pneumococcal disease accounted for 29,382 cases and 3,254 deaths.
- However, the introduction of the seven-valent pneumococcal vaccination for infants and children in 2000 has directly and indirectly (through *herd immunity*) reduced pneumococcal infections among children and adults.

Since 2010, infants younger than age 2 years have routinely been vaccinated with the 13-valent pneumococcal conjugate vaccine (PCV13). In 2014, the ACIP recommended vaccinating adults aged ≥65 years using the PCV13 along with the 23-valent inactivated pneumococcal polysaccharide vaccine (PPSV23), as shown in Box 6-16. *The vaccines should not be co-administered.* Adults in this age range who never received the PPSV23 should first receive the PCV13 followed 12 months later by the PPSV23. Adults aged ≥65 years previously vaccinated with PPSV23 should receive a dose of PCV13 no earlier than 1 year following the most recent PPSV23 vaccination.

BOX 6-16. Pneumococcal Vaccine Recommendations for High-Risk Adults

Risk Group	Medical Condition	PCV13 Recommended	PPSV23 Recommended	PPSV23 Revaccination 5 Years After First Dose
Immunocompetent persons	Chronic heart disease		✓	
	Chronic lung disease		✓	
	Diabetes mellitus		✓	
	Cerebrospinal fluid leak	✓	✓	
	Cochlear implant	✓	✓	
	Alcoholism		✓	
	Chronic liver disease, cirrhosis		✓	
	Cigarette smoking		✓	

continued

Persons with functional or anatomic asplenia	Sickle cell disease	✓	✓	✓
	Congenital or acquired asplenia	✓	✓	✓
Immuno-compromised persons	Congenital or acquired immunodeficiency	✓	✓	✓
	HIV infection	✓	✓	✓
	Chronic renal failure	✓	✓	✓
	Nephrotic syndrome	✓	✓	✓
	Leukemia	✓	✓	✓
	Lymphoma	✓	✓	✓
	Hodgkin disease	✓	✓	✓
	Generalized malignancy	✓	✓	✓
	Iatrogenic immuno-suppression	✓	✓	✓
	Solid-organ transplants	✓	✓	✓
	Multiple myeloma	✓	✓	✓

Tetanus, Diphtheria, Pertussis Vaccine

- Tetanus, or "lockjaw," caused by the anaerobic bacterium *Clostridium tetani*, which enters the body through broken skin, is a neurologic disorder that causes intense painful muscle contractions that can affect swallowing and breathing.
- Diphtheria is caused by *Corynebacterium diphtheriae* and is usually spread through respiratory droplets. The infection causes a "pseudo-membrane" of dead respiratory tissue that can extend throughout the respiratory tract. Complications can include pneumonia, myocarditis, neurologic toxicities, and kidney failure.
- Pertussis, or "whooping cough" is a contagious respiratory disease caused by *Bordetella pertussis*.

All adults aged 19 and older who have not previously received a tetanus-diphtheria-acellular pertussis (Tdap) vaccine should receive one dose followed by a tetanus-diphtheria (Td) booster every 10 years.

Varicella Vaccine

- *Varicella* infection, or *chicken pox*, usually occurs in childhood and causes an itchy rash. Infections can also occur in adults, particularly immuno-compromised patients who are at risk for disseminated disease.

- Before the varicella vaccination program was implemented in the United States in 2006, an estimated 4 million cases occurred each year. By 2014, the annual incidence of varicella had declined by nearly 85%.

The CDC recommends the vaccine to adults born in the United States in 1980 or later who have not received two doses of chicken pox vaccine or never had chicken pox.

A two-dose series of varicella vaccine is recommended for children under age 13 and those aged 13 and older who were previously unvaccinated and who have no evidence of immunity. Live vaccines should not be given to pregnant women or people who have a very weakened immune system which includes people with HIV infection and a CD4 count less than 200.

Herpes Zoster Vaccine

- *Herpes zoster*, which results from reactivation of latent varicella (chicken pox) virus infection within the sensory ganglia, usually causes painful unilateral vesicular rashes in a dermatomal distribution.
- The lifetime risk of herpes zoster infection is about one in three and is higher for women than for men.
- Up to one in four adults experience complications following infection, including postherpetic neuralgia (persistent pain in the area of the rash), bacterial skin infections, ophthalmic complications, cranial and peripheral neuropathies, encephalitis, pneumonitis, and hepatitis. Herpes zoster risk is increased in immunocompromised conditions including cancer, HIV, bone marrow or organ transplantation, and immunosuppressive therapies.
- Increasing age is also strongly associated with developing both herpes zoster infection and postherpetic neuralgia.

The herpes zoster vaccine effectively reduces the short-term risks for zoster and postherpetic neuralgia in adults ≥50 years. The ACIP currently recommends offering the two-dose series of recombinant zoster vaccine (RZV) for immunocompetent adults aged ≥50 years including adults who have had shingles or received the previous shingles vaccine (ZVL). **Doses should be 2 to 6 months apart.**

PREVENTIVE CARE IN SPECIAL POPULATIONS

For screening, counseling, and immunization recommendations for special population groups, see children (pp. 486–487), older adults (pp. 548–551), and pregnant women (pp. 519–524).

Evaluating Clinical Evidence

Clinical decision making requires integrating clinical expertise, patient preferences, and the best available clinical evidence. Carefully study the clear descriptions of how the history and physical examination can be viewed as diagnostic tests; how to assess the accuracy of laboratory tests, radiographic imaging, and diagnostic procedures; and how to evaluate clinical research studies and disease prevention guidelines. Throughout the regional examination chapters, you will encounter current evidence in the use of elements of the history and physical examination to support diagnostic reasoning.

USING ELEMENTS OF THE HISTORY AND PHYSICAL EXAMINATION AS DIAGNOSTIC TESTS

The process of diagnostic reasoning begins with the generation of a list of potential causes for the patient's problems (*differential diagnosis*). As you learn more about your patient, you will assign probabilities to various diagnoses that correspond to how likely you view them as explanations of the patient's problem, with the goal of determining the need to perform additional testing or initiate treatment (Fig. 7-1).

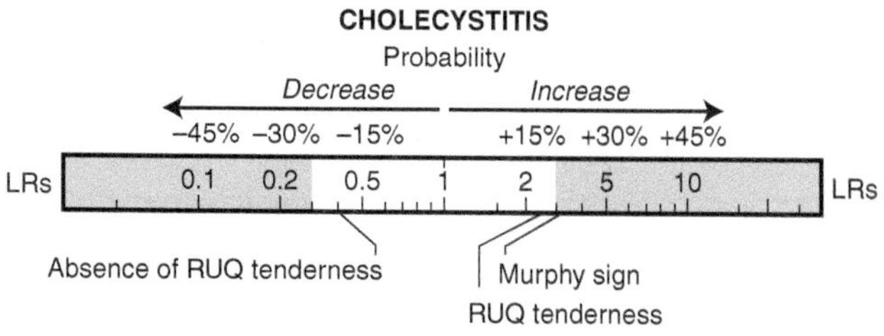

FIGURE 7-1. Revising probabilities for acute cholecystitis. (Reprinted from McGee S. Abdominal pain and tenderness. In: McGee S, ed. *Evidence-Based Physical Diagnosis*. 4th ed. Elsevier; 2018:445–456.e444. Copyright © 2018 Elsevier. With permission.)

EVALUATING DIAGNOSTIC TESTS

Two concepts in evaluating diagnostic tests will be explored: the *validity* of the findings and the *reproducibility* of the test results.

Validity

Does the test accurately identify whether a patient has a disease? This involves comparing the test against a *gold standard*—the best measure of whether a patient has disease.

The *2 × 2 table* is the basic format for evaluating the performance characteristics of a diagnostic test, which means how well the test is able to accurately identify diseased and non-diseased patients (Box 7-1). There are two columns—patients with disease present and patients with disease absent. These categorizations are based on the gold standard test. The two rows correspond to positive and negative test results. The four cells (a, b, c, d) correspond to true positives, false positives, false negatives, and true negatives, respectively.

BOX 7-1. Setting up the 2 × 2 Table

History or Physical Examination Element	Gold Standard: Disease Present	Gold Standard: Disease Absent
Present (test positive)	a True positive	b False positive
Absent (test negative)	c False negative	d True negative

Sensitivity and Specificity

- *Sensitivity* is the probability that a person with disease has a positive test. This is represented as $a/(a + c)$ in the disease present column of the 2 × 2 table. Sensitivity is also known as the *true positive rate*.
- *Specificity* is the probability that a nondiseased person has a negative test, represented as $d/(b + d)$ in the disease absent column of the 2 × 2 table. Specificity is also known as the *true negative rate*.

A negative result from a test with a high sensitivity (i.e., a very low false-negative rate) usually excludes disease. This is represented by the mnemonic *SnNOUT*—a **Sen**sitive test with a **N**egative result rules **out** disease. Conversely, a positive result in a test with high specificity (e.g., a very low false-positive rate) usually indicates disease. This is represented by the mnemonic *SpPIN*—a **Sp**ecific test with a **P**ositive result rules **in** disease.

Predictive Values. To determine the probability that a patient actually has disease based on a test result that is either positive or negative, calculate positive and negative predictive values (Box 7-2).

BOX 7-2. Positive and Negative Predictive Values

- The *positive predictive value (PPV)* is the probability that a person with a positive test has disease, represented as a/(a + b) from the test positive row in the 2 × 2 table.
- The *negative predictive value (NPV)* is the probability that a person with a negative test does not have disease, represented as d/(c + d) in the test negative row in 2 × 2 table.

Prevalence of Disease. Predictive value statistics vary substantially according to the prevalence of disease (i.e., the proportion of patients in the disease present column), which is based on the characteristics of the patient population and the clinical setting. Box 7-3 shows a 2 × 2 table where both the sensitivity and specificity of the diagnostic test are 90% and the prevalence is 10%. The positive predictive value (PPV) calculated from the test positive row of the table would be 90/180 = 50%. This means that half of the people with a positive test have disease.

BOX 7-3. Predictive Values: Prevalence of 10% with Sensitivity and Specificity = 90%

	Disease Present	Disease Absent	Total
Test positive	a	b	
	90	90	180
Test negative	c	d	
	10	810	820
Total	100	900	1,000

Sensitivity = a/(a + c) = 90/100 or 90%; specificity = d/(b + d) = 810/900 $$= 90\%$$

Positive predictive value = a/(a + b) = 90/180 = 50%

However, if the sensitivity and specificity of the diagnostic test remained the same, but prevalence of the disease was only 1%, then the cells would look very different (Box 7-4).

BOX 7-4. Predictive Values: Prevalence of 1% with Sensitivity and Specificity = 90%

	Disease Present	Disease Absent	Total
Test positive	a 9	b 99	108
Test negative	c 1	d 891	892
Total	10	990	1,000

Sensitivity = a/(a + c) = 9/10 or 90%; specificity = d/(b + d) = 891/990
$$= 90\%$$

Positive predictive value = a/(a + b) = 9/108 = 8.3%

Likelihood Ratios. To evaluate how well a diagnostic test accounts for the varying disease prevalence observed in different patient populations, you can use *likelihood ratio* statistics. These are defined as the probability of obtaining a given test result in a diseased patient divided by the probability of obtaining a given test result in a nondiseased patient. The likelihood ratio tells us how much a test result changes the pretest disease probability (prevalence) to the posttest disease probability (Box 7-5).

▪ The *likelihood ratio for a positive test* is the ratio of getting a positive test result in a diseased person divided by the probability of getting a positive test result in a nondiseased person.

From the 2 × 2 table, we see that this is the same as saying the ratio of the true positive rate (sensitivity) over the false positive rate (1 − specificity). A higher value (much >1) indicates that a positive test is much more likely to be coming from a diseased person than from a nondiseased person, increasing our confidence that a person with a positive result has disease.

▪ The *likelihood ratio for a negative test* is the ratio of the probability of getting a negative test result in a diseased person divided by the probability of getting a negative test result in a nondiseased person.

From the 2 × 2 table, we see that this is the same as saying the ratio of the false negative rate (1 − sensitivity) divided by the true negative rate (specificity). A lower value (much <1) indicates that the negative test is much more likely to be coming from a nondiseased person than from a diseased person, increasing our confidence that a person with a negative result does not have disease.

BOX 7-5. Interpreting Likelihood Ratios

Likelihood Ratios[a]	Effect on Pre- to Posttest Probability
LRs >10 or <0.1	Generate large changes
LRs 5–10 or 0.1–0.2	Generate moderate changes
LRs 2–5 and 0.5–0.2	Generate small (sometimes important) changes
LRs 1–2 and 0.5–1	Alter the probability to a small degree (rarely important)

[a]Likelihood ratios >1 are associated with positive results and an increased probability for disease. Likelihood ratios <1 are associated with negative results and a decreased probability of disease. A test with a likelihood ratio of 1 provides no additional information about the probability of disease.

Fagan Nomogram. The Fagan nomogram is a graphical way to show how the likelihood ratios for a given test result can change the probability of disease (Fig. 7-2). With this nomogram, you set the pretest probabilities (based on disease prevalence) on the vertical line on the left, then take a straight edge and draw a line from the pretest probability through the likelihood ratio in the middle line, and then read the posttest probability on the vertical line on the right.

Figure 7-2 shows how the Fagan nomogram displays probability revisions. The likelihood ratio for a positive test = sensitivity/(1-specificity) = 90%/9% = 10. The likelihood ratio for a negative test = (1 – sensitivity)/specificity = 10%/91% = 0.11. In this example, the diagnostic test has a sensitivity of 90% and specificity of 91%. With a pretest probability (prevalence) of 1%, a positive test result (blue line) leads to a posttest probability of 9%. A negative test result (red line) leads to a posttest probability of 0.1%.

Reproducibility

An important aspect of evaluating diagnostic elements of the history or physical examination is determining the reproducibility of the findings for diagnosing a clinical disorder.

Kappa Score. Two clinicians examining a patient may not always agree upon the presence of a given finding. Understanding whether there is

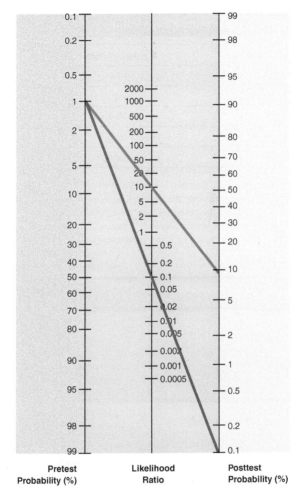

FIGURE 7-2. Fagan nomogram. (Adapted from Fagan TJ. Letter: nomogram for Bayes theorem. *N Engl J Med*. 1975;293(5):257. Copyright © 1975 Massachusetts Medical Society. Reprinted with permission from Massachusetts Medical Society.)

agreement well beyond chance is important in knowing whether the finding is useful enough to support clinical decision making. The *kappa score* measures the amount of agreement that occurs beyond chance. Box 7-6 shows how to interpret Kappa values.

BOX 7-6. **Interpreting Kappa Values**	
Value of Kappa	**Strength of Agreement**
<0.20	Poor
0.21–0.40	Fair
0.41–0.60	Moderate
0.61–0.80	Good
0.81–1.00	Excellent

For example, although clinicians agree 75% of the time that a patient has an abnormal physical finding, the expected agreement based on chance is 50%. This means that the potential agreement beyond chance is 50% and the actual observer agreement beyond chance is 25%. The kappa level is then 25%/50% = 0.5, which indicates moderate agreement (Fig. 7-3).

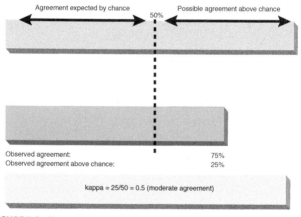

FIGURE 7-3. Kappa scores. (Reprinted with permission from McGinn T, et al. Tips for learners of evidence-based medicine: 3. Measures of observer validity (kappa statistic). *CMAJ.* 2004;171(11):1369–1373.)

Precision. In the context of reproducibility, *precision* refers to being able to apply the same test to the same unchanged person and obtain the same result. Precision is often used when referring to laboratory tests. A statistical test used to characterize precision is the coefficient of variation, defined as the standard deviation divided by the mean value. Lower values indicate greater precision.

CRITICAL APPRAISAL OF THE CLINICAL EVIDENCE

Learn the process of critically appraising the clinical literature in order to interpret new studies and guidelines as they appear throughout your professional career. The Evidence-Based Working Group, which consists of experts in epidemiology, has created a rigorous and standardized approach for evaluating studies that has been applied to a wide range of clinical topics, including therapeutic and prevention trials, diagnostic tests, meta-analyses, cost-effectiveness analyses, and practice guidelines. This approach asks three basic questions:

1. Are the results valid (can you believe them)?
2. What are the results (magnitude and precision)?
3. How can you apply the results to patient care?

Are the Results Valid?

When evaluating results of studies on treatment or a prevention intervention, it is important to have a thorough understanding of bias. The key sources of bias in clinical research are selection bias, performance bias, detection bias, and attrition bias (Box 7-7).

BOX 7-7. Types of Biases Affecting Evidence

Bias	Description
Selection bias	■ Occurs when comparison groups have systematic differences in their baseline characteristics that can affect the outcome of the study ■ Creates problems in interpreting observed differences in outcomes because they could result from the interventions or the baseline differences between groups ■ Randomly allocating subjects to the intervention is the best approach to minimizing this bias
Performance bias	■ Occurs when there are systematic differences in the care received between comparison groups (other than the intervention) ■ Creates problems in interpreting outcome differences ■ Blinding subjects and providers to the intervention is the best approach to minimizing this bias

continued

Detection bias	■ Occurs when there are systematic differences in efforts to diagnose or ascertain an outcome ■ Blinding outcomes assessors (ensuring that they are unaware of the intervention received by the subject) is the best approach to minimizing this bias.
Attrition bias	■ Occurs when there are systematic differences in the comparison groups in the number of subjects who do not complete the study ■ Failing to account for these differences can lead to incorrectly estimating the effectiveness of an intervention ■ Using an intention-to-treat analysis, where all outcome analyses consider all subjects who were assigned to a comparison group, regardless of whether they received or completed the intervention, can minimize this bias

What Are the Results?

The statistics used to characterize the results of the performance of a treatment or prevention intervention include *relative risks, relative risk differences* (can be a reduction or increase, reflecting benefit or harm), *absolute risk differences* (can be a reduction or increase, reflecting benefit or harm), *numbers needed to treat*, and *numbers needed to harm* (Boxes 7-8 and 7-9).

BOX 7-8. 2 × 2 Tables for Evaluating Studies of Treatment or Prevention

	Event Occurred	No Event	Total
Experimental group	a	b	a + b
Control group	c	d	c + d

BOX 7-9. Statistics Used to Characterize the Performance of a Treatment or Prevention Intervention

Statistics	Definition	Calculation
Experimental event rate (EER)	■ The probability that an *intervention* subject had the outcome	a/(a + b) From row 1 of table (experimental group)

Control event rate (CER)	▪ The probability that a *control* subject had the outcome	$c/(c + d)$ From row 2 of table (control group)
Relative risk	▪ The probability of an outcome in the intervention group compared to the probability of an outcome in the control group ▪ Can be a reduction or increase, reflecting benefit or harm	EER/CER
Relative risk difference	▪ The proportion of baseline risk is reduced or increased by the therapy	$\lvert CER - EER \rvert/CER \times 100\%$ or $(1 - \text{relative risk}) \times 100\%$
Absolute risk difference	▪ The difference in outcome rates between the comparisons groups	$\lvert CER - EER \rvert$
Number needed to treat (NNT)[a]	▪ The number of subjects who need to be treated over a specific period of time to prevent one outcome ▪ In many studies these calculations are used to measure treatment effectiveness between control and treatment interventions comparing medications, procedures, or diagnostic tests	The reciprocal of the absolute risk difference (reported as a fraction)

[a]If the intervention actually increases the risk for a bad outcome, then this statistic becomes the *number needed to harm (NNH)*.

Can You Apply the Results to Patient Care?

To make a generalizability determination, you need to first look at the demographics of the study subjects (e.g., age, sex, race/ethnicity, socio-economic status, clinical conditions). Then, you need to determine: Are the study demographics applicable to your patient? Is the intervention feasible in your clinical setting? And, most importantly, is the range of potential benefits and harm of the intervention acceptable for your patient?

General Survey, Vital Signs, and Pain

HEALTH HISTORY

This chapter focuses on common manifestations of illness, collectively known as *constitutional symptoms*. These symptoms are often not confined to a single organ system, but broadly affect a patient's "constitution," or their physical state with regard to vitality, health, and strength.

Common or Concerning Symptoms

- Fatigue and weakness
- Fever, chills, and night sweats
- Weight change
- Pain

Fatigue and Weakness

Fatigue is a nonspecific symptom with many causes. Use open-ended questions to explore the attributes of the patient's fatigue and encourage the patient to fully describe what he or she is experiencing. See Algorithm 8-1, Approach to the patient with fatigue, p. 126.

Weakness differs from fatigue. It denotes a demonstrable loss of muscle power and will be discussed later with other neurologic symptoms.

Fever, Chills, and Night Sweats

Ask about fever if the patient has an acute or chronic illness. Find out whether the patient has used a thermometer to measure the temperature. Distinguish between *feeling cold* and a *shaking chill*, with shivering throughout the body and chattering of teeth. *Night sweats* raise concerns about tuberculosis or malignancy.

Focus your questions on the timing of the illness and its associated symptoms. Become familiar with patterns of infectious diseases that may affect your patient. Inquire about travel, contact with sick people, or other unusual exposures. Be sure to inquire about medications, as they may cause fever. In contrast, recent ingestion of aspirin, acetaminophen, corticosteroids, and nonsteroidal anti-inflammatory drugs may mask fever.

Weight Change

Good opening questions include "How often do you check your weight?" and "How is it compared to a year ago?"

▪ *Weight gain* occurs when caloric intake exceeds caloric expenditure over time. It also may reflect abnormal accumulation of body fluids.
▪ *Weight loss* has many causes: decreased food intake, dysphagia, vomiting, and insufficient supplies of food; defective absorption of nutrients; increased metabolic requirements; and loss of nutrients through the urine, feces, or injured skin. Also consider chronic illnesses, malignancy, and abuse of alcohol, cocaine, amphetamines, or opiates, or withdrawal from marijuana. Be alert for signs of malnutrition.

Pain

Pain is one of the most common presenting symptoms in clinical practice and is often underassessed (Fig. 8-1 and Box 8-1).

▪ *Acute pain* is the normal, predicted physiologic response to an adverse stimulus that typically lasts less than 3 to 6 months and is commonly associated with surgery, trauma, and acute illness.
▪ *Chronic pain* is pain associated with cancer or other medical conditions that persists for more than 3 to 6 months; pain lasting more than 1 month beyond the course of an acute illness or injury; or pain recurring at intervals of months or years.

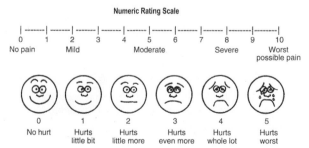

FIGURE 8-1. Numeric Rating Scale (NRS) and the Wong-Baker FACES Pain Rating Scale. (From King MS, et al. *Step-Up to Geriatrics.* Wolters Kluwer; 2017. Figure 5-5.)

BOX 8-1. Pain Assessment

- Adopt a multidisciplinary measurement-based approach to assessing pain, carefully listening to the patient's story, and any contributing factors.
- Accept the *patient's self-report*, which experts state is *the most reliable indicator of pain*.
- Pursue the attributes of pain, as you would with any symptom.
- Ask the patient to point to the pain. Lay terms may not be specific enough to localize the site of origin.
- Use a consistent method to determine *severity*.

Be sure to ask about any treatments that the patient has tried, including medications, physical therapy, and alternative medicines. Identify any comorbid conditions such as arthritis, diabetes, HIV/AIDS, substance abuse, sickle cell disease, or psychiatric disorders that can significantly affect the patient's experience of pain.

TECHNIQUES OF EXAMINATION

Key Components of the General Survey, Vital Signs, and Pain Assessment

- Perform a general survey
- Measure height and weight and calculate body mass index (BMI)
- Measure blood pressure using a sphygmomanometer
- Measure orthostatic blood pressure (if indicated)
- Examine arterial pulses, heart rate, and rhythm
- Observe rate, rhythm, depth, and effort of breathing
- Measure core body temperature
- Assess acute and chronic pain (if indicated)

General Survey

Apparent State of Health   Acutely or chronically ill, frail, robust, vigorous

Level of Consciousness. Is the patient awake, alert, and interactive?   If not, promptly assess level of consciousness (see p. 133)

Signs of Distress

- Cardiac or respiratory distress

  Clutching the chest, pallor, diaphoresis; labored breathing, wheezing, cough

- Pain

  Wincing, sweating, protecting painful area

- Anxiety or depression

  Anxious face, fidgety movements, cold and moist palms; inexpressive or flat affect, poor eye contact, psychomotor slowing

Skin Color and Obvious Lesions. See Chapter 10, *Skin, Hair, and Nails*, for details.

Pallor, cyanosis, jaundice, rashes, bruises

Dress, Grooming, and Personal Hygiene

- How is the patient dressed? Is the clothing suitable for the temperature and weather? Is it clean and appropriate to the setting?

  Body piercing or tattoos can be associated with alcohol and drug use.

- Note patient's hair, fingernails, and use of makeup.

  These may be clues to the patient's personality, mood, lifestyle, and self-regard.

Facial Expression. Watch for eye contact. Is it natural? Sustained and unblinking? Averted quickly? Absent?

Stare of hyperthyroidism; flat or sad affect of depression. Decreased eye contact may be cultural or may suggest anxiety, fear, or sadness.

Odors of Body and Breath. Odors can be important diagnostic clues.

Breath odor of alcohol, acetone (diabetes), uremia, or liver failure. Fruity odor of diabetes. (Never assume that alcohol on a patient's breath explains changes in mental status or neurologic findings.)

Posture, Gait, and Motor Activity

Preference to sit up in left-sided heart failure and to lean forward with arms braced in chronic obstructive pulmonary disease (COPD).

Height and Weight

Height. Measure the patient's height. Note the build—muscular or deconditioned, tall or short. Observe the body proportions.

Short stature in Turner syndrome; elongated arms in Marfan syndrome; loss of height in osteoporosis.

Weight. Is the patient emaciated? If obese, is there central or dispersed distribution of fat? Weigh the patient with shoes off.

Obesity (BMI ≥30 kg/m²) increases risk of diabetes, heart disease, stroke, hypertension, osteoarthritis, sleep apnea syndrome, and some forms of cancer.

As shown in Box 8-2, calculate the *body mass index* (BMI), which incorporates estimated but more accurate measurements of body fat than weight alone (see classification on p. 82).

BOX 8-2. Methods to Calculate Body Mass Index (BMI)

Unit of Measure	Method of Calculation
Weight in pounds, height in inches	(1) Standard BMI Chart (2) $\dfrac{\text{Weight (lb)} \times 700^{a}}{\text{height (inches)}}$
Weight in kilograms, height in meters squared	(3) $\dfrac{\text{Weight (kg)}}{\text{height (m}^2)}$
Either unit of measure	(4) "BMI Calculator" at http://www.nhlbi. nih.gov/health/educational/lose_wt/BMI/ bmicalc.htm

[a]Several organizations use 704.5, but the variation in BMI is negligible. Conversion formula: 2.2 lb = 1 kg; 1 in = 2.54 cm; 100 cm = 1 m.
Source: National Institutes of Health–National Heart, Lung, and Blood Institute. *Calculate your body mass index.* Available at http://www.nhlbi.nih.gov/health/educational/lose_wt/BMI/bmicalc.htm. Accessed June 9, 2019.

Vital Signs: Blood Pressure, Heart Rate, Respiratory Rate, and Temperature

Blood Pressure

Methods for Measuring Blood Pressure. Office screening with *manual* and *automated cuffs* remains common, but elevated readings increasingly require confirmation with *home* and *ambulatory monitoring*, which are more predictive of cardiovascular disease and end-organ damage than manual and automated measurements in the office. Automated ambulatory blood pressure monitoring measures blood pressure at preset intervals over 24 to 48 hours, usually every 15 to 20 minutes during the day and 30 to 60 minutes during the night. Be familiar with these different methods of blood pressure measurement and their varying criteria for hypertension.

Types of Hypertension. Three types of hypertension are especially import-ant to recognize (Box 8-3). Suspicion of these entities and assessing the effects of treatment are indications for ambulatory blood pressure moni-toring. Box 8-4 offers guidelines for selecting the correct size blood pres-sure cuff. Boxes 8-5 through 8-7 offer additional information on blood pressure measurement.

BOX 8-3. Types of Hypertension

White-coat hypertension (isolated clinic hypertension)	■ Blood pressure ≥140/90 in medical settings and mean awake ambulatory readings <135/85
	■ Reported in up to 20% of patients with elevated office blood pressure
	■ Carries normal to slightly increased cardiovascular risk and does not require treatment; attributed to a conditioned anxiety response
Masked hypertension	■ Blood pressure <140/90, but an elevated daytime blood pressure of >135/85 on home or ambulatory testing
	■ Reported in an estimated 10% to 30% of the general population
	■ If untreated, it increases risk of cardiovascular disease and end-organ damage
Nocturnal hypertension	■ Physiologic blood pressure "dipping" occurs in most patients as they shift from wakefulness to sleep
	■ A nocturnal fall of <10% of daytime values is associated with poor cardiovascular outcomes and can only be identified on 24-hour ambulatory blood pressure monitoring
	■ Two other patterns have poor cardiovascular outcomes, a nocturnal *rising* pattern and a marked nocturnal *fall* of >20% of daytime values

---

BOX 8-4. Selecting the Correct Size Blood Pressure Cuff

It is important for clinicians and patients to use a cuff that fits the patient's arm. Follow the guidelines outlined here for selecting the correct size:

■ Width of the inflatable bladder of the cuff should be about 40% of upper arm circumference (about 12 to 14 cm in the average adult).
■ Length of the inflatable bladder should be about 80% of upper arm circumference (almost long enough to encircle the arm).
■ The standard cuff is 12 × 23 cm, appropriate for arm circumferences up to 28 cm.

BOX 8-5. Steps to Ensure Accurate Blood Pressure Measurement

1. The patient should avoid smoking or drinking caffeinated beverages for 30 minutes before the blood pressure is taken and rest for at least 5 minutes.
2. Make sure the examining room is quiet and comfortably warm.
3. Make sure the arm selected is *free of clothing*. There should be no arteriovenous fistulas for dialysis, scarring from prior brachial artery cutdowns, or signs of lymphedema (seen after axillary node dissection or radiation therapy).
4. Palpate the brachial artery to confirm that it has a viable pulse.
5. Position the arm so that the brachial artery, at the antecubital crease, is *at heart level*—roughly level with the 4th interspace at its junction with the sternum.
6. If the patient is seated, rest the arm on a table a little above the patient's waist; if standing, try to support the patient's arm at the midchest level.

BOX 8-6. Potential Sources of Inaccuracy in the Measurement of Adult Blood Pressure in Clinical Settings

	Effect on Systolic BP	Effect on Diastolic BP
Patient-Related Factors		
Acute meal ingestion	↓	↓
Acute alcohol ingestion	↓	↓
Acute caffeine use	↑	↑
Acute nicotine use or exposure	↑	↑
Bladder distention	↑	↑
Cold exposure	↑	↑
Paretic arm	↑	↑
White-coat effect	↑	↑

Procedure-Related Factors		
Insufficient rest period	↑	↑
Legs crossed at knees	↑	↑
Unsupported arm	↑	↑
Arm lower than heart level	↑	↑
Talking during measurement	↑	↑
Incorrect smaller cuff size	↑	↑
Incorrect larger cuff size	↓	↓
Stethoscope under cuff	↑	↓
Fast cuff deflation rate (>3 mm Hg/sec)	↑	↓
Unsupported back	no effect	↑
Excessive pressure on stethoscope head	no effect	↑

BOX 8-7. Measuring Blood Pressure

- Center the inflatable bladder over the brachial artery. The lower border of the cuff should be about 2.5 cm above the antecubital crease. Secure the cuff snugly. Position the patient's arm so that it is slightly flexed at the elbow.
- To determine how high to raise the cuff pressure, first estimate the systolic pressure by palpation. As you feel the radial artery with the fingers of one hand, rapidly inflate the cuff until the radial pulse disappears. Read this pressure on the manometer and add 30 mm Hg to it. Use of this sum as the target for subsequent inflations prevents discomfort from unnecessarily high cuff pressures. It also avoids the occasional error caused by an auscultatory gap—a silent interval between the systolic and diastolic pressures.
- Deflate the cuff promptly.
- Now place the bell of a stethoscope lightly over the brachial artery, taking care to make an air seal with its full rim. Because the sounds to be heard (*Korotkoff sounds*) are relatively low in pitch, they are heard better with the *bell*.
- Inflate the cuff rapidly again to the level just determined, and then deflate it slowly, at a rate of about 2 to 3 mm Hg per second.

continued

Note the level at which you hear the sounds of at least two consecutive beats. This is the *systolic pressure*.

- Continue to lower the pressure slowly. The disappearance point, usually only a few mm Hg below the muffling point, is the best estimate of *diastolic pressure*.
- Read both the systolic and diastolic levels to the nearest 2 mm Hg. Wait 2 or more minutes and repeat. Average your readings. If the first two readings differ by more than 5 mm Hg, take additional readings.
- Take blood pressure in both arms at least once.
- In patients taking antihypertensive medications or with a history of fainting, postural dizziness, or possible depletion of blood volume, take the blood pressure in two positions—supine and standing (unless contraindicated).

In 2013, the Joint National Committee on Detection, Evaluation, and Treatment of High Blood Pressure (JNC) updated the classification of systolic blood pressure (SBP) and diastolic blood pressure (DBP), as shown in Box 8-8.

BOX 8-8. Blood Pressure Categories for Adults (JNC 8)

Category[a]	Systolic (mm Hg)		Diastolic (mm Hg)
Normal	<120	and	<80
Elevated	120–129	and	<80
Stage 1 hypertension	130–139	or	80–89
Stage 2 hypertension	≥140	or	≥90

[a]BP indicates blood pressure (based on an average of ≥2 careful readings obtained on ≥2 occasions). Patients with SBP and DBP in two categories should be designated to the higher BP category.

When the systolic and diastolic levels fall in different categories, use the higher category. For example, 170/92 mm Hg is stage 2 hypertension; 135/100 mm Hg is stage 1 hypertension. In *isolated systolic hypertension*, SBP is ≥140 mm Hg, and DBP is <90 mm Hg.

A fall in systolic pressure of 20 mm Hg or more within 3 minutes after standing up, especially when accompanied by symptoms, indicates *orthostatic (postural) hypotension*.

Heart Rate. The radial pulse is used commonly to count the heart rate. With the pads of your index and middle fingers, compress the radial artery until you detect a maximal pulsation (Fig. 8-2). If the rhythm is regular, count the rate for 15 seconds and multiply by 4. If the rate is unusually fast or slow, count it for 60 seconds. When the rhythm is irregular, evaluate the rate by auscultation at the cardiac apex (the apical pulse).

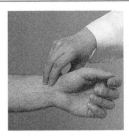

FIGURE 8-2. Palpating the radial pulse.

Rhythm. Palpate the radial pulse. Check the rhythm again by listening with your stethoscope at the cardiac apex. Is the rhythm regular or irregular? If irregular, try to identify a pattern: (1) Do early beats appear in a basically regular rhythm? (2) Does the irregularity vary consistently with respiration? (3) Is the rhythm totally irregular?

Palpation of an irregularly irregular rhythm may likely indicate atrial fibrillation. For all irregular patterns, an ECG is needed to identify the arrhythmia.

Respiratory Rate and Rhythm. Observe the *rate, rhythm, depth,* and *effort of breathing.* Count the number of respirations in 1 minute either by visual inspection or by subtly listening over the patient's trachea with your stethoscope during examination of the head and neck or chest. *Normally, adults take 14 to 20 breaths per minute in a quiet, regular pattern.*

See Table 15-3, p. 239, Abnormalities in Rate and Rhythm of Breathing.

Temperature. Average *oral temperature,* usually 37°C (98.6°F), fluctuates considerably from the early morning to the late afternoon or evening. *Rectal temperatures are higher* than oral temperatures by about 0.4 to 0.5°C (0.7 to 0.9°F) but also vary. *Axillary temperatures* are *lower* than oral temperatures by approximately 1°C but take 5 to 10 minutes to register and are considered less accurate than other measurements.

Fever or *pyrexia* refers to an elevated body temperature. *Hyperpyrexia* refers to extreme elevation in temperature, above 41.1°C (106°F), whereas *hypothermia* refers to an abnormally low temperature, below 35°C (95°F) rectally.

Causes of fever include infection, trauma (such as surgery or crush injuries), malignancy, blood disorders (such as acute hemolytic anemia), drug reactions, and immune disorders such as collagen vascular disease.

Tympanic membrane temperature is more variable than oral or rectal temperatures. Studies suggest that in adults, *oral* and *temporal artery temperatures* correlate more closely with the pulmonary artery temperature but are about 0.5°C lower. See Box 8-9 for temperature sources.

The chief cause of hypothermia is exposure to cold. Other causes include reduced movement as in paralysis, interference with vasoconstriction as from sepsis or excess alcohol, starvation, hypothyroidism, and hypoglycemia. Older adults are especially susceptible to hypothermia and also less likely to develop fever.

BOX 8-9. Various Temperature Sources

Temperature Source	Directions
Oral temperature	Choose either glass or electronic thermometer.
■ Glass thermometer	■ Shake the thermometer down to 35°C (96°F) or below, insert it under the tongue, instruct the patient to close both lips, and wait 3 to 5 minutes. Then read the thermometer, reinsert for 1 minute, and read it again. ■ Avoid breakage.
■ Electronic thermometer	■ Carefully place the disposable cover over the probe and insert the thermometer under the tongue for about 10 seconds.
Rectal temperature	■ Position the patient on one side with the hip flexed. ■ Select a rectal thermometer with a stubby tip, lubricate it, and insert it about 3 to 4 cm (1.5") into the anal canal, in a direction pointing to the umbilicus. Remove it after 3 minutes, then read. ■ Alternatively, use an electronic thermometer after lubricating the probe cover. Wait about 10 seconds for the digital temperature recording to appear.
Tympanic membrane temperature	■ Make sure the external auditory canal is free of cerumen. Position the probe in the canal. Wait 2 to 3 seconds until the digital reading appears. ■ This method measures core body temperature, which is higher than the normal oral temperature by approximately 0.8°C (11.4°F).
Temporal artery temperature	■ Place the probe against the center of the forehead, depress the infrared scanning button, and brush the device across the forehead, down the cheek, and behind an earlobe. Read the display, which records the highest measure temperature. ■ Industry information suggests that combined forehead and behind-the-ear contact is more accurate than scanning only the forehead.

Pain Management. Managing pain is a complex clinical challenge. Experts recommend a stepped-care approach, with an emphasis on measurement and tracking tools to follow responses to treatment and referrals to specialists (Boxes 8-10 and 8-11).

BOX 8-10. Addiction, Physical Dependence, and Tolerance

- *Tolerance:* A state of adaptation in which exposure to a drug induces changes that result in a diminution of one or more of the drug's effects over time.
- *Physical dependence:* A state of adaptation that is manifested by a drug class–specific withdrawal syndrome that can be produced by abrupt cessation, rapid dose reduction, decreasing blood level of the drug, and/or administration of an antagonist.
- *Addiction:* A primary, chronic, neurobiologic disease, with genetic, psychosocial, and environmental factors influencing its development and manifestations. It is characterized by behaviors that include one or more of the following: impaired control over drug use, compulsive use, continued use despite harm, and craving.

Source: American Pain Society. Definitions Related to the Use of Opioids for the Treatment of Pain. A consensus statement from the American Academy of Pain Medicine, the American Pain Society, and the American Society of Addiction Medicine, 2001. Available at https://www.asam.org/docs/default-source/public-policy-statements/1opioid-definitions-consensus-2-011.pdf. Accessed June 7, 2019. Reprinted with permission from American Society of Addiction Medicine.

BOX 8-11. Managing Chronic Pain: Steps for Measurement-Based Care

Step 1: *Measure pain intensity and pain interference.* A validated two-item questionnaire is available for primary care asking patients to rate pain in the past month and interference with daily activities on a scale of 1 to 10.

Step 2: *Measure mood.* Treatable depression, anxiety, and posttraumatic stress disorder (PTSD) frequently accompany chronic pain. The PHQ-4 is a four-item questionnaire for detecting anxiety and depression. The Primary Care-PTSD is a four-question screen for PTSD.

Step 3: *Measure the effect of pain on sleep.* Opioid doses correlate with sleep-disordered breathing and sleep apnea.

continued

Step 4: *Measure risk of co-occurring substance abuse*, estimated at 18% to 30%.

Step 5: *Measure the opioid dose* and calculate the opioid dose equivalency using available web-based calculators.

Source: Tauben D. Chronic pain management: measurement-based stepped care solutions. *Pain: Clinical Updates*. International Association for the Study of Pain. December 2012. Available at http://www.iasp-pain.org/PublicationsNews/NewsletterIssue.aspx?ItemNumber=2064. Accessed June 9, 2019. These steps have been reproduced with permission of the International Association for the Study of Pain® (IASP). The steps may not be reproduced for any other purpose without permission.

Be aware of the well-documented health disparities in pain treatment and delivery of care, which range from lower use of analgesics in emergency rooms for African American and Hispanic patients to disparities in use of analgesics for cancer, postoperative, and low back pain. Clinician stereotypes, language barriers, and unconscious clinician biases in decision making all contribute to these disparities. Critique your own communication style, seek information and best practice standards, and improve your techniques of patient education and empowerment.

RECORDING YOUR FINDINGS

Initially you may use sentences to describe your findings; later you will use phrases. The style in the next box contains phrases appropriate for most write-ups. Common abbreviations for blood pressure, heart rate, and respiratory rate are self-explanatory.

Recording the Physical Examination—General Survey and Vital Signs

"Mrs. Cortez is a young, healthy-appearing woman, well-groomed, fit, and in good spirits. Height is 5′4″, weight 135 lb, BP 120/80, HR 72 and regular, RR 16, temperature 37.5°C."

OR

"Mr. Robinson is an elderly man who looks pale and chronically ill. He is alert, with good eye contact, but cannot speak more than two or three words at a time because of shortness of breath. He has intercostal muscle retraction when breathing and sits upright in bed. He is thin, with diffuse muscle wasting. Height is 6′2″, weight 175 lb, BP 160/95, HR 108 and irregular, RR 32 and labored, temperature 101.2°F."

These findings suggest COPD exacerbation.

HEALTH PROMOTION AND COUNSELING: EVIDENCE AND RECOMMENDATIONS

Important Topics for Health Promotion and Counseling

- Hypertension
- Blood pressure and dietary sodium

Screening for Hypertension

Hypertension is an important public health problem in the United States.

- *Primary (essential) hypertension* is the most common cause of hypertension: risk factors include age, genetics, black race, obesity and weight gain, excessive salt intake, physical inactivity, and excessive alcohol use.
- *Secondary hypertension* accounts for <5% of hypertension cases. Causes include obstructive sleep apnea, chronic kidney disease, renal artery stenosis, medications, thyroid disease, parathyroid disease, Cushing syndrome, hyperaldosteronism, pheochromocytoma, and coarctation of the aorta.

The U.S. Preventive Services Task Force (USPSTF) has issued a grade A recommendation strongly encouraging annual BP screening of adults aged 40 years and older and those at increased risk for high BP. It has consistently found good-quality evidence that screening provides substantial benefits for reducing cardiovascular disease events

In 2017, the American College of Cardiology (ACC) and American Heart Association (AHA) recommended obtaining automated BP measurements in the clinic and confirming hypertension with ABPM and HBPM. The ACC/AHA defined hypertension as SBP >130 mm Hg or DBP >80 mm Hg with stage I versus stage II hypertension as being 130–139/80–89 mm Hg and >140/>90 mm Hg, respectively. Adults with SBP between 120 mm Hg and 129 mm Hg and DBP <80 mm Hg were classified as having elevated BP. A 1-year reassessment was recommended for adults with normal BP, while those with elevated BP should be reassessed in 3 to 6 months.

Blood Pressure and Dietary Sodium

The Institute of Medicine (IOM) recommends a maximum daily dietary intake of 2,300 mg of sodium for adults to reduce risk of hypertension. Advise patients to read the Nutrition Facts panel on food labels to help them adhere to the 2,300 mg/day guideline and to consider adopting the well-investigated Dietary Approaches to Stop Hypertension, or DASH Eating Plan (see Table 8-1, Patients with Hypertension: Recommended Changes in Diet, p. 127).

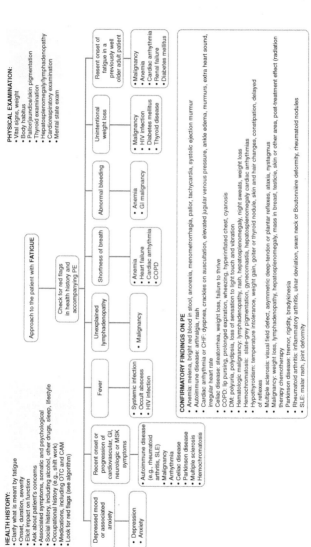

HEALTH HISTORY:
- Clarify what is meant by fatigue
- Onset, duration, severity
- Elicit impact on function
- Ask about patient's concerns
- Associated symptoms, somatic and psychological concerns
- Social history, including alcohol, other drugs, sleep, lifestyle
- Occupational history (e.g., shift work)
- Medications, including OTC and CAM
- Look for red flags (see algorithm)

PHYSICAL EXAMINATION:
- Vital signs, weight
- Body habitus
- Pallor/jaundice/skin pigmentation
- Thyroid examination
- Hepatosplenomegaly/lymphadenopathy
- Cardiorespiratory examination
- Mental state exam

Approach to the patient with FATIGUE

Check for red flags in health history and accompanying PE

Depressed mood or associated anxiety
- Depression
- Anxiety

Recent onset or progression of cardiovascular, GI, neurologic or MSK symptoms
- Autoimmune disease (e.g., rheumatoid arthritis, SLE)
- Malignancy
- Arrhythmia
- Celiac disease
- Parkinson disease
- Multiple sclerosis
- Hemochromatosis

Fever
- Systemic infection
- Occult abscess
- HIV infection

Unexplained lymphadenopathy
- Malignancy

Shortness of breath
- Anemia
- Heart failure
- Cardiac arrhythmia
- COPD

Abnormal bleeding
- Anemia
- GI malignancy

Unintentional weight loss
- Malignancy
- HIV infection
- Diabetes mellitus
- Thyroid disease

Recent onset of fatigue in a previously well older adult patient
- Malignancy
- Anemia
- Cardiac arrhythmia
- Renal failure
- Diabetes mellitus

CONFIRMATORY FINDINGS ON PE
- Anemia: melena, bright red blood in stool, anorexia, menometrorrhagia, pallor, tachycardia, systolic ejection murmur
- Autoimmune disease: arthralgia, rash
- Cardiac arrhythmia or CHF: dyspnea, crackles on auscultation, elevated jugular venous pressure, ankle edema, murmurs, extra heart sound, irregular heart rate
- Celiac disease: steatorrhea, weight loss, failure to thrive
- COPD: lip pursing, prolonged expiration, wheezing, hyperinflated chest, cyanosis
- DM: polyuria, polydipsia, loss of sensation to light touch and vibration
- Hematologic malignancy: lymphadenopathy, rash, hepatosplenomegaly, night sweats, weight loss
- Hemochromatosis: slate-grey pigmentation, gynecomastia, hepatosplenomegaly cardiac arrhythmias
- Hypothyroidism: temperature intolerance, weight gain, goiter or thyroid nodule, skin and hair changes, constipation, delayed of reflexes
- Multiple sclerosis: visual field defect, asymmetric deep-tendon or plantar reflexes, ataxia, nystagmus
- Malignancy: weight loss, lymphadenopathy, hepatosplenomegaly, mass in breast, testicle, skin or other area, post-treatment effect (radiation therapy chemotherapy
- Parkinson disease: tremor, rigidity, bradykinesia
- Rheumatoid arthritis: inflammatory arthritis, ulnar deviation, swan neck or Boutonnière deformity, rheumatoid nodules
- SLE: malar rash, joint deformity

Algorithm 8-1. Approach to the patient with fatigue. (Note: Although it is not comprehensive, this algorithm may be a helpful starting approach.) CAM, complementary and alternative medicine; CHF, congestive heart failure; COPD, chronic obstructive pulmonary disease; DM, diabetes mellitus; GI, gastrointestinal; HIV, human immunodeficiency virus; MSK, musculoskeletal; OTC, over the counter; PE, physical examination; SLE, systemic lupus erythematosus.

INTERPRETATION AIDS

TABLE 8-1. Patients with Hypertension: Recommended Changes in Diet

Dietary Change	Food Source
Increase foods high in potassium	Baked white or sweet potatoes, white beans, beet greens, soybeans, spinach, lentils, kidney beans
	Yogurt
	Tomato paste, juice, puree, and sauce
	Bananas, plantains, many dried fruits, orange juice
Decrease foods high in sodium	Canned foods (soups, tuna fish)
	Pretzels, potato chips, pizza, pickles, olives
	Many processed foods (frozen dinners, ketchup, mustard)
	Batter-fried foods
	Table salt, including for cooking

Adapted from U.S. Department of Agriculture and U.S. Department of Health and Human Services. *Dietary Guidelines for Americans, 2010*. Washington, DC: U.S. Government Printing Office; 2010; *Choose MyPlate.gov*. Available at http://www.choosemyplate.gov/index.html. Accessed December 15, 2014; Office of Dietary Supplements, National Institutes of Health. Dietary Supplement fact sheets: calcium; vitamin D. Available at http://ods.od.nih.gov/factsheets/list-all/. Accessed June 9, 2019.

Cognition, Behavior, and Mental Status

HEALTH HISTORY

This chapter uses *mental disorder* to denote any condition or syndrome whose clinical manifestations are characterized by significant impairment in cognition, emotion regulation, or behavior that is measured in terms of deviation from some normative concept and leads to significant distress and/or disability in social, occupational, or other important activities of daily life. This is also the term used in the current *Diagnostic and Statistical Manual of Mental Disorders*, Fifth Edition (*DSM-5*), the diagnostic manual used by psychiatrists and other mental health professionals in the United States. However, there are inherent issues with this nomenclature and terms such as *mental illness* or *psychiatric illness* may be preferred. In fact, *DSM-5* acknowledges that the term maybe misleading since it implies a distinction between mental disorders and physical disorders but continues its use because there is no appropriate substitute as of the present time.

Common or Concerning Symptoms

- Anxiety, excessive worrying
- Depressed mood
- Memory problems
- Medically unexplained symptoms

Anxiety, Excessive Worrying

Try to explore with an open-ended question like "Can you tell me how things have been going with you recently?" See Box 9-1 for more.

Common risk factors in patients with anxiety and related disorders include family history of anxiety, personal history of mood disorder, childhood stressful life events or trauma, being female, chronic medical illness, and behavioral inhibition.

BOX 9-1. High-Yield Screening Questions for Anxiety

- Over the past 2 weeks, have you been feeling nervous, anxious, or on edge?

- Over the past 2 weeks, have you been unable to stop or control worrying?

Worrying that predominates as the nature of the complaint may lead one to suspect a generalized anxiety disorder or panic disorder.

- Over the past 4 weeks, have you had an anxiety attack— suddenly feeling fear or panic?

Excessive worry persisting over a 4-week period suggests a possible generalized anxiety disorder.

Depressed Mood

As with anxiety, it is important to start out open-ended. "How have you been feeling?" or "How your mood has been?" can be helpful ways to start screening for depression (Box 9-2).

See Algorithm 9-1, Approach to the patient with depression, p. 143.

Ask about a personal history of a depressive episode, a family history of first-degree family members with depression, history of recent stressful life events or significant childhood adversity, chronic and/or disabling medical illness.

Sadness after a recent loss of a loved one is common and expected, and it may be part of normal bereavement rather than depression.

BOX 9-2. High-Yield Screening Questions for Depression

Over the past 2 weeks, have you:

- felt down, depressed, or hopeless?
- felt little interest or pleasure in doing things (anhedonia)?
- had trouble falling or staying asleep, or sleeping too much?
- been feeling bad about yourself, or that you're a failure or have let your family down?
- felt tired or having little energy?
- had poor appetite or overeating?

continued

- had trouble concentrating on things, such as reading the newspaper or watching television? - been moving or speaking so slowly that other people could have noticed? Or been so fidgety or restless that you have been moving a lot more than usual? - had thoughts that you would be better off dead or thoughts of hurting yourself in some way?	Major depressive disorder (MDD) is characterized by at least 2 weeks of depressed/irritable mood. Persistent depressive disorder (PDD) is characterized by depressive/irritable mood lasting for at least 2 years.

Memory Problems

In the *DSM-5*, *delirium* and *dementia* fall under the new category of *neurocognitive disorders*, based on consultation with expert groups. Dementia is classified as a major cognitive disorder; a less severe level of cognitive impairment is now *mild neurocognitive disorder*, which applies to younger individuals with impairment from traumatic brain injury or HIV infection. The *DSM-5* retains the term *dementia*, however, due to widespread clinical usage. See Table 9-2, Neurocognitive Disorders: Delirium and Dementia, and Algorithm 9-2, Approach to the patient with memory impairment, p. 144.

Ask "Have you or anyone you know expressed concerns about your memory?"	Patients with milder forms of dementia may be able to acknowledge their forgetfulness. Patients with more severe forms may be more likely to remember other people worrying about their memory than episodes of forgetfulness.
Ask "When did you first notice the forgetfulness?" "Did it happen over time, or was it sudden?"	Sudden-onset memory problems is concerning for major vascular neurocognitive disorder. Rapid-onset memory problems after a head injury should raise suspicion for major neurocognitive disorder due to traumatic brain injury. Most other dementias have an insidious onset.

Patients with Medically Unexplained Symptoms

Physical symptoms account for approximately 50% of office visits. Approximately 25% of these patients may present with persisting and recurrent symptoms that elude assessment and fail to improve. Overall, 30% of these symptoms are considered to be *medically unexplained*.

Failure to recognize the admixture of physical symptoms, functional syndromes, and common mental disorders—anxiety, depression, unexplained and somatoform symptoms, and substance abuse—adds to the burden of patient undertreatment and poor quality of life. See Table 9-1, Somatoform Disorders: Types and Approach to Symptoms, p. 145.

MENTAL HEALTH SCREENING

Unexplained conditions lasting more than 6 weeks are increasingly recognized as chronic disorders that should prompt screening for depression, anxiety, or both (Box 9-3). Because screening all patients is time consuming and expensive, experts recommend a *two-tiered approach*: brief screening questions with high sensitivity and specificity for patients at risk, followed by more detailed investigation when indicated.

BOX 9-3. Patient Identifiers for Mental Health Screening

- Medically unexplained physical symptoms
- Multiple physical or somatic symptoms or "high symptom count"
- High severity of the presenting somatic symptom
- Chronic pain
- Symptoms for more than 6 weeks
- Physician rating as a "difficult encounter"
- Recent stress
- Low self-rating of overall health
- High use of health care services
- Substance abuse

More than half have a depressive or anxiety disorder.

See Table 9-1, Somatoform Disorders: Types and Approach to Symptoms, p. 145.

TECHNIQUES OF EXAMINATION

Key Components of the Mental Status Examination

- Assess *appearance* and *behavior* including *level of consciousness, posture* and *motor behavior, dress, grooming, personal hygiene, facial expression, affect,* and *manner*
- Assess *speech* and *language* including *quantity, rate, volume, articulation,* and *fluency*
- Assess *mood*
- Assess *thoughts* and *perceptions*
- Assess *insight* and *judgment*
- Assess *cognition*, including *orientation, attention, memory,* and *higher cognitive functions*

Many of the terms used to describe the mental status examination are familiar to you from social conversation. Take the time to learn their precise meanings in the context of the formal evaluation of mental status (Box 9-4).

BOX 9-4. Terminology: Mental Status Examination

Level of consciousness	Alertness or state of awareness of the environment
Attention	Ability to focus or concentrate over time on one task or activity
Memory	Process of registering or recording information. Recent or short-term memory covers minutes, hours, or days; remote or long-term memory refers to intervals of years.
Orientation	Awareness of personal identity, place, and time; requires both memory and attention
Perceptions	Sensory awareness of objects in the environment and their interrelationships; also refers to internal stimuli (e.g., dreams)
Thought processes	Logic, coherence, and relevance of the patient's thoughts, or how people think
Thought content	What the patient thinks about, including level of insight and judgment
Insight	Awareness that symptoms or disturbed behaviors are normal or abnormal

Judgment	Process of comparing and evaluating alternatives; reflects values that may or may not be based on reality and social conventions or norms
Affect	Observable, usually episodic, feeling tone expressed through voice, facial expression, and demeanor
Mood	More sustained emotion that may color a person's view of the world (*affect is to mood as weather is to climate*)
Language	Complex symbolic system for expressing, receiving, and comprehending words; essential for assessing other mental functions
Higher cognitive functions	Assessed by vocabulary, fund of information, abstract thinking, calculations, construction of objects with two or three dimensions

The Mental Status Examination consists of six components: appearance and behavior, speech and language, mood, thoughts and perceptions, insight and judgment, and cognitive function. Each of these components will be discussed in the following sections.

Appearance and Behavior

Assess the following:

- *Level of Consciousness.* Observe alertness and response to verbal and tactile stimuli (Box 9-5).

  Normal consciousness, lethargy, obtundation, stupor, coma

- *Posture and Motor Behavior.* Observe pace, range, character, and appropriateness of movements.

  Restlessness, agitation, bizarre postures, immobility, involuntary movements

- *Dress, Grooming, and Personal Hygiene*

  Fastidiousness, neglect

- *Facial Expressions.* Assess during rest and interaction.

  Anxiety, depression, elation, anger, and facial immobility of parkinsonism

- *Manner, Affect, and Relation to People and Things*

  Anger, hostility, suspiciousness, or evasiveness in patients with paranoia; the elation and euphoria of mania; the flat affect and remoteness of schizophrenia; the apathy and dulled affect of depression and dementia

BOX 9-5. Levels of Consciousness

Level	Patient Response
Alertness	The alert patient has eyes open, looks at you when spoken to in a *normal tone of voice*, and responds fully and appropriately to stimuli.
Lethargy	The lethargic patient appears drowsy but opens the eyes when spoken to in a *loud voice* and looks at you, responds to questions, and then falls asleep.
Obtundation	The obtunded patient opens the eyes when *tactile* stimulus is applied and looks at you but responds to you slowly and is somewhat confused.
Stupor	The stuporous patient arouses only after *painful* stimuli. Verbal responses are slow or even absent. The patient lapses into an unresponsive state when the stimulus ceases.
Coma	A comatose patient remains unarousable with eyes closed. There is no evident response to inner need or external stimuli.

Speech and Language

Note quantity, rate, loudness, clarity, and fluency of speech. If indicated, test for aphasia. A person who can write a correct sentence does not have aphasia.

Aphasia, dysphonia, dysarthria, changes with mood disorders.

Mood

Ask about the patient's spirits. Note nature, intensity, duration, and stability of any abnormal mood. If indicated, assess risk of suicide.

Happiness, elation, depression, anxiety, anger, indifference.

Thought and Perceptions

Thought Processes. Assess logic, relevance, organization, and coherence.

Derailments, flight of ideas, incoherence, confabulation, blocking

Thought Content. Ask about and explore any unusual or unpleasant thoughts.

Obsessions, compulsions, delusions, feelings of unreality

Perceptions. Ask about any unusual perceptions (e.g., seeing or hearing things).

Illusions, hallucinations

TECHNIQUES OF EXAMINATION	POSSIBLE FINDINGS
Insight and Judgment. Assess patient's insight into the illness and level of judgment used in making decisions or plans.	Recognition or denial of mental cause of symptoms; bizarre, impulsive, or unrealistic judgment

Cognitive Functions

If indicated, assess:

Orientation to time, place, and person	Disorientation

Attention

- *Digit span*—ability to repeat a series of numbers forward and then backward

- *Serial 7s*—ability to subtract 7 repeatedly, starting with 100

- *Spelling backward* of a five-letter word, such as W-O-R-L-D

Poor performance of digit span, serial 7s, and spelling backward are common in dementia and delirium but have other causes, too.

Remote Memory (e.g., birthdays, anniversaries, social security number, schools, jobs, wars)	Impaired in late stages of dementia
Recent Memory (e.g., events of the day) and *New Learning Ability*—ability to repeat three or four words after a few minutes of unrelated activity	Recent memory and new learning ability impaired in dementia, delirium, and amnestic disorders

Higher Cognitive Functions

If indicated, assess:

Information and Vocabulary. Note range and depth of patient's information, complexity of ideas expressed, and vocabulary used. For the fund of information, ask names of presidents, other political figures, or large cities.	These attributes reflect intelligence, education, and cultural background. They are limited by mental retardation but are fairly well preserved in early dementia.
Calculating Abilities, such as addition, subtraction, and multiplication	Poor calculation in mental retardation and dementia
Abstract Thinking—ability to respond abstractly to questions about:	Concrete responses (observable details rather than concepts) are common in mental retardation, dementia, and delirium. Responses are sometimes bizarre in schizophrenia.

- The meaning of *proverbs*, such as "A stitch in time saves nine."

- The *similarities* of beings or things, such as a cat and a mouse or a piano and a violin

Constructional Ability. Ask the patient:

To copy figures such as circle, cross, diamond, and box, and two intersecting pentagons, or to draw a clock face with numbers and hands

Impaired ability is common in dementia and with parietal lobe damage.

RECORDING YOUR FINDINGS

Initially you may use sentences to describe your findings; later you will use phrases. The style in the next box contains phrases appropriate for most write-ups.

Recording the Behavior and Mental Status Examination

"Mental Status: The patient is alert, well groomed, and cheerful. Speech is fluent and words are clear. Thought processes are coherent, insight is good. The patient is oriented to person, place, and time. Serial 7s accurate; recent and remote memory intact. Calculations intact."

OR

"Mental Status: The patient appears sad and fatigued; clothes are wrinkled. Speech is slow and words are mumbled. Thought processes are coherent, but insight into current life reverses is limited. The patient is oriented to person, place, and time. Digit span, serial 7s, and calculations accurate, but responses delayed. Clock drawing is good."

These findings suggest depression.

HEALTH PROMOTION AND COUNSELING: EVIDENCE AND RECOMMENDATIONS

Important Topics for Health Promotion and Counseling

- Screening for depression
- Assessing for suicide risk
- Screening for neurocognitive disorders: dementia and delirium

Screening for Depression

The U.S. Preventive Services Task Force (USPSTF) issued a grade B recommendation in 2016 for depression screening in clinical settings that can provide "accurate diagnosis, effective treatment, and appropriate follow-up." Responding "Yes" to two simple questions about mood and anhedonia has a sensitivity of 83% and a specificity of 92% for detecting major depression and appears to be as effective as using more detailed instruments (see Box 9-2).

▪ "Over the past 2 weeks, have you felt down, depressed, or hopeless?" (screens for *depressed mood*)
▪ "Over the past 2 weeks, have you felt little interest or pleasure in doing things?" (screens for *anhedonia*)

These screening questions are also used in the Patient Health Questionnaire (PHQ-9), as shown in Box 9-6. All positive screening tests warrant full diagnostic interviews.

Assessing for Suicide Risk

Suicide ranks as the 10th leading cause of death in the United States, accounting for nearly 45,000 deaths annually, and is the second leading cause of death among 15- to 24-year-olds. Suicide rates are highest among those ages 45 to 54 years, followed by elderly adults age ≥85 years. Men have suicide rates nearly four times higher than women, although women are three times more likely to attempt suicide. Risk factors include suicidal or homicidal ideation, intent, or plan; access to the means for suicide; current symptoms of psychosis or severe anxiety; any history of psychiatric illness (especially linked to a hospital admission); substance abuse; personality disorder; and prior history or family history of suicide.

Despite the public health burden of suicide, the USPSTF has concluded that the current evidence is insufficient to assess the balance of benefits and harms of screening for suicide risk in a primary care setting (I statement), but clinicians should be aware of patient clues and risk factors.

Screening for Neurocognitive Disorders

Dementia. The *Mini Mental State Examination* is the best-known screening test for dementia but is now copyrighted for commercial use, so is less accessible. Recommended screening tests now include the Mini-Cog and the Montreal Cognitive Assessment (MoCA). The *Mini-Cog* has a sensitivity and a specificity as high as 91% and 86%, respectively, and is shorter to administer—about 3 minutes (Box 9-7).

BOX 9-6. Screening for Depression: The Patient Health Questionnaire (PHQ-9)

Administration

The PHQ-9 should be completed by the patient and scored by a staff person or clinician.

Patient Health Questionnaire (PHQ-9)
Nine Symptom Depression Checklist

Name: _____ Date: _____

Over the *last 2 weeks*, how often have you been bothered by any of the following problems?
(Please circle your answer.)

	Not at All	Several Days	More than Half the Days	Nearly Every Day
1. Little interest or pleasure in doing things	0	1	2	3
2. Feeling down, depressed, or hopeless	0	1	2	3
3. Trouble falling or staying asleep, or sleeping too much	0	1	2	3
4. Feeling tired or having little energy	0	1	2	3
5. Poor appetite or overeating	0	1	2	3
6. Feeling bad about yourself—or that you are a failure or have let yourself or your family down	0	1	2	3
7. Trouble concentrating on things, such as reading the newspaper or watching television	0	1	2	3
8. Moving or speaking so slowly that other people could have noticed. Or the opposite—being so fidgety or restless that you have been moving around a lot more than usual	0	1	2	3
9. Thoughts that you would be better off dead or of hurting yourself in some way	0	1	2	3

Add Columns, [____] + [____] + [____]

Total Score*, [____]   *Score is for healthcare provider incorporation

10. If you circled *any* problems, how *difficult* have these problems made it for you to do your work, take care of things at home, or get along with other people? (Please circle your answer.)	Not Difficult at All	Somewhat Difficult	Very Difficult	Extremely Difficult

A score of: 0–4 is considered non-depressed; 5–9 mild depression; 10–14 moderate depression; 15–19 moderately severe depression; and 20–27 severe depression.

PHQ-9 is adapted from PRIME ME TODAY™.
PHQ Copyright © 1999 Pfizer Inc. All rights reserved. Reproduced with permission. PRIME ME TODAY is a trademark of Pfizer Inc.

Scoring

Count the number (#) of boxes checked in a column. Multiply that number by the value indicated below, then add the subtotal to produce a total score. The possible range is 0–27. Use the table below to interpret the PHQ-9 score.

- Not at all (#) _____ × 0 = _____
- Several days (#) _____ × 1 = _____
- More than half the days (#) _____ × 2 = _____
- Nearly every day (#) _____ × 3 = _____

Total score: _____

Total Score	Depression Severity	Proposed Treatment Action
0–4	None–Minimal	None
5–9	Mild	Watchful waiting; repeat PHQ-9 at follow-up
10–14	Moderate	Treatment plan, consider counseling, follow-up, and/or pharmacotherapy
15–19	Moderately severe	Active treatment with pharmacotherapy and/or psychotherapy
20–27	Severe	Immediate initiation of pharmacotherapy and, if severe impairment or poor response to therapy, expedited referral to a mental health specialist for psychotherapy and/or collaborative management

Note: Perform suicide risk assessment in patients who respond positively to item 9 "Thoughts that you would be better off dead or of hurting yourself in some way."

Additional information on administering the PHQ-2 and PHQ-9 can be found at www.phqscreeners.com

BOX 9-7. Screening for Dementia: Mini-Cog

Administration

The test is administered as follows:

1. Instruct the patient to listen carefully to and remember three unrelated words and then to repeat the words.
2. Instruct the patient to draw the face of a clock, either on a blank sheet of paper or on a sheet with the clock circle already drawn on the page. After the patient puts the numbers on the clock face, ask him or her to draw the hands of the clock to read a specific time.
3. Ask the patient to repeat the three previously stated words.

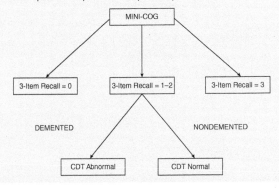

continued

Scoring

Give 1 point for each recalled word after the clock drawing test (CDT) distractor.

Patients recalling none of the three words are classified as demented (Score = 0).

Patients recalling all three words are classified as nondemented (Score = 3).

Patients with intermediate word recall of one to two words are classified based on the CDT (Abnormal = demented; Normal = nondemented).

Note: The CDT is considered normal if all numbers are present in the correct sequence and position, and the hands readably display the requested time.

From Borson S, Scanlan JM, Chen P, et al. The Mini-Cog as a screen for dementia: validation in a population-based sample. *J Am Geriatr Soc*. 2003;51(10):1451–1454.

The *MoCA* has comparable sensitivity and specificity, 91% and 81% in recent studies, and takes 10 minutes to administer (Box 9-8). However, the USPSTF issued an I statement on screening for cognitive impairment because it did not find convincing evidence that pharmacologic or non-pharmacologic interventions could benefit patients with mild to moderate cognitive impairment.

Box 9-8. Screening for Dementia: The Montreal Cognitive Assessment (MoCA)

Administration

The Montreal Cognitive Assessment (MoCA) was designed as a rapid screening instrument for mild cognitive dysfunction. It assesses different cognitive domains: attention and concentration, executive functions, memory, language, visuoconstructional skills, conceptual thinking, calculations, and orientation. Time to administer the MoCA is approximately 10 minutes.

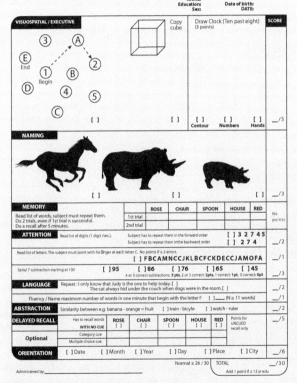

Scoring

Sum all subscores listed on the right-hand side. Add one point for an individual who has 12 years or fewer of formal education, for a possible maximum of 30 points. A final total score of 26 and above is considered normal.

Delirium. The Confusion Assessment Method (CAM) is recommended for screening at-risk patients (Box 9-9). The CAM instrument can quickly and accurately detect delirium at the bedside. Note the features that differentiate dementia from delirium (Table 9-1).

BOX 9-9. The Confusion Assessment Method (CAM) Diagnostic Algorithm

Acute change in mental status and fluctuating course

- Is there evidence of an acute change in cognition from baseline?
- Does the abnormal behavior fluctuate during the day?

Inattention

- Does the patient have difficulty focusing attention?

Disorganized Thinking

- Does the patient have rambling or irrelevant conversations, unclear or illogic flow of ideas, or unpredictable switching from subject to subject?

Abnormal Level of Consciousness

- Is the patient anything besides alert—hyperalert, lethargic, stuporous, or comatose?

Scoring: Diagnosing delirium requires features 1 and 2 and either 3 or 4.

Mental Disorders and Substance Use Disorders

The harmful interactions between mental disorders and substance use disorders also present a major public health problem. The 2017 National Survey on Drug Use and Health showed that 24.5% of the U.S. population ages 12 years or older reported binge drinking, and about 6% reported heavy drinking. Over 30 million Americans reported using an illicit drug during the month before the survey, including nearly 26 million marijuana users, 2.2 million cocaine users, and 6.0 million misusers of psychotherapeutic drugs. Nearly 20 million persons aged 12 years or older were classified as having a substance use disorder based on *DSM-IV* criteria. See Chapter 6, Health Maintenance and Screening for additional information on screening for substance use disorders including misuse of alcohol and prescription and illicit drugs, p. 82.

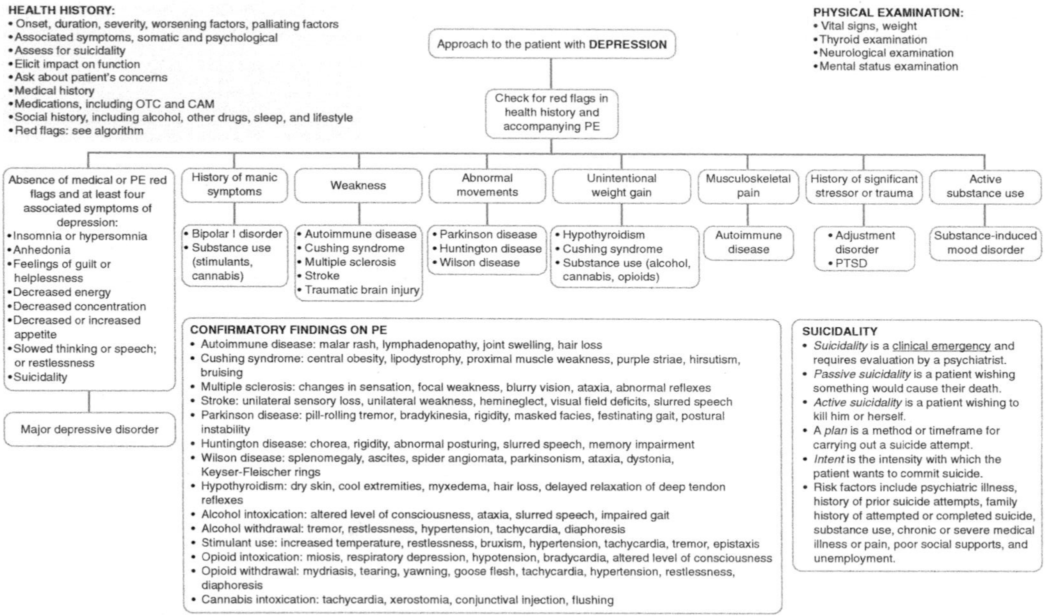
HEALTH HISTORY:
• Onset, duration, severity, worsening factors, palliating factors
• Associated symptoms, somatic and psychological
• Assess for suicidality
• Elicit impact on function
• Ask about patient's concerns
• Medical history
• Medications, including OTC and CAM
• Social history, including alcohol, other drugs, sleep, and lifestyle
• Red flags: see algorithm
Approach to the patient with DEPRESSION
PHYSICAL EXAMINATION:
• Vital signs, weight
• Thyroid examination
• Neurological examination
• Mental status examination
Check for red flags in health history and accompanying PE
Absence of medical or PE red flags and at least four associated symptoms of depression:
• Insomnia or hypersomnia
• Anhedonia
• Feelings of guilt or helplessness
• Decreased energy
• Decreased concentration
• Decreased or increased appetite
• Slowed thinking or speech; or restlessness
• Suicidality
Major depressive disorder
History of manic symptoms
• Bipolar I disorder
• Substance use (stimulants, cannabis)
Weakness
• Autoimmune disease
• Cushing syndrome
• Multiple sclerosis
• Stroke
• Traumatic brain injury
Abnormal movements
• Parkinson disease
• Huntington disease
• Wilson disease
Unintentional weight gain
• Hypothyroidism
• Cushing syndrome
• Substance use (alcohol, cannabis, opioids)
Musculoskeletal pain
Autoimmune disease
History of significant stressor or trauma
• Adjustment disorder
• PTSD
Active substance use
Substance-induced mood disorder
CONFIRMATORY FINDINGS ON PE
• Autoimmune disease: malar rash, lymphadenopathy, joint swelling, hair loss
• Cushing syndrome: central obesity, lipodystrophy, proximal muscle weakness, purple striae, hirsutism, bruising
• Multiple sclerosis: changes in sensation, focal weakness, blurry vision, ataxia, abnormal reflexes
• Stroke: unilateral sensory loss, unilateral weakness, hemineglect, visual field deficits, slurred speech
• Parkinson disease: pill-rolling tremor, bradykinesia, rigidity, masked facies, festinating gait, postural instability
• Huntington disease: chorea, rigidity, abnormal posturing, slurred speech, memory impairment
• Wilson disease: splenomegaly, ascites, spider angiomata, parkinsonism, ataxia, dystonia, Keyser-Fleischer rings
• Hypothyroidism: dry skin, cool extremities, myxedema, hair loss, delayed relaxation of deep tendon reflexes
• Alcohol intoxication: altered level of consciousness, ataxia, slurred speech, impaired gait
• Alcohol withdrawal: tremor, restlessness, hypertension, tachycardia, diaphoresis
• Stimulant use: increased temperature, restlessness, bruxism, hypertension, tachycardia, tremor, epistaxis
• Opioid intoxication: miosis, respiratory depression, hypotension, bradycardia, altered level of consciousness
• Opioid withdrawal: mydriasis, tearing, yawning, goose flesh, tachycardia, hypertension, restlessness, diaphoresis
• Cannabis intoxication: tachycardia, xerostomia, conjunctival injection, flushing
SUICIDALITY
• Suicidality is a clinical emergency and requires evaluation by a psychiatrist.
• Passive suicidality is a patient wishing something would cause their death.
• Active suicidality is a patient wishing to kill him or herself.
• A plan is a method or timeframe for carrying out a suicide attempt.
• Intent is the intensity with which the patient wants to commit suicide.
• Risk factors include psychiatric illness, history of prior suicide attempts, family history of attempted or completed suicide, substance use, chronic or severe medical illness or pain, poor social supports, and unemployment.

Algorithm 9-1. Approach to the patient with depression. (Note: Although it is not comprehensive, this algorithm may be a helpful starting approach.) CAM, complementary and alternative medicine; OTC, over the counter; PE, physical examination; PTSD, posttraumatic stress disorder.

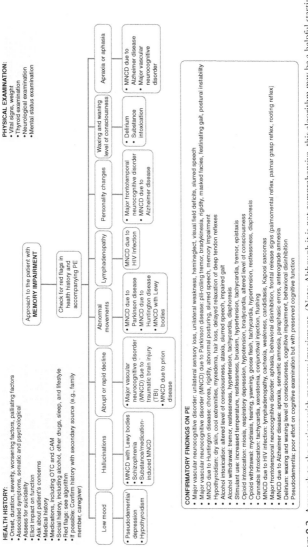

HEALTH HISTORY:
- Onset, duration, severity, worsening factors, palliating factors
- Associated symptoms, somatic and psychological
- Assess for suicidality
- Elicit impact on function
- Ask about patient's concerns
- Medical history
- Medications, including OTC and CAM
- Social history, including alcohol, other drugs, sleep, and lifestyle
- Red flags: see algorithm
- If possible: Confirm history with secondary source (e.g., family member, caregiver)

PHYSICAL EXAMINATION:
- Vital signs, weight
- Thyroid examination
- Neurological examination
- Mental status examination

Approach to the patient with
MEMORY IMPAIRMENT

Check for red flags in
health history and
accompanying PE

Low mood	Hallucinations	Abrupt or rapid decline	Abnormal movements	Lymphadenopathy	Personality changes	Waxing and waning level of consciousness	Apraxia or aphasia
• Pseudodementia/ depression • Hypothyroidism	• MNCD with Lewy bodies • Schizophrenia • Substance/medication-induced MNCD	• Major vascular neurocognitive disorder (MNCD) due to traumatic brain injury (TBI) • MNCD due to prion disease	• MNCD due to Parkinson disease • MNCD due to Huntington disease • MNCD with Lewy bodies	• MNCD due to HIV infection	• Major frontotemporal neurocognitive disorder • MNCD due to Alzheimer disease	• Delirium • Substance intoxication	• MNCD due to Alzheimer disease • Major vascular neurocognitive disorder

CONFIRMATORY FINDINGS ON PE
- Major vascular neurocognitive disorder: unilateral sensory loss, unilateral weakness, hemineglect, visual field deficits, slurred speech
- Major vascular neurocognitive disorder (MNCD) due to Parkinson disease: pill-rolling tremor, bradykinesia, rigidity, masked facies, festinating gait, postural instability
- MNCD due to Huntington disease: chorea, rigidity, abnormal posturing, slurred speech, memory impairment
- Hypothyroidism: dry skin, cool extremities, myxedema, hair loss, delayed relaxation of deep tendon reflexes
- Alcohol intoxication: altered level of consciousness, ataxia, slurred speech, impaired gait
- Alcohol withdrawal: tremor, restlessness, hypertension, tachycardia, diaphoresis
- Stimulant user: increased temperature, restlessness, bruxism, tachycardia, tremor, epistaxis
- Opioid intoxication: miosis, respiratory depression, hypotension, bradycardia, altered level of consciousness
- Opioid withdrawal: mydriasis, tearing, yawning, goose flesh, tachycardia, hypertension, restlessness, diaphoresis
- Cannabis intoxication: tachycardia, xerostomia, conjunctival injection, flushing
- MNCD due to HIV infection: lymphadenopathy, cachexia, weakness, candidiasis, Kaposi sarcomas
- Major frontotemporal neurocognitive disorder: aphasia, behavioral disinhibition, frontal release signs (palmomental reflex, palmar grasp reflex, rooting reflex)
- MNCD due to Alzheimer disease: apraxia, semantic amnesia, paraphasic errors, anterograde amnesia
- Delirium: waxing and waning level of consciousness, cognitive impairment, behavioral disinhibition
- Pseudodementia: poor effort on cognitive examination but with preserved cognitive function

Algorithm 9-2. Approach to the patient with memory impairment. (Note: Although it is not comprehensive, this algorithm may be a helpful starting approach.) CAM, complementary and alternative medicine; HIV, human immunodeficiency virus; OTC, over the counter; PE, physical examination.

INTERPRETATION AIDS

TABLE 9-1. Somatoform Disorders: Types and Approach to Symptoms

Type of Disorder	Diagnostic Features
Somatic symptom disorder	Somatic symptoms are either very distressing or result in significant disruption of functioning, as well as excessive and disproportionate thoughts, feelings, and behaviors related to those symptoms. Symptoms should be specific if with predominant pain.
Illness anxiety disorder	Preoccupation with having or acquiring a serious illness where somatic symptoms, if present, are only mild in intensity.
Conversion disorder	Syndrome of symptoms of deficits mimicking neurologic or clinical illness in which psychological factors are judged to be of etiologic importance.
Psychological factors affecting other clinical conditions	Presence of one or more clinically significant psychological or behavioral factors that adversely affect a clinical condition by increasing the risk for suffering, death, or disability
Factitious disorder	Falsification of physical or psychological signs or symptoms, or induction of injury or disease, associated with identified deception. The individual presents him- or herself as ill, impaired, or injured even in the absence of external rewards.
Other Related Disorders or Behaviors	
Body dysmorphic disorder	Preoccupation with one or more perceived defects or flaws in physical appearance that are not observable or appear only slight to others
Dissociative disorder	Disruption of and/or discontinuity in the normal integration of consciousness, memory, identity, emotion, perception, body representation, motor control, and behavior

Note to readers: Regarding tables in past editions on mood, anxiety, and psychotic disorders, per current *DSM-5* copyright, readers are referred to the *DSM-5* for further diagnostic information.

TABLE 9-2. Neurocognitive Disorders: Delirium and Dementia

	Delirium	Dementia
Mental Status		
Level of Consciousness	Disturbed. Person less alert to clearly aware of the environment and less able to focus, sustain, or shift attention	Usually normal until late in the course of the illness
Behavior	Activity often abnormally decreased (somnolence) or increased (agitation, hypervigilance)	Normal to slow; may become inappropriate
Speech	May be hesitant, slow or rapid, incoherent	Difficulty in finding words, aphasia
Mood	Fluctuating, labile, from fearful or irritable to normal or depressed	Often flat, depressed
Thought Processes	Disorganized, may be incoherent	Impoverished. Speech gives little information
Thought Content	Delusions common, often transient	Delusions may occur
Perceptions	Illusions, hallucinations, most often visual	Hallucinations may occur
Judgment	Impaired, often to a varying degree	Increasingly impaired over the course of the illness
Orientation	Usually disoriented, especially for time. A known place may seem unfamiliar.	Fairly well maintained, but becomes impaired in the later stages of illness

TABLE 9-2. Neurocognitive Disorders: Delirium and Dementia *(continued)*

	Delirium	Dementia
Attention	Fluctuates, with inattention. Person easily distracted, unable to concentrate on selected tasks	Usually unaffected until late in the illness
Memory	Immediate and recent memory impaired	Recent memory and new learning especially impaired
Examples of Cause	Delirium tremens (due to withdrawal from alcohol) Uremia Acute hepatic failure Acute cerebral vasculitis Atropine poisoning	*Reversible:* Vitamin B_{12} deficiency, thyroid disorders *Irreversible:* Alzheimer disease, vascular dementia (from multiple infarcts), dementia due to head trauma

10

Skin, Hair, and Nails

HEALTH HISTORY

Common or Concerning Symptoms

- Lesions
- Rashes
- Itching or pruritus
- Hair loss or nail changes

Lesions

A *lesion* is any single area of altered skin. It may be solitary or multiple. Start by asking if the patient is concerned about any new lesions: "Have you noticed any changes in your skin? . . . your hair? . . . your nails?" "Have you had any growths? . . . sores? . . . lumps?" Pursue the personal and family history of skin cancer and note the type, location, and date of occurrence. Ask about regular self-skin examination and use of sunscreen. See Algorithm 10-1, Approach to the patient with a primary lesion, p. 161.

Rashes and Itching (Pruritus)

A *rash* is a widespread eruption of lesions. For complaints of rash, ask about itching (*pruritus*), the most important symptom when assessing rashes. Does itching precede the rash or follow the rash? For itchy rashes, ask about seasonal allergies with itching and watery eyes, asthma, and atopic dermatitis. Can the patient sleep all night or does itching wake up the patient?

Causes of generalized itching, without apparent rash, include dry skin; pregnancy; uremia; jaundice; lymphomas and leukemia; drug reactions; and, less commonly, polycythemia vera and thyroid disease.

Hair Loss or Nail Changes

Ask if there is hair thinning or hair shedding and, if so, where. If shedding, does the hair come out at the roots or break along the hair shafts?

Hair shedding at the roots is common in telogen effluvium and alopecia areata. Hair breaks along the shaft suggest damage from hair care or tinea capitis.

TECHNIQUES OF EXAMINATION

Key Components of the Full-Body Skin Examination

Patient Position—Seated

- Inspect hair and scalp
- Inspect head and neck, including forehead, eyebrows, eyelids, eyelashes, conjunctivae, sclerae nose, ears, cheeks, lips, oral cavity, chin, and beard
- Inspect upper back
- Inspect shoulders, arms, and hands including palpation of fingernails
- Inspect chest and abdomen
- Inspect anterior thighs and legs
- Inspect feet and toes including soles, interdigital areas, and toenails

Patient Position—Standing

- Inspect lower back
- Inspect posterior thighs and legs
- Inspect breasts, axillae, and genitalia including axillary and pubic hair

Alternative positioning is having the patient supine then prone. The systematic flow of examination from head to foot anteriorly to posteriorly remains.

Standard Technique: Patient Position—Seated then Standing

Choose one of two patient positions for performing the full-body skin examination. The patient can be seated or lie supine then prone. Plan to examine the skin in the same order every time, so you are less likely to skip part of the examination.

Stand in front of the patient and adjust the table to a comfortable height. Start by examining the hair and scalp (Fig. 10-1).

Alopecia, or hair loss, can be diffuse, patchy, or total. Male and female pattern hair loss are normal with aging. Focal patches may be lost suddenly in alopecia areata. Refer scarring alopecia to a dermatologist.

Sparse hair is seen in hypothyroidism; fine, silky hair in hyperthyroidism.

See Table 10-7, Hair Loss, pp. 171–173.

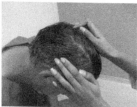

FIGURE 10-1. Parting the hair to expose the scalp.

Inspect the head and neck, including the forehead; eyes including eyelids, conjunctivae, sclerae, eyelashes, and eyebrows; nose, cheeks, lips, oral cavity, and chin; and anterior neck (Figs. 10-2 to 10-4).

Look for signs of basal cell carcinoma on the face. See Table 10-4, Pink Lesions: Basal Cell Carcinoma and Its Mimics, p. 166.

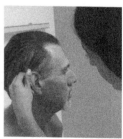

FIGURE 10-3. Inspecting the face and ears.

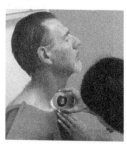

FIGURE 10-4. Inspecting an anterior neck lesion with a dermoscope.

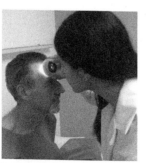

FIGURE 10-2. Inspecting a lesion in the forehead with a dermoscope (or dermatoscope).

Move the gown to see each area. Ask permission first.

Inspect the shoulders, arms, and hands (Fig. 10-5). Inspect and palpate the fingernails. Note their color, shape, and any lesions.

See Table 10-8, Findings in or near the Nails, pp. 174–175.

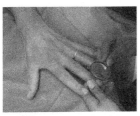

FIGURE 10-5. Inspecting the hands with a magnifying lens and palpating the fingernails.

Inspect the chest and abdomen (Fig. 10-6). Lower or raise the gown to expose these areas and cover up when you are finished.

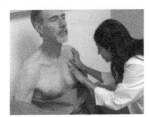

FIGURE 10-6. Inspecting the chest.

Inspect the thighs and lower legs (Fig. 10-7). Inspect and palpate the toenails and inspect the soles and between the toes (Fig. 10-8).

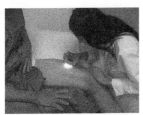

FIGURE 10-7. Inspecting a thigh lesion with a dermoscope.

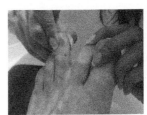

FIGURE 10-8. Inspecting the interdigital areas between toes.

Ask the patient to stand so that you inspect the lower back and posterior legs (Fig. 10-9). If needed, uncover the buttocks. Examination of the breasts and genitalia may be saved for last.

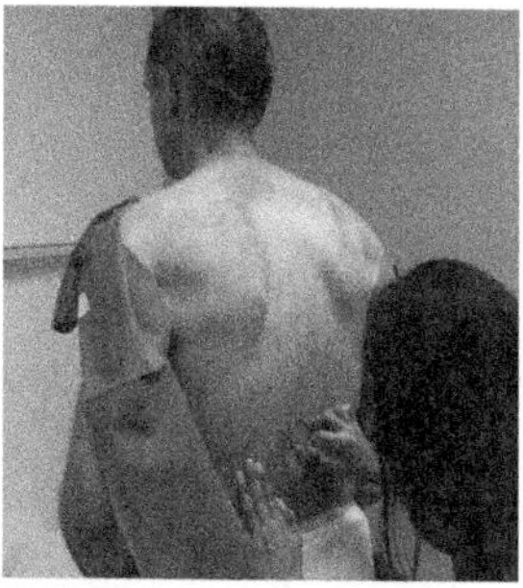

Alternative Technique: Patient Position—Supine then Prone

Some clinicians prefer this positioning for more thorough examinations (Fig. 10-10). With the patient supine, inspect the scalp, face, and anterior neck; the shoulders, arms, and hands; the chest and abdomen; anterior thighs; and lower legs, feet, and, if appropriate, the genitalia. Ask permission when moving the gown to expose different areas, and let the patient know which areas you will be examining next.

Ask the patient to turn over to the *prone* position, lying face down. Look at the posterior scalp, posterior neck, back, posterior thighs, legs, soles of the feet, and buttocks (if appropriate).

Integrated Skin Examinations

Try to integrate certain aspects of the full-body skin examination into your routine physical examination. You can pursue an integrated skin examination as you examine areas on the head and neck, arms and hands, and over the back as you listen to the lungs that are already easily accessible. Integrating the skin examination into the physical examination and routinely recording your findings as part of the general write-up saves time and contributes to earlier detection of skin cancers, when they are easier to treat. Systemic illnesses also have many associated skin findings.

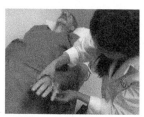

FIGURE 10-9. Inspecting the back with the patient standing.

FIGURE 10-10. Skin examination with the patient supine.

See Tables 10-1 to 10-6, pp. 162–171, for examples of primary lesions (flat, raised, and fluid-filled; pustules, furuncles, nodules, cysts, wheals, and burrows); rough, pink, and brown lesions ; and vascular and purpuric lesions.

Special Techniques

Patient Instructions for the Skin Self-Examination. The patient will need a full-length mirror, a handheld mirror, and a well-lit room that provides privacy. Teach patients the ABCDE-EFG method for assessing moles (Box 10-1). Help them and to identify melanomas by looking at photographs of benign and malignant nevi on easy-to-access websites, handouts, or tables in this chapter.

BOX 10-1. Patient Instructions for Skin Self-Examination

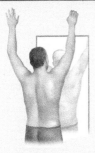

Examine your body front and back in the mirror, then look at right and left sides with your arms raised.

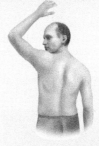

Bend elbows and look carefully at forearms, underarms, and palms.

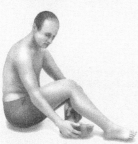

Look at the backs of your legs and feet, the spaces between your toes, and the soles.

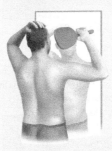

Examine the back of your neck and scalp with a hand mirror. Part hair for a closer look.

continued

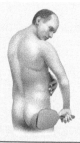

Finally, check your back and buttocks with a hand mirror.

Source: Adapted from American Academy of Dermatology, Inc. How to SPOT Skin Cancer™. Available at https://www.aad.org/public/spot-skin-cancer/learn-about-skin-cancer/detect/how-to-spot-skin-cancer. Accessed October 23, 2018.

Examining the Patient with Hair Loss. Examine the hair to determine the overall pattern of hair loss or hair thinning. Inspect the scalp for erythema, scaling, pustules, tenderness, bogginess, and scarring. Look at the width of the hair part in various sections of the scalp. For shedding from the roots, perform a *hair pull test* by gently grasping 50 to 60 hairs with your thumb and index and middle fingers, pulling firmly away from the scalp (Fig. 10-11).

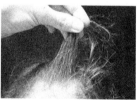

If all the hairs have telogen bulbs, the most likely diagnosis is telogen effluvium.

FIGURE 10-11. Examining the hair for shredding from the roots (hair pull test).

For fragility, perform the *tug test* by holding a group of hairs in one hand, pulling along the hair shafts with the other (Fig. 10-12); if any hairs break, it is abnormal.

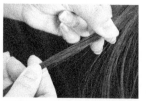

Possible internal causes of diffuse nonscarring hair shedding in young women are iron-deficiency anemia and hyper- or hypothyroidism.

FIGURE 10-12. Examining the hair for fragility (tug test).

Evaluating the Bedbound Patient. People confined to beds, especially when they are emaciated, elderly, or neurologically impaired, are particularly susceptible to *pressure injuries* or *ulcers* (Box 10-2). Carefully inspect the skin that overlies the sacrum, buttocks, greater trochanters, knees, and heels. Roll the patient onto one side to see the low back and gluteal area best.

Local redness of the skin warns of impending necrosis, although some deep pressure sores develop without antecedent redness. Inspect closely for skin breaks and ulcers.

BOX 10-2. Revised Pressure Injury Staging System

The new revised staging system uses the term *injury* instead of *ulcer* and denotes stages using Arabic numerals rather than Roman numerals (Fig. 10-13).

- **Stage 1:** Intact skin with a localized area of nonblanchable erythema, which may appear differently in darkly pigmented skin.
- **Stage 2:** Partial-thickness loss of skin with exposed dermis.
- **Stage 3:** Full-thickness skin loss, in which adipose (fat) is visible in the ulcer and granulation tissue and rolled wound edges, is often present.
- **Stage 4:** Full-thickness skin and tissue loss with exposed or directly palpable fascia, muscle, tendon, ligament, cartilage, or bone in the ulcer.
- **Unstageable:** Full-thickness skin and tissue loss in which the extent of tissue damage within the ulcer cannot be confirmed because it is obscured by slough or *eschar*.
- **Deep tissue pressure injury:** Persistent nonblanchable deep red, maroon, or purple discoloration.

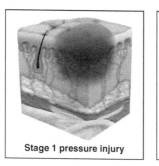

Stage 1 pressure injury

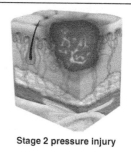

Stage 2 pressure injury

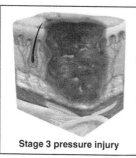

Stage 3 pressure injury

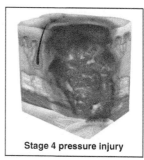

Stage 4 pressure injury

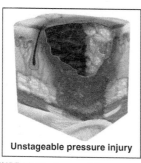

Unstageable pressure injury

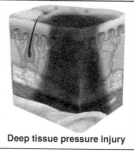

Deep tissue pressure injury

FIGURE 10-13. Pressure injury stages. (Modified from Nettina SM. *Lippincott Manual of Nursing Practice.* 11th ed. Wolters Kluwer; 2019. Figure 9-3.)

RECORDING YOUR FINDINGS

Use specific terms to describe skin lesions and rashes, including number of lesions, size, color, shape, texture, location, configuration, and whether a primary lesion.

Recording the Skin, Hair, and Nails Examination

"Skin warm and dry. Nails without clubbing or cyanosis. Approximately 20 brown, round macules on upper back, chest, and arms, are all symmetric in pigmentation, none suspicious. No rash, petechiae, or ecchymoses."

These findings suggest normal nevi and perfusion without any rashes or suspicious lesions.

OR

"Scattered stuck-on verrucous plaques on back and abdomen. Over 30 small round brown macules with symmetric pigmentation on back, chest, and arms. Single 1.2- × 1.6-cm asymmetric dark brown and black plaque with erythematous, uneven border, on left upper arm."

These findings suggest normal seborrheic keratoses and benign nevi, but also a possible malignant melanoma.

HEALTH PROMOTION AND COUNSELING: EVIDENCE AND RECOMMENDATIONS

Important Topics for Health Promotion and Counseling

- Skin cancer prevention
- Skin cancer screening including melanoma

Skin Cancer Prevention

Skin cancers affect an estimated one in five Americans during their lifetime. The most common skin cancer is *basal cell carcinoma (BCC)*, followed by *squamous cell carcinoma (SCC)*, and then *melanoma*. Although it is the least common skin cancer, melanoma is the most lethal due to its high rate of metastasis and high mortality at advanced stages, causing over 70% of skin cancer deaths. Nonmelanoma skin cancers are rarely fatal.

Melanoma. The incidence of melanoma has the most rapid increase of any cancer and is now the fifth most frequently diagnosed cancer in men and the sixth most frequently diagnosed in women.

Use of the *Melanoma Risk Assessment Tool* developed by the National Cancer Institute, available at http://www.cancer.gov/melanomarisktool/ to assess an individual's 5-year risk of melanoma based on geographic location, gender, race, age, history of blistering sunburns, complexion, number and size of moles, freckling, and sun damage.

Avoiding Ultraviolet Radiation and Tanning Beds. Increasing lifetime sun exposure correlates directly with increasing risk of skin cancer. Intermittent sun exposure appears to be more harmful than chronic exposure. The best defense against skin cancers is to avoid ultraviolet radiation exposure by limiting time in the sun, avoiding midday sun, using sunscreen, and wearing sun-protective clothing with long sleeves and hats with wide brims. Advise patients to avoid indoor tanning, especially children, teens, and young adults. Use of indoor tanning beds, especially before age 35 years, increases risk of melanoma by as much as 75%. In 2009, the International Agency for Research on Cancer classified ultraviolet-emitting tanning devices as "carcinogenic to humans."

Regular Use of Sunscreen. A landmark study in 2011 demonstrated that the regular use of sunscreen decreases the incidence of melanoma. Advise patients to use at least sun-protective factor (SPF) 30 and broad-spectrum protection. For water exposure, patients should use water-resistant sunscreens. The U.S. Preventive Services Task Force (USPSTF) has issued a grade B recommendation supporting behavioral counseling to minimize ultraviolet radiation exposure in fair-skinned persons aged 6 months to 24 years.

Skin Cancer Screening

Although the USPSTF found insufficient evidence (grade I) to recommend routine skin cancer screening, it does advise clinicians to "remain alert for skin lesions with malignant features" during routine physical examinations and reference the ABCDE criteria. The American Cancer Society (ACS) and the AAD recommend full-body examinations for patients over age 50 years or at high risk, because melanoma can appear in any location. High-risk patients are those with a personal or family history of multiple or dysplastic nevi or previous melanoma. Both new and changing nevi should be closely examined, as at least half of melanomas arise de novo from isolated melanocytes rather than pre-existing nevi.

Screening for Melanoma: ABCDEs. Clinicians should apply the ABC-DE-EFG method when screening moles for melanoma (this does not apply for nonmelanocytic lesions like seborrheic keratoses) (Box 10-3). The sensitivity of this tool for detecting melanoma ranges from 43% to 97%, and specificity from 36% to 100%; diagnostic accuracy depends on how many criteria are used to define abnormality.

BOX 10-3. The ABCDE Rule

If two or more of the ABCDE criteria are present, the risk of melanoma increases, and biopsy should be considered. Some have suggested adding EFG to help detect aggressive nodular melanomas.

	Melanoma	Benign Nevus
Asymmetry Of one side of mole compared to the other	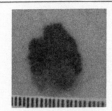	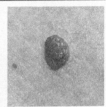
Border irregularity Especially if ragged, notched, or blurred	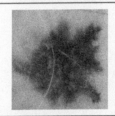	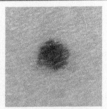
Color variations[a] More than two colors, especially blue-black, white (loss of pigment due to regression), or red (inflammatory reaction to abnormal cells)	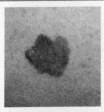	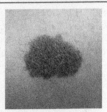
Diameter >6 mm[b] Approximately the size of a pencil eraser	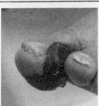	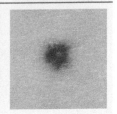

continued

Evolving[c]
Or changing rapidly in
size, symptoms, or
morphology

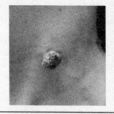
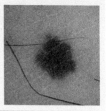

Some have suggested adding **EFG** to help detect aggressive nodular melanomas.
- **E**levated
- **F**irm to palpation
- **G**rowing progressively over several weeks

[a]With the exception of a homogeneous blue color in a blue nevus, blue or black color within a larger pigmented lesion is especially concerning for melanoma.

[b]Early melanomas may be <6 mm, and many benign lesions are >6 mm.

[c]Evolution, or change, is the most sensitive of these criteria. A reliable history of change may prompt biopsy of a benign-appearing lesion.

Patient Screening: The Skin Self-Examination. The AAD and the ACS recommend regular self-skin examination. Instruct patients with risk factors for skin cancer and melanoma, especially those with a history of high sun exposure, prior or family history of melanoma, and ≥50 moles or >5 to 10 atypical moles, to perform regular self-skin examinations.

Approximately half of melanomas are initially detected by patients or their partners.

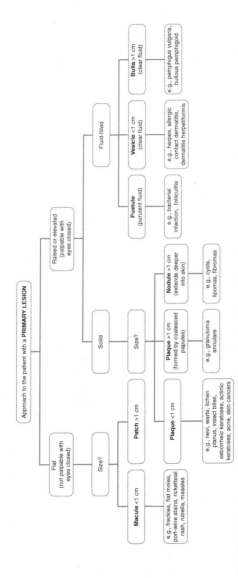

Algorithm 10-1. Approach to the patient with a primary lesion. (Note: Although it is not comprehensive, this algorithm may be a helpful starting approach.)

INTERPRETATION AIDS

TABLE 10-1. Describing Primary Skin Lesions: Flat, Raised, and Fluid-Filled

Describe skin lesions accurately, including number, size, color, texture, shape, primary lesion, location, and configuration. This table identifies common primary skin lesions and includes classic descriptions of each lesion with the diagnosis in italics.

Flat spots: If you run your finger over the lesion but do not feel the lesion, the lesion is flat. If a flat spot is small (<1 cm), it is a macule. If a flat spot is larger (>1 cm), it is a patch.

Macules (flat, small)

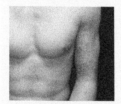

Multiple 3–8-mm erythematous confluent round macules on chest, back, and arms; *morbilliform drug eruption*

Patches (flat, large)

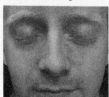

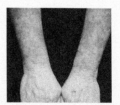

Bilaterally symmetric erythematous patches on central cheeks and eyebrows, some with overlying greasy scale; *seborrheic dermatitis*

Large confluent completely depigmented patches on dorsal hands and distal forearms; *vitiligo*

Raised spots: If you run your finger over the lesion and it is palpable above the skin, it is *raised*. If a raised spot is small (<1 cm), it is a papule. If a raised spot is larger (>1 cm), it is a plaque.

TABLE 10-1. Describing Primary Skin Lesions: Flat, Raised, and Fluid-Filled *(continued)*

Papules (raised, small)

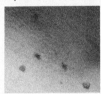

Multiple 2–4-mm soft, fleshy skin-colored to light brown papules on lateral neck and axillae in skin folds; *skin tags*

Scattered erythematous round drop-like, flat-topped well-circumscribed scaling papules and plaques on trunk; *guttate psoriasis*

Plaques (raised, large)

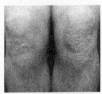

Scattered erythematous to bright pink well-circumscribed flat-topped plaques on extensor knees and elbows, with overlying silvery scale; *plaque psoriasis*

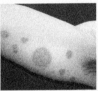

Multiple round coin-like eczematous plaques on arms, legs, and abdomen, with overlying dried transudate crust; *nummular dermatitis*

Fluid-filled lesions: If the lesion is raised, filled with fluid, and small (<1 cm), it is a vesicle. If a fluid-filled spot is larger (>1 cm), it is a bulla.

Vesicles (fluid-filled, small)

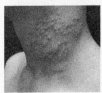

Multiple 2–4-mm vesicles and pustules on erythematous base, grouped together on left neck; *herpes simplex virus*

Bullae (fluid-filled, large)

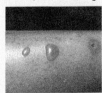

Several tense bullae on lower legs; *insect bites*

> ### TABLE 10-2. Additional Primary Lesions: Pustules, Furuncles, Nodules, Cysts, Wheals, Burrows

Pustule: Small palpable collection of neutrophils or keratin that appears white

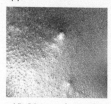

~15–20 pustules and acneiform papules on buccal and parotid cheeks bilaterally; *acne vulgaris*

Furuncle: Inflamed hair follicle; multiple furuncles together form a carbuncle

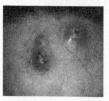

Two large (2-cm) furuncles on forehead, without fluctuance; *furunculosis* (Note: fluctuant deep infections are *abscesses*)

Nodule: Larger and deeper than a papule

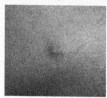

Solitary blue-brown 1.2-cm firm nodule with positive dimple sign and hyperpigmented rim on left lateral thigh; *dermatofibroma*

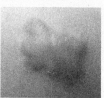

Solitary 4-cm pink and brown scar-like nodule on central chest at site of previous trauma; *keloid*

Subcutaneous mass/cyst: Whether mobile or fixed, cysts are encapsulated collections of fluid or semisolid

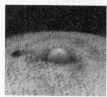

Three 6–8-mm mobile subcutaneous cysts on vertex scalp, that on excision reveal pearly white balls; *pilar cysts*

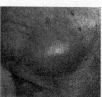

Solitary 9-cm mobile rubbery subcutaneous mass on left temple; *lipoma*

TABLE 10-2. Additional Primary Lesions: Pustules, Furuncles, Nodules, Cysts, Wheals, Burrows *(continued)*

Wheal: Area of localized dermal edema that evanesces (comes and goes) within a period of 1–2 days; this is the essential primary lesion of *urticaria*

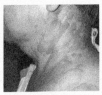

Many variably sized (1–10-cm) wheals on lateral neck, shoulders, abdomen, arms, and legs; *urticaria*

Burrow: Small linear or serpiginous pathways in the epidermis created by the scabies mite

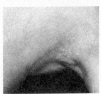

Multiple small (3–6-mm) erythematous papules on abdomen, buttocks, scrotum, and shaft and head of penis, with four burrows noted on interdigital web spaces; *scabies*

TABLE 10-3. Rough Lesions: Actinic Keratoses and Squamous Cell Carcinoma

Patients commonly report feeling rough lesions. Many are benign, like seborrheic keratoses or warts, but squamous cell carcinoma (SCC) and its precursor actinic keratosis can also feel rough or keratotic.

Actinic keratosis

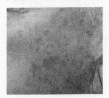

- Often easier to feel than to see
- Superficial keratotic papules that "come and go," on sun-damaged skin

Warts

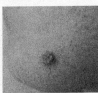

- Usually skin-colored to pink, texture more verrucous than keratotic
- May be filiform
- Often have hemorrhagic punctate that can be seen with a magnifying glass or dermoscope

continued

TABLE 10-3. Rough Lesions: Actinic Keratoses and Squamous Cell Carcinoma *(continued)*

Squamous cell carcinoma

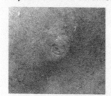

- Keratoacanthomas are SCCs that arise rapidly and have a crateriform center
- Often have a smooth but firm border
- SCCs can become quite large if left untreated (Note: *highest sites of metastasis are the scalp, lips, and ears*)

TABLE 10-4. Pink Lesions: Basal Cell Carcinoma and Its Mimics

Basal cell carcinoma (BCC) is the most common cancer in the world. Fortunately, it rarely spreads to other parts of the body. Nonetheless, it can invade and destroy local tissues, causing significant morbidity to the eye, nose, or brain.

Basal Cell Carcinoma
Superficial basal cell carcinoma

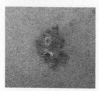

Nodular basal cell carcinoma

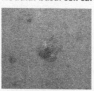
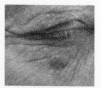

- Pink patch that does not heal
- May have focal scaling

- Pink papule, often with translucent or pearly appearance and overlying telangiectasias
- May have focal pigmentation
- Dermoscopy shows arborizing vessels, focal pigment globules, and other specific patterns

TABLE 10-5. Brown Lesions: Melanoma and Its Mimics

Most patients have brown spots on their body surface. Although these are usually freckles, benign nevi, solar lentigines, or seborrheic keratoses, you and the patient must look closely for any that stand out as a possible *melanoma*. With enough practice, when you see a melanoma, it will stick out as the "ugly duckling." Review the ABCDE rule and photographs on pp. 158–160.

Melanoma	Mimics
Amelanotic melanoma	*Skin tags or intradermal nevi*

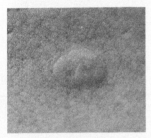

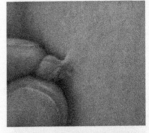

■ Usually in very fair-skinned people
■ Evolution or rapid change is the most important feature, because variegation or dark pigment is missing in this type

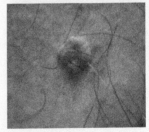

■ Soft and fleshy
■ Often around neck, axillae, or back
■ Sessile nevi may have a hint of brown pigmentation

continued

TABLE 10-5. Brown Lesions: Melanoma and Its Mimics *(continued)*

Melanoma	Mimics
Melanoma in situ	*Solar lentigo*

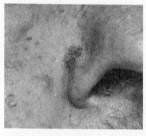

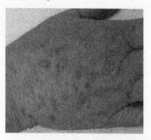

■ On sun-exposed or sun-protected skin ■ Look for ABCDE features	■ On sun-exposed skin ■ Light brown and uniform in color but may be asymmetric

Melanoma	*Dysplastic nevus*

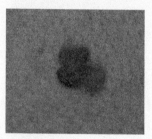

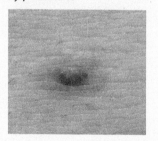

■ May arise de novo or in existing nevi and exhibits ABCDEs ■ Patients with many dysplastic nevi have increased risk of melanoma	■ May have macular base and papular central "fried egg" component ■ Compare to the patient's other nevi and monitor changes

TABLE 10-5. Brown Lesions: Melanoma and Its Mimics *(continued)*

Melanoma	Mimics

Melanoma

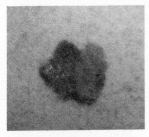

Inflamed seborrheic keratosis

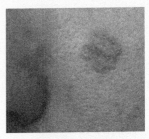

- May have variegated color (browns, red)
- Has melanocytic features on dermoscopy

- Can sometimes mimic a melanoma if it has an erythematous base
- Dermoscopy helps the trained eye distinguish these

Melanoma

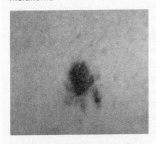

Seborrheic keratosis

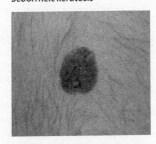

- May be uniform in color but asymmetric; key feature is rapid change or evolution

- Stuck-on and verrucous, may be darkly pigmented

TABLE 10-6. Vascular and Purpuric Lesions of the Skin

Lesions	Features: Appearance, Distribution, Significance
Cherry Angioma 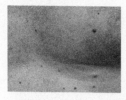	▪ Bright or ruby red, may become purplish with age; 1–3 mm; round, flat, sometimes raised; may be surrounded by a pale halo ▪ Found on trunk or extremities ▪ Not significant; increase in size and number with aging
Spider Angioma^a 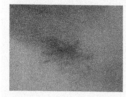	▪ Fiery red; very small to 2 cm; central body, sometimes raised, radiating with erythema ▪ Face, neck, arms, and upper trunk, but almost never below the waist ▪ Seen in liver disease, pregnancy, vitamin B deficiency; normal in some people
Spider Vein^a 	▪ Bluish; varies from very small to several inches; may resemble a spider or be linear, irregular, or cascading ▪ Most often on the legs, near veins; also on anterior chest ▪ Often accompanies increased pressure in the superficial veins, as in varicose veins
Petechia/Purpura 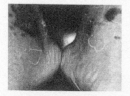	▪ Deep red or reddish purple; fades over time; 1–3 mm or larger; rounded, sometimes irregular, flat ▪ Varied distribution ▪ Seen if blood outside the vessels; may suggest a bleeding disorder or, if petechiae, emboli to skin

TABLE 10-6. Vascular and Purpuric Lesions of the Skin *(continued)*

Lesions	Features: Appearance, Distribution, Significance
Ecchymosis 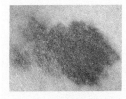	■ Purple or purplish blue, fading to green, yellow, and brown over time; larger than petechiae; rounded, oval, or irregular ■ Varied distribution ■ Seen if blood outside the vessels; often secondary to bruising or trauma; also seen in bleeding disorders

^aThese are telangiectasias, or dilated small vessels that look red or bluish.

Sources of photos: Spider Angioma—Image provided by Stedman's; Petechia/Purpura—Kelley WN. *Textbook of Internal Medicine*. JB Lippincott; 1989.

TABLE 10-7. Hair Loss

Generalized or Diffuse Hair Loss

In men, look for frontal hairline regression and thinning on the posterior vertex; in women look for thinning that spreads from the crown down without hairline regression.

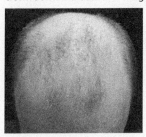

Male pattern hair loss (MPHL)

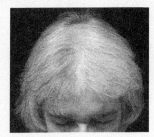

Female pattern hair loss (FPHL)

continued

TABLE 10-7. Hair Loss *(continued)*

Telogen Effluvium and Anagen Effluvium

In *telogen effluvium* overall the patient's scalp and hair distribution appear normal, but a positive *hair pull test* reveals most hairs have telogen bulbs. In *anagen effluvium* there is diffuse hair loss from the roots. The *hair pull test* shows few if any hairs with telogen bulbs.

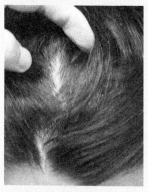

Normal hair part width in telogen effluvium

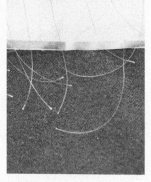

Positive hair pull test in telogen effluvium showing all hairs have telogen bulbs

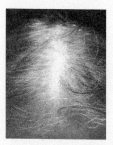

Anagen effluvium

TABLE 10-7. Hair Loss *(continued)*

Focal Hair Loss

Alopecia Areata

There is sudden onset of clearly demarcated, usually localized, round or oval patches of hair loss leaving smooth skin without hairs, in children and young adults. There is no visible scaling or erythema.

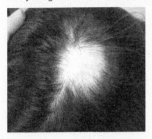

Tinea Capitis ("Ringworm")

There are round scaling patches of alopecia, usually caused by *Trichophyton tonsurans* from humans, and less commonly, *Microsporum canis* from dogs or cats.

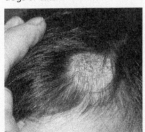
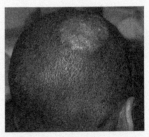

For a complete guide to evaluation of hair loss, review Mubki T, Rucnicka L, Olszewska M, et al. Evaluation and diagnosis of the hair loss patient: Part I. History and Clinical Examination. *J Am Acad Dermatol.* 2014;71(3):415.e1–415.e15.

Source of photo: Alopecia Areata—Goodheart HP, Gonzalez M. *Goodheart's Photoguide to Common Pediatric and Adult Skin Disorders.* 4th ed. Wolters Kluwer; 2016. Appendix Figure 10.

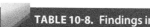

TABLE 10-8. Findings in or Near the Nails

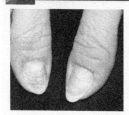

Paronychia
A superficial infection of the proximal and lateral nail folds adjacent to the nail plate. The nail folds are often red, swollen, and tender. Represents the most common infection of the hand, usually from *Staphylococcus aureus* or *Streptococcus*. Creates a *felon* (infection of the finger pad) if it extends into the pulp space of the finger.

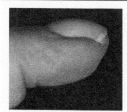

Clubbing of the Fingers
Clinically a bulbous swelling of the soft tissue at the nail base, with loss of the normal angle between the nail and the proximal nail fold. The angle increases to 180° or more, and the nail bed feels spongy or floating. The mechanism is still unknown. Seen in congenital heart disease, interstitial lung disease and lung cancer, inflammatory bowel diseases, and malignancies.

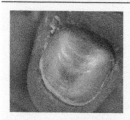

Habit Tic Deformity
There is depression of the central nail with regular radiating ridges in a "Christmas tree"-like pattern from small horizontal depressions, resulting from repetitive trauma from rubbing the index finger over the thumb or vice versa.

Melanonychia
Caused by increased pigmentation in the nail matrix, leading to a streak as the nail grows out. This may be a normal ethnic variation if found in multiple nails. A wide streak, especially if growing or irregular, could represent a subungual melanoma.

TABLE 10-8. Findings in or Near the Nails *(continued)*

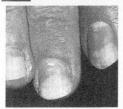

Onycholysis
A painless separation of the whitened opaque nail plate from the pinker translucent nail bed.

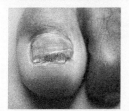

Onychomycosis
The most common cause of nail thickening and subungual debris is onychomycosis, most often from the dermatophyte *Trichophyton rubrum*.

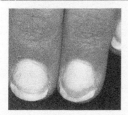

Terry Nails
Nail plate turns white with a ground-glass appearance, a distal band of reddish brown, and obliteration of the lunula. Seen in liver disease, usually cirrhosis, heart failure, and diabetes.

Head and Neck

HEALTH HISTORY

Common or Concerning Symptoms

- Neck mass or lump
- Thyroid mass, nodule, or goiter

Neck Mass or Lump

Assess any lumps or swollen glands in the neck. Ask for onset, discharge, pain in swallowing (*dysphagia*), difficulty breathing (*dyspnea*).

A persistent neck mass in an adult older than 40 years should raise a suspicion of malignancy; see Algorithm 11-1, Approach to the patient with a neck mass, p. 181.

Enlarged tender lymph nodes commonly accompany pharyngitis.

Thyroid Mass, Nodule, or Goiter

Assess thyroid function. Ask about enlargement of the thyroid gland (*goiter*), temperature intolerance, and sweating.

With goiter, thyroid function may be increased, decreased, or normal. Cold intolerance in hypothyroidism; heat intolerance, palpitations, and involuntary weight loss in hyperthyroidism

TECHNIQUES OF EXAMINATION

Key Components of the Head and Neck Examination

- Examine the hair
- Examine scalp
- Examine the skull

- Inspect skin in the head and face
- Palpate cervical lymph nodes
- Examine trachea
- Examine thyroid gland

ℍ Head

Examine the:

- Hair, including quantity, distribution, and texture

  Coarse and sparse in hypothyroidism, fine in hyperthyroidism

- Scalp, including lumps or lesions

  Pilar cysts, psoriasis, seborrheic dermatitis, pigmented nevi

- Skull, including size and contour

  Hydrocephalus, skull depression from trauma

- Face, including symmetry and facial expression

  Facial paralysis; flat affect of depression, moods such as anger, sadness

- Skin, including color, texture, hair distribution, and lesions

  Pale, fine, hirsute, acne, skin cancer

Neck

Inspect the neck.

Scars, masses, torticollis

Palpate cervical lymph nodes

Cervical lymphadenopathy from HIV or AIDS, infectious mononucleosis, lymphoma, leukemia, and sarcoidosis. Enlarged supraclavicular node from possible abdominal malignancy

- Submental—palpate in the midline a few centimeters behind the tip of the mandible.

- Submandibular—midway between the angle and the tip of the mandible.

- Preauricular—palpate in front of the ear.

- Posterior auricular—palpate behind the ear and superficial to the mastoid process.

- Tonsillar (jugulodigastric)—palpate at the angle of the mandible.

- Occipital—palpate at the base of the skull posteriorly.

- Anterior superficial cervical—palpate for these nodes anterior and superficial to the sternocleidomastoid (SCM)

- Posterior cervical—palpate along the anterior edge of the trapezius

- Deep cervical chain—deep in the SCM muscle and often inaccessible to examination.

- Supraclavicular—palpate deep in the angle formed by the clavicle and the SCM muscle.

Inspect and palpate the position of the trachea.

Deviated trachea from neck mass or pneumothorax

Inspect the thyroid gland:

- At rest

- As patient swallows water

From behind patient, palpate the thyroid gland, including the isthmus, and first one then the opposite lobe:

Goiter, nodules, tenderness of thyroiditis. See Table 11-1, Abnormalities of the Thyroid Gland, p. 182.

- At rest

- As patient swallows water (Fig. 11-1)

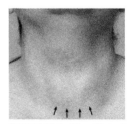

FIGURE 11-1. Thyroid gland with goiter while swallowing.

RECORDING YOUR FINDINGS

Initially you may use sentences to describe your findings; later you will use phrases. The style in the next box contains phrases appropriate for most write-ups.

Recording the Head, Eyes, Ears, Nose, and Throat (HEENT) Examination

HEENT: Head—**The skull is normocephalic/atraumatic (NC/AT). Hair with average texture.** Eyes—Visual acuity 20/20 bilaterally. Sclera white, conjunctiva pink. Pupils are 4 mm constricting to 2 mm, equally round and reactive to light and accommodations. Disc margins sharp; no hemorrhages or exudates, no arteriolar narrowing. Ears—Acuity good to whispered voice. Tympanic membranes (TMs) with good cone of light. Weber midline. AC > BC. Nose—Nasal mucosa pink, septum midline; no sinus tenderness. Throat (or Mouth)—Oral mucosa pink, dentition good, pharynx without exudates.

Neck—**Trachea midline. Neck supple; thyroid isthmus palpable, lobes not felt.**

Lymph Nodes—**No cervical, axillary, epitrochlear, inguinal adenopathy.**

OR

Head—**The skull is normocephalic/atraumatic. Frontal balding.**

Eyes—Visual acuity 20/100 bilaterally. Sclera white; conjunctiva injected. Pupils constrict 3 to 2 mm, equally round and reactive to light and accommodation. Disc margins sharp; no hemorrhages or exudates. Arteriolar-to-venous ratio (AV ratio) 2:4; no AV nicking. *Ears*—Acuity diminished to whispered voice; intact to spoken voice. TMs clear. *Nose*—Mucosa swollen with erythema and clear drainage. Septum midline. Tender over maxillary sinuses. *Throat*—Oral mucosa pink, dental caries in lower molars, pharynx erythematous, no exudates.

Neck—**Trachea midline. Neck supple; thyroid isthmus midline, lobes palpable but not enlarged.**

Lymph Nodes—**Submandibular and anterior cervical lymph nodes tender, 1 cm × 1 cm, rubbery and mobile; no posterior cervical, epitrochlear, axillary, or inguinal lymphadenopathy.**

HEALTH PROMOTION AND COUNSELING: EVIDENCE AND RECOMMENDATIONS

Important Topics for Health Promotion and Counseling

- Screening for thyroid dysfunction
- Screening for thyroid cancer
- Oral health

Screening for Thyroid Dysfunction

The U.S. Preventive Services Task Force (USPSTF) found evidence that treating subclinical hypothyroidism was associated with a decreased risk for coronary disease events. However, they concluded that evidence was insufficient to recommend for or against screening asymptomatic non-pregnant adults.

Screening for Thyroid Cancer

Although neck palpation and ultrasound could potentially be used as *thyroid cancer* screening tests, the USPSTF found inadequate evidence that screening was beneficial.

Oral Health

Be sure to promote *oral health:* 19% of children aged 2 to 19 years have untreated cavities, and about 5% of adults aged 40 to 59 years and 25% of those older than age 60 years have no teeth at all.

Inspect the oral cavity for decayed or loose teeth, inflammation of the gingiva, signs of periodontal disease (bleeding, pus, receding gums, and bad breath), and oral cancers. Counsel patients to use fluoride-containing toothpastes, brush, floss, and seek dental care at least annually.

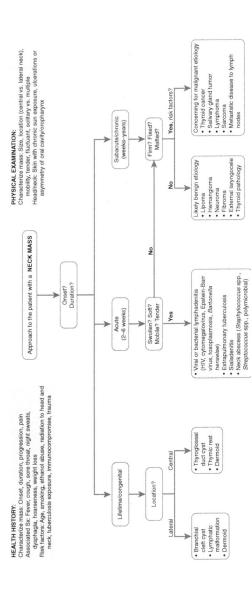

HEALTH HISTORY:
Characterize mass: Onset, duration, progression, pain
Associated Sx: Fever, cough, sore throat, night sweats,
  dysphagia, hoarseness, weight loss
Risk factors: Age, smoking, ethanol abuse, radiation to head and
  neck, tuberculosis exposure, immunocompromise, trauma

PHYSICAL EXAMINATION:
Characterize mass: Size, location (central vs. lateral neck),
  mobility, tender, fluctuant, solitary vs. multiple
Head/neck: Skin with chronic sun exposure, ulcerations or
  asymmetry of oral cavity/oropharynx

Approach to the patient with a **NECK MASS**

Onset? Duration?

Lifetime/congenital

Location?

Lateral
• Branchial cleft cyst
• Lymphatic malformation
• Dermoid

Central
• Thyroglossal duct cyst
• Thymic rest
• Dermoid

Acute (2–6 weeks)

Swollen? Soft? Mobile? Tender?

Yes
• Viral or bacterial lymphadenitis (HIV, cytomegalovirus, Epstein-Barr virus, toxoplasmosis, *Bartonella henselae*)
• Extrapulmonary tuberculosis
• Sialadenitis
• Neck abscess (*Staphylococcus* spp., *Streptococcus* spp., polymicrobial)

No

Subacute/chronic (weeks–years)

Firm? Fixed? Matted?

No
Likely benign etiology
• Lipoma
• Hemangioma
• Neuroma
• Fibroma
• External laryngocele
• Thyroid pathology

Yes, risk factors?

Concerning for malignant etiology
• Thyroid cancer
• Salivary gland tumor
• Lymphoma
• Sarcoma
• Metastatic disease to lymph nodes

Algorithm 11-1. Approach to the patient with a neck mass. (Note: Although it is not comprehensive, this algorithm may be a helpful starting approach.)

INTERPRETATION AIDS

TABLE 11-1. Abnormalities of the Thyroid Gland

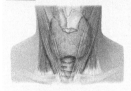

Diffuse enlargement. May result from Graves disease, Hashimoto thyroiditis, endemic goiter (iodine deficiency), or sporadic goiter

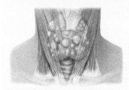

Multinodular goiter. An enlargement with two or more identifiable nodules, usually metabolic in cause

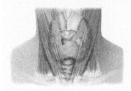

Single nodule. May result from a cyst, a benign tumor, or cancer of the thyroid, or may be one palpable nodule in a clinically unrecognized multinodular goiter

Eyes

HEALTH HISTORY

Common or Concerning Symptoms

- Change in vision: blurred vision, loss of vision, floaters, flashing lights
- Eye pain, redness, or tearing
- Double vision (diplopia)

Change in Vision

Ask "How is your vision?" If the patient reports a change in vision, pursue the related details:

Gradual blurring, often from refractive errors; also occurs in hyperglycemia.

- Is the problem worse during close work or at distances?

  Difficulty with close work suggests *hyperopia* (farsightedness) or *presbyopia* (aging vision); difficulty with distances suggests *myopia* (nearsightedness).

- Is the onset sudden or gradual?

  Sudden visual loss suggests retinal detachment, vitreous hemorrhage, or occlusion of the central retinal artery.

- Is there blurring of the entire field of vision or only parts? Is blurring central, peripheral, or only on one side?

  Slow central loss occurs in nuclear cataract and macular degeneration; peripheral loss in advanced open-angle glaucoma; one-sided loss in hemianopsia and quadrantic defects (p. 195).

- Has the patient seen lights flashing across the field of vision? Vitreous floaters?

  These symptoms suggest detachment of vitreous from the retina. Prompt eye consultation is indicated.

Eye Pain, Redness, or Tearing

Ask about pain in or around the eyes, redness, and excessive tearing or watering.

Eye pain in acute glaucoma and optic neuritis; see Algorithms 12-1, Approach to the patient with bilateral red eyes, p. 192, and 12-2, Approach to the patient with unilateral red eye, p. 193.

Double Vision (Diplopia)

Check for *diplopia*, or double vision.

Diplopia in brainstem or cerebellar lesions, also from weakness or paralysis of one or more extraocular muscles.

TECHNIQUES OF EXAMINATION

Key Components of the Ophthalmologic Examination

- Test visual acuity using a Snellen eye chart
- Test visual fields by confrontation
- Test color vision and contrast sensitivity
- Assess position and alignment of the eyes
- Inspect eyebrows
- Inspect eyelids and eyelashes
- Assess lacrimal apparatus
- Inspect conjunctivae and sclerae
- Inspect cornea, iris, and lens
- Inspect pupils
- Test for pupillary reaction to light
- Inspect light reflection in the corneas
- Test extraocular muscle movements
- Perform ophthalmoscopic (funduscopic) examination including optic disc and cup, retina, and retinal vessels

⊙ Visual Acuity

Test visual acuity in each eye with a Snellen wall chart or handheld card.

Vision of 20/200 means that at 20 ft, the patient can read print that a person with normal vision could read at 200 ft.

Visual Fields by Confrontation

Assess visual fields by confrontation with the *static finger wiggle test*, if indicated (Fig. 12-1).

See Table 12-1, Visual Field Defects, p. 195.

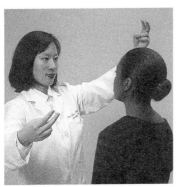

FIGURE 12-1. Testing visual fields using static finger wiggle technique.

Inspect the:

- Position and alignment of eyes

  Exophthalmos, strabismus

- Eyebrows

  Seborrheic dermatitis

- Eyelids

  Sty, chalazion, ectropion, ptosis, xanthelasma, blepharitis. See Table 12-2, Physical Findings in Eyelids, p. 196 and Algorithm 12-3, Approach to the patient with swollen eyelids, p. 194.

- Lacrimal apparatus

  Swollen lacrimal sac, excessive tearing

- Conjunctiva and sclera

  Red eye, conjunctivitis, jaundice, episcleritis

- Cornea, iris, and lens

  Cataract, crescentic shadow of acute angle glaucoma. See Table 12-3, Physical Findings in and around the Eye

Inspect pupils for:

- Size, shape, and symmetry

  Miosis, mydriasis, anisocoria

- Reactions to light, direct and consensual

  Absent in paralysis of CN III

- The *near reaction*, namely pupillary constriction with gaze shift to near object; note the accompanying convergence of the eyes and accommodation of the lens (becomes more convex) (Fig. 12-2)

Constriction slows in tonic (*Adie*) pupil and is absent in Argyll Robertson pupils of syphilis; poor convergence in hyperthyroidism

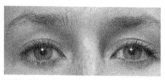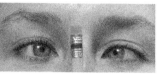

FIGURE 12-2. The pupils constrict when the focus shifts to a close object (*near reaction*).

Assess the extraocular muscles by observing:

- The symmetry of corneal reflections from a midline light

Asymmetric reflection if deviation in ocular alignment

- The six cardinal directions of gaze (Fig. 12-3)

Cranial nerve palsy, strabismus, nystagmus, lid lag of hyperthyroidism

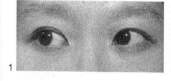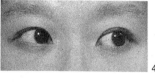
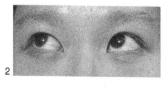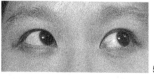
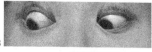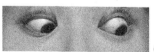

1   4
2   5
3   6

FIGURE 12-3. Test extraocular movements.

Inspect the fundi with an ophthalmoscope (Box 12-1).

BOX 12-1. Steps for Using the Ophthalmoscope

- Darken the room. Switch on the ophthalmoscope light and turn the lens disc until you see the large round beam of white light. Shine the light on the back of your hand to check the type of light, its desired brightness, and the electrical charge of the ophthalmoscope.

- Turn the focusing wheel to the 0 diopter. (A *diopter* is a unit that measures the power of a lens to converge or diverge light.) At this diopter, the lens neither converges nor diverges light. Keep your finger on the edge of the lens disc so that you can turn the focusing wheel to focus the lens when you examine the fundus.

- Hold the ophthalmoscope in your right hand and *use your right eye to examine the patient's right eye*; hold it in your left hand and *use your left eye to examine the patient's left eye*. This keeps you from bumping the patient's nose and gives you more mobility and closer range for visualizing the fundus. With practice, you will become accustomed to using your nondominant eye.

- Hold the ophthalmoscope firmly braced against the medial aspect of your bony orbit, with the handle tilted laterally at about 20° slant from the vertical. Check to make sure you can see clearly through the aperture. *Instruct the patient to look slightly up and over your shoulder at a point directly ahead on the wall.*

- Place yourself about 15 in away from the patient and at an angle *15° lateral to the patient's line of vision.* Shine the light beam on the pupil and look for the orange glow in the pupil—the *red reflex*. Note any opacities interrupting the red reflex. If you are nearsighted and have taken off your glasses, you may need to adjust the focusing wheel toward the minus/red diopters until the structures you see at a distance is in focus.

- Now *place the thumb of your other hand across the patient's eyebrow*, which steadies your examining hand. Keeping the light beam focused on the red reflex, move in with the ophthalmoscope on the 15° angle toward the pupil until you are very close to it, almost touching the patient's eyelashes and the thumb of your other hand.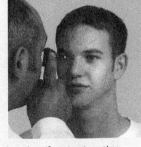

- Try to keep both eyes open and relaxed, as if gazing into the distance, to help minimize any fluctuating blurriness as your eyes attempt to accommodate.

Inspect the fundi for the following:

- Red reflex

  Cataracts, artificial eye

- Optic disc (Fig. 12-4 and Boxes 12-2 and 12-3)

  Papilledema, glaucomatous cupping, optic atrophy.

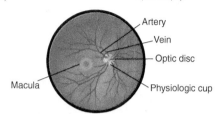

FIGURE 12-4. Optic disc.

BOX 12-2. Abnormalities of the Optic Disc

	Process	Appearance
Normal 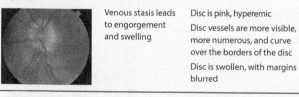	Tiny disc vessels give normal color to the disc	Disc is yellowish orange to creamy pink Disc vessels are tiny Disc margins are sharp (except perhaps nasally)
Papilledema	Venous stasis leads to engorgement and swelling	Disc is pink, hyperemic Disc vessels are more visible, more numerous, and curve over the borders of the disc Disc is swollen, with margins blurred
Glaucomatous Cupping 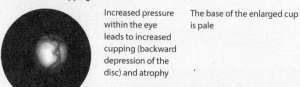	Increased pressure within the eye leads to increased cupping (backward depression of the disc) and atrophy	The base of the enlarged cup is pale

Optic Atrophy

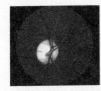

Death of optic nerve fibers leads to loss of the tiny disc vessels

Disc is white
Disc vessels are absent

- Arteries, veins, and AV crossings

  AV nicking, copper wiring in hypertensive changes

- Adjacent retina (note any lesions)

  Hemorrhages, exudates, cotton-wool patches, microaneurysms, pigmentation. See changes with diabetic retinopathy in Table 12-4, p. 198.

- Macular area

  Macular degeneration

- Anterior structures

  Vitreous floaters, cataracts

BOX 12-3. Tips for Examining the Optic Disc and Retina

- *Locate the optic disc.* Look for the round yellowish-orange structure.
- Now, *bring the optic disc into sharp focus.* If structures are blurred, rotate the focusing wheel until you find the sharpest focus.
- *Inspect the optic disc.* Note the following features:
  - *The sharpness or clarity of the disc outline*
  - *The color of the disc*
  - *The size of the central physiologic cup* (an enlarged cup suggests chronic open-angle glaucoma)
  - *Venous pulsations* in the retinal veins as they emerge from the central portion of the disc (loss of venous pulsations from elevated intracranial pressure may occur in head trauma, meningitis)
- *Inspect the retina.* Distinguish arteries from veins based on the features listed below.

	Arteries	Veins
Color	Light red	Dark red
Size	Smaller (2/3 to 3/4 the diameter of veins)	Larger
Light Reflex (reflection)	Bright	Inconspicuous or absent

continued

- *Follow the vessels peripherally in each of four directions.*
- Inspect the *fovea* and surrounding *macula.* Macular degeneration types include *dry atrophic* (more common but less severe) and *wet exudative* (neovascular). Undigested cellular debris, called drusen, may be hard or soft.
- Assess for any *papilledema* from increased intracranial pressure leading to swelling of the optic nerve head.

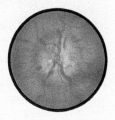

RECORDING YOUR FINDINGS

Initially you may use sentences to describe your findings; later you will use phrases. The style in the next box contains phrases appropriate for most write-ups.

Recording the Head, Eyes, Ears, Nose, and Throat (HEENT) Examination

Head—The skull is normocephalic/atraumatic. Frontal balding. *Eyes*—Visual acuity 20/100 bilaterally. Sclera white; conjunctiva injected. Pupils constrict from 3 to 2 mm, equally round and reactive to light and accommodation. Disc margins sharp; no hemorrhages or exudates. Arteriolar-to-venous ratio (AV ratio) 2:4; no AV nicking. *Ears*—Acuity diminished to whispered voice; intact to spoken voice. TMs clear. *Nose*—Mucosa swollen with erythema and clear drainage. Septum midline. Tender over maxillary sinuses. *Throat*—Oral mucosa pink, dental caries in lower molars, pharynx erythematous, no exudates.

Neck—Trachea midline. Neck supple; thyroid isthmus midline, lobes palpable but not enlarged.

Lymph Nodes—Submandibular and anterior cervical lymph nodes tender, 1 × 1 cm, rubbery and mobile; no posterior cervical, epitrochlear, axillary, or inguinal lymphadenopathy.

These findings suggest myopia and mild arteriolar narrowing as well as upper respiratory infection.

HEALTH PROMOTION AND COUNSELING: EVIDENCE AND RECOMMENDATIONS

Important Topics for Health Promotion and Counseling

- Visual impairment: cataracts, macular degeneration, diabetic retinopathy
- Screening for glaucoma

Visual Impairment

Visual impairment is defined as having corrected visual acuity of only 20/40 or worse in the better eye while corrected visual acuity of only 20/200 or worse in the better eye defines *legal blindness.* The major causes of visual impairment are *cataracts, age-related macular degeneration, glaucoma,* and *diabetic retinopathy.*

Although acknowledging that numerous treatments can improve visual acuity with only small risks of harm, in 2009, the U.S. Preventive Services Task Force (USPSTF) found insufficient evidence to recommend screening for impaired visual acuity in older adults, issuing an I statement.

Screening for Glaucoma

Primary open-angle glaucoma (POAG) is a leading cause of visual impairment and blindness in the United States overall. Glaucoma causes gradual vision loss, with damage to the optic nerve, loss of visual fields, beginning usually at the periphery.

In 2013, the USPSTF found insufficient evidence for general glaucoma screening by primary care physicians due to the complexities of diagnosis and treatment, issuing an I statement. However, the American Academy of Ophthalmology strongly recommends periodic glaucoma testing, with a baseline exam starting at the age of 40, but possibly earlier for at-risk patients.

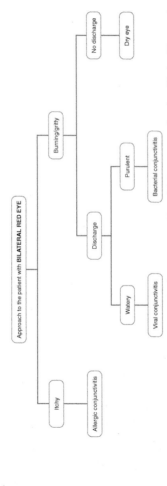

Algorithm 12-1. Approach to the patient with bilateral red eyes. (Note: Although it is not comprehensive, this algorithm may be a helpful starting approach.)

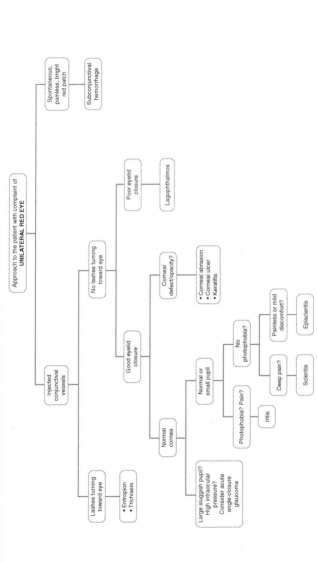

Algorithm 12-2. Approach to the patient with unilateral red eye. (Note: Although it is not comprehensive, this algorithm may be a helpful starting approach.)

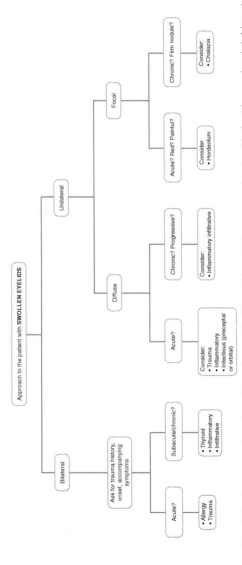

Algorithm 12-3. Approach to the patient with swollen eyelids. (Note: Although it is not comprehensive, this algorithm may be a helpful starting approach.)

INTERPRETATION AIDS

TABLE 12-1. Visual Field Defects

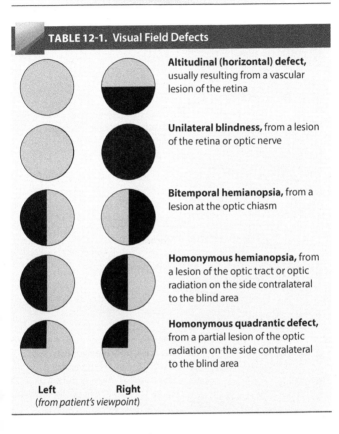

Altitudinal (horizontal) defect, usually resulting from a vascular lesion of the retina

Unilateral blindness, from a lesion of the retina or optic nerve

Bitemporal hemianopsia, from a lesion at the optic chiasm

Homonymous hemianopsia, from a lesion of the optic tract or optic radiation on the side contralateral to the blind area

Homonymous quadrantic defect, from a partial lesion of the optic radiation on the side contralateral to the blind area

Left　　　　**Right**
(from patient's viewpoint)

TABLE 12-2. Physical Findings in Eyelids

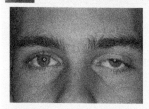

Ptosis. A drooping upper eyelid that narrows the palpebral fissure from a muscle or nerve disorder

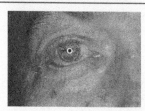

Ectropion. Outward turning of the margin of the lower lid, exposing the palpebral conjunctiva

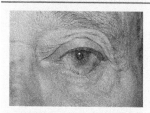

Entropion. Inward turning of the lid margin, causing irritation of the cornea or conjunctiva

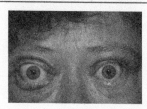

Lid retraction and exophthalmos. A wide-eyed stare suggests hyperthyroidism. Note the rim of sclera between the upper lid and the iris. Retracted lids and "lid lag" when eyes move from up to down markedly increase the likelihood of hyperthyroidism, especially when accompanied by fine tremor, moist skin, and heart rate >90 beats per minute. Exophthalmos describes protrusion of the eyeball, a common feature of Graves ophthalmopathy, triggered by autoreactive T lymphocytes

Source of photos: Ptosis, Ectropion, Entropion—Tasman W, et al., eds. *The Wills Eye Hospital Atlas of Clinical Ophthalmology.* 2nd ed. Lippincott Williams & Wilkins; 2001.

TABLE 12-3. Physical Findings in and around the Eye

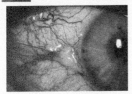

Pinguecula. Harmless yellowish nodule in the bulbar conjunctiva on either side of the iris; associated with aging

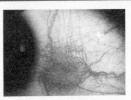

Episcleritis. A localized ocular redness from inflammation of the episcleral vessels. Seen in rheumatoid arthritis, Sjögren syndrome, and herpes zoster

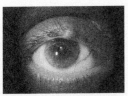

Sty. A pimple-like infection around a hair follicle near the lid margin, usually from *Staphylococcus aureus*

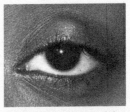

Chalazion. A beady nodule in either eyelid caused by a chronically inflamed meibomian gland

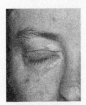

Xanthelasma. Yellowish plaque seen in lipid disorders. Half of affected patients have *hyperlipidemia;* also common in *primary biliary cirrhosis*

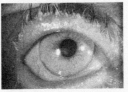

Blepharitis. Chronic inflammation of the eyelids at the base of the hair follicles, often from *S. aureus.* A scaling seborrheic variant also exists.

Source of photos: Pinguecula—Shields JA, Shields CL, eds. *Eyelid, Conjunctival, and Orbital Tumors: An Atlas and Textbook*. 3rd ed. Wolters Kluwer; 2016. Figure 24-67. Episcleritis, Sty, Xanthelasma, Blepharitis—Tasman W, et al., eds. *The Wills Eye Hospital Atlas of Clinical Ophthalmology*. 2nd ed. Lippincott Williams & Wilkins; 2001. Chalazion—Bagheri N, Wajda BN. *The Wills Eye Manual: Office and Emergency Room Diagnosis and Treatment of Eye Disease*. 7th ed. Wolters Kluwer; 2017. Figure 6-2.

TABLE 12-4. Ocular Fundi: Diabetic Retinopathy

Nonproliferative Retinopathy, Moderately Severe

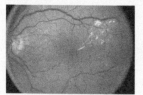

Note tiny red dots or microaneurysms, also the ring of hard exudates (white spots) located superotemporally. Retinal thickening or edema in the area of hard exudates can impair visual acuity if it extends to center of macula. Detection requires specialized stereoscopic examination.

Nonproliferative Retinopathy, Severe

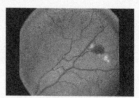

In superior temporal quadrant, note large retinal hemorrhage between two cotton-wool patches, beading of the retinal vein just above, and tiny tortuous retinal vessels above the superior temporal artery, termed *intraretinal microvascular abnormalities.*

Proliferative Retinopathy, with Neovascularization

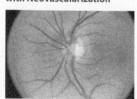

Note new preretinal vessels arising on disc and extending across disc margins. Visual acuity is still normal, but the risk of severe visual loss is high. Photocoagulation can reduce this risk by >50%.

Proliferative Retinopathy, Advanced

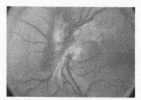

Same eye as above, but 2 years later and without treatment. Neovascularization has increased, now with fibrous proliferations, distortion of the macula, and reduced visual acuity.

Source of photos: Nonproliferative Retinopathy, Moderately Severe; Proliferative Retinopathy, With Neovascularization; Nonproliferative Retinopathy, Severe; Proliferative Retinopathy, Advanced—Early Treatment Diabetic Retinopathy Study Research Group. Courtesy of MF Davis, MD, University of Wisconsin, Madison. Source: Frank RB. Diabetic retinopathy. *N Engl J Med.* 2004;350(1):48–58.

Ears and Nose

HEALTH HISTORY

Common or Concerning Symptoms

- Hearing loss
- Earache and ear discharge
- Ringing in the ears (*tinnitus*)
- Dizziness and vertigo
- Nasal discharge (*rhinorrhea*) and nasal congestion
- Nosebleed (epistaxis)

Ears

Ask "How is your hearing?" Does the patient have special difficulty understanding people as they talk? Does a noisy environment make a difference?

Sensorineural loss (inner ear) leads to difficulty understanding speech, with complaints that others mumble; noisy environments worsen hearing. In *conductive loss* (external or middle ear), noisy environments may help.

For complaints of *earache*, or *pain in the ear*, ask about associated fever, sore throat, cough, and concurrent upper respiratory infection.

Consider otitis externa if pain in the ear canal; *otitis media* if pain associated with respiratory infection.

Tinnitus is an internal musical ringing or rushing or roaring noise, often unexplained.

When associated with hearing loss and vertigo, tinnitus suggests Ménière disease.

Ask about dizziness which may be:

- Perception that the patient or the environment is rotating or spinning (*vertigo*) often accompanied by nystagmus and ataxia (Box 13-1)

Vertigo in labrynthitis (inner ear), CN VII lesions, brainstem lesions; see Algorithm 13-1, Approach to the patient with dizziness, p. 207.

BOX 13-1. Peripheral and Central Vertigo

	Onset	Duration and Course	Hearing	Tinnitus	Additional Features
Peripheral vertigo					
Benign positional vertigo	Sudden, often when rolling onto the affected side or tilting up the head	Lasts a few weeks, may recur	Not affected	Absent	Sometimes nausea, vomiting, nystagmus
Vestibular neuronitis	Sudden	May recur over 12–18 months	Not affected	Absent	Nausea, vomiting, nystagmus
Acute labyrinthitis	Sudden	May recur over 12–18 months	Sensorineural hearing loss—unilateral	May be present	Nausea, vomiting, nystagmus
Ménière disease	Sudden	Recurrent	Sensorineural hearing loss—fluctuating, recurs, eventually progresses	Present, fluctuating	Pressure or fullness in affected ear, nausea, vomiting, nystagmus
Drug toxicity	Insidious or acute—linked to loop diuretics, aminoglycosides, salicylates, alcohol	May or may not be reversible Partial adaptation occurs	May be impaired	May be present	Nausea, vomiting
Acoustic neuroma	Insidious from CN VIII compression, vestibular branch	Variable	Impaired, one side	Present	May involve CN V and VII
Central vertigo	Often sudden (see causes above)	Variable but rarely continuous	Not affected	Absent	Usually with other brainstem deficits—dysarthria, ataxia, crossed motor and sensory deficits

- Feeling faint or light-headed (*pre-syncope*)

Causes include orthostatic hypotension, especially from medication, arrhythmias, and vasovagal attacks (~5%).

- Unsteadiness or imbalance when walking (dysequilibrium) especially in older patients

Causes include fear of falling, visual loss, weakness from musculoskeletal problems, and peripheral neuropathy (up to 15%).

Psychiatric causes include anxiety, panic disorder, hyperventilation, depression, somatization disorder, alcohol, and substance abuse (~10%).

Nose and Sinuses

Rhinorrhea, or drainage from the nose, frequently accompanies nasal congestion. Ask further about *sneezing*, watery eyes, throat discomfort, and *itching* in the eyes, nose, and throat (Algorithm 13-2).

Causes include viral infections, allergic rhinitis ("hay fever"), and vasomotor rhinitis. Itching favors an allergic cause; see Algorithm 13-2, Approach to the patient with rhinitis, p. 208.

For *epistaxis*, or bleeding from the nose, identify the source carefully. Is the bleeding actually from the nose, or has the patient coughed up or vomited blood? Assess the site of bleeding, its severity, and associated symptoms.

Local causes of epistaxis include trauma (especially nose-picking), inflammation, drying and crusting of the nasal mucosa, tumors, and foreign bodies. Anticoagulants, NSAIDs, and coagulopathies may contribute.

TECHNIQUES OF EXAMINATION

Key Components of the Ear Examination

- Inspect auricle and surrounding tissue (deformities, lumps, pits, or skin lesions)
- Palpate auricle, tragus, and mastoid (tenderness)
- Examine ear canals and tympanic membranes with an otoscope
- Test auditory acuity or gross hearing with whispered voice test
- If hearing loss or difficulty is present, determine sensorineural versus conductive hearing loss with tuning fork tests

ᖾ Ears

Examine on each side:

Auricle. Inspect the auricle.

Keloid, epidermoid cyst

If you suspect otitis:

- Move the auricle up and down and press on the tragus.

  Pain in otitis externa ("tug test")

- Press firmly behind the ear.

  Possible tenderness in otitis media and mastoiditis

Ear Canal and Tympanic Membrane. Pull the auricle up, back, and slightly out. Inspect, through an otoscope with speculum:

- Ear canal

  Cerumen; swelling and erythema in otitis externa

- Eardrum/tympanic membrane (Fig. 13-1)

  Red bulging drum in acute otitis media; serous otitis media, tympanosclerosis, perforations. See Table 13-1, Abnormalities of the Tympanic Membrane, p. 210.

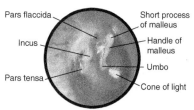

Pars flaccida

Incus

Pars tensa

Short process of malleus

Handle of malleus

Umbo

Cone of light

FIGURE 13-1. Right tympanic membrane.

Hearing. "Do you feel you have a hearing loss or difficulty hearing?" is a sensitive screening question. Assess auditory acuity to spoken or whispered voice or with a handheld audiometer (Box 13-2). The whispered voice test detects significant hearing loss of greater than 30 decibels. A formal hearing test is still the reference standard.

BOX 13-2. Whispered Voice Test for Auditory Acuity

- Inform the patient that you will be whispering a combination of numbers and letters and then asking him/her to repeat the sequence.
- Then stand at arm's length (2 ft) behind the seated patient so that the patient cannot read your lips.
- Each ear is tested individually. Occlude the nontest ear with a finger and gently rub the tragus in a circular motion to prevent transfer of sound to the nontest ear.
- Exhale a full breath before whispering to ensure a quiet voice.
- Whisper a combination of three words of numbers and letters, such as 4-K-2 or 5-B-6.
- If the patient responds correctly, then hearing is considered normal for that ear.
- If the patient responds incorrectly or not at all, the test is repeated once more using a different three numeral/letter combination. It is important to use a different combination each time to exclude the effect of learning.
- If the patient repeats at least three out of a possible total of six letters or numerals correctly, then they have passed the screening test.
- If the patient repeats less than three words correctly then conduct further testing by audiometry.
- Using a different number/letter combination, the other ear is then tested in a similar manner.

If hearing is diminished, use a 512-Hz tuning fork to:

- Test *lateralization* (Weber test), but only in patients with unilateral hearing loss. Place vibrating and tuning fork on vertex of skull and check hearing. See Algorithm 13-3.

  In unilateral *conductive hearing loss*, sound is heard in (lateralized to) the impaired ear; see Algorithm 13-3, Approach to the patient with hearing loss, p. 209.

- Compare *air and bone conduction* (Rinne test). Place vibrating and tuning fork on mastoid bone, then remove and check hearing.

  In *conductive hearing loss*, sound is heard through bone longer than through air (BC = AC or BC > AC). In *sensorineural hearing loss*, sound is heard longer through air (AC > BC). See Box 13-3.

BOX 13-3. Patterns of Hearing Loss

	Conductive Loss	Sensorineural Loss
Impaired Understanding of Words	Minor	Often troublesome
Effects	Noisy environment may improve hearing	Noisy environment worsens hearing
	Voice remains soft since cochlear nerve intact	Voice may be loud due to nerve damage
Usual Age of Onset	Childhood, young adulthood	Middle and later years
Ear Canal and Drum	Often a visible abnormality	Problem not visible
Weber Test (in Unilateral Hearing Loss)	Lateralizes to the impaired ear	Lateralizes to the good ear
Rinne Test	BC ≥ AC	AC > BC
Causes	Plugged ear canal, *otitis media,* immobile or perforated drum, otosclerosis, foreign body	Sustained loud noise, drugs, inner ear infections, trauma, hereditary disorder, aging, acoustic neuroma

Key Components of the Nose and Paranasal Sinus Examination

- Inspect anterior and inferior surfaces of the nose
- Test for nasal obstruction on each ala nasi (if indicated)
- Inspect nasal mucosa, nasal septum, inferior and middle turbinates, and corresponding meatuses with a light source or otoscope with large speculum
- Palpate frontal sinuses
- Palpate maxillary sinuses

☌ Nose and Sinuses

Inspect and palpate:

- External nose

Tenderness of the nasal tip or ala suggests local infection such as a furuncle, particularly if there is a small erythematous and swollen area.

Inspect, through a speculum, the:

- Nasal mucosa that covers the septum and turbinates, noting its color and any swelling

Swollen and red in viral rhinitis, swollen and pale in allergic rhinitis; polyps (Fig. 13-2); ulcer from cocaine use

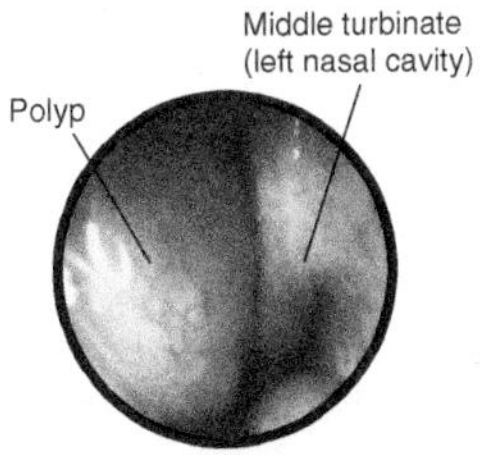

FIGURE 13-2. Nasal polyp.

- Nasal septum for position and integrity

Deviation, perforation

- Palpate the frontal and maxillary sinuses

Tender in acute sinusitis

RECORDING YOUR FINDINGS

Initially you may use sentences to describe your findings; later you will use phrases. The style in the next box contains phrases appropriate for most write-ups.

Recording the Head, Eyes, Ears, Nose, and Throat (HEENT) Examination

Head—The skull is normocephalic/atraumatic. Frontal balding.
Eyes—Visual acuity 20/100 bilaterally. Sclera white; conjunctiva injected. Pupils constrict from 3 to 2 mm, equally round and reactive to light and accommodation. Disc margins sharp; no hemorrhages or exudates. Arteriolar-to-venous ratio (AV ratio) 2:4; no AV nicking.

continued

Ears—**Acuity diminished to whispered voice; intact to spoken voice. TMs clear.** *Nose*—**Mucosa swollen with erythema and clear drainage. Septum midline. Tender over maxillary sinuses.** *Throat*—Oral mucosa pink, dental caries in lower molars, pharynx erythematous, no exudates.

Neck—Trachea midline. Neck supple; thyroid isthmus midline, lobes palpable but not enlarged.

Lymph Nodes—Submandibular and anterior cervical lymph nodes tender, 1 × 1 cm, rubbery and mobile; no posterior cervical, epitrochlear, axillary, or inguinal lymphadenopathy.

These findings suggest myopia and mild arteriolar narrowing as well as upper respiratory infection.

HEALTH PROMOTION AND COUNSELING: EVIDENCE AND RECOMMENDATIONS

Important Topics for Health Promotion and Counseling

- Hearing loss

Hearing Loss

Hearing loss is frequently considered the inability to hear tones at frequencies between 500 Hz and 4,000 Hz, the most important for speech processing. More than a third of adults older than 65 years have *detectable hearing deficits*. Questionnaires and handheld audioscopes work well for periodic screening.

The U.S. Preventive Services Task Force (USPSTF) pointed out that the effectiveness of any hearing screening strategy will depend on how likely those who might benefit from hearing aids are to actually use them. Consequently, it concluded that evidence was insufficient to make a determination about screening adults 50 years of age and older for hearing loss (I statement). However, noise reduction and avoidance are recommended strategies for preventing or delaying hearing loss.

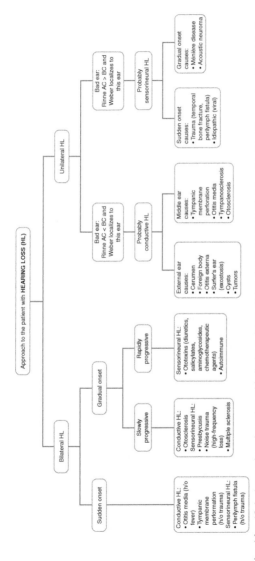

Algorithm 13-1. Approach to the patient with dizziness. (Note: Although it is not comprehensive, this algorithm may be a helpful starting approach.)

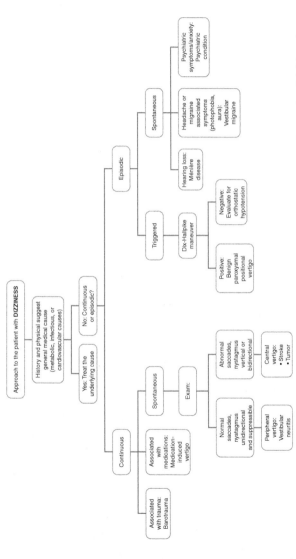

Algorithm 13-2. Approach to the patient with rhinitis. (Note: Although it is not comprehensive, this algorithm may be a helpful starting approach.)

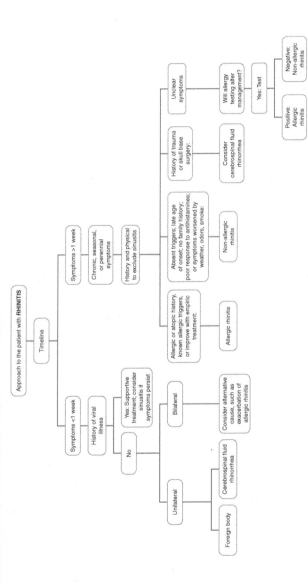

Algorithm 13-3. Approach to the patient with hearing loss. (Note: Although it is not comprehensive, this algorithm may be a helpful starting approach.)

INTERPRETATION AIDS

TABLE 13-1. Abnormalities of the Tympanic Membrane

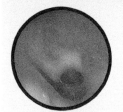

Perforation

Hole in the eardrum that may be central or marginal

Usually from *otitis media* or trauma

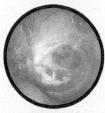

Tympanosclerosis

A chalky white patch

Scarring process of the middle ear from otitis media with deposition of hyaline and calcium and phosphate crystals in the eardrum and middle ear. When severe, it may entrap the ossicles and cause conductive hearing loss

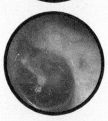

Serous Effusion

Amber fluid behind the eardrum, with or without air bubbles

Associated with viral upper respiratory infections or sudden changes in atmospheric pressure (diving, flying)

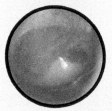

Acute Otitis Media with Purulent Effusion

Red, bulging drum, loss of landmarks

Painful hemorrhagic vesicles appear on the tympanic membrane and/or ear canal causing earache, blood-tinged discharge from the ear, and conductive hearing loss. Seen in mycoplasma and viral infections and bacterial otitis media

Sources of photos: Perforation—Courtesy of Michael Hawke, MD, Toronto, Canada. Serous Effusion—Reprinted from Hawke M, Keene M, Alberti PW. *Clinical Otoscopy: A Text and Colour Atlas*. Churchill Livingstone; 1984. Copyright © 1984 Elsevier. With permission. Acute Otitis Media—Johnson JT. *Bailey's Head and Neck Surgery*. 5th ed. Wolters Kluwer; 2014. Figure 99-1.

Throat and Oral Cavity

HEALTH HISTORY

Common or Concerning Symptoms

- Sore throat
- Gum swelling/bleeding gums
- Hoarseness
- Malodorous breath (*halitosis*)

Sore Throat

Sore throat or pharyngitis is a frequent complaint. Ask about fever, swollen glands, and any associated cough.

Fever, pharyngeal exudates, and anterior cervical lymphadenopathy, especially without cough, suggest streptococcal pharyngitis, or "*strep throat*" (p. 473).

Gum Bleeding

Gum bleeding, especially when brushing teeth, is a common symptom. Ask about local lesions and any tendency to bleed or bruise elsewhere.

Bleeding gums are usually caused by gingivitis.

Hoarseness

Hoarseness may arise from overuse of the voice, allergies, smoking, or inhaled irritants.

If present more than 2 weeks, refer for laryngoscopy; consider hypothyroidism, reflux, vocal cord nodules, head and neck cancers, thyroid masses, and neurologic disorders (Parkinson disease, amyotrophic lateral sclerosis, or myasthenia gravis). See Algorithm 14-1, Approach to the patient with hoarseness, p. 215.

Malodorous Breath

Malodorous breath (*halitosis*) is an unpleasant or offensive odor emanating from the breath.

Common oral causes of breath malodor include poor oral hygiene, tobacco smoking, plaque retention on teeth, and mouth appliances. Causes of breath malodor may also be systemic.

TECHNIQUES OF EXAMINATION

Key Components of the Mouth and Pharynx Examination

- Inspect lips
- Inspect oral mucosa
- Palpate oral mucosa (if indicated)
- Inspect gingiva
- Inspect gum margins and interdental papillae
- Inspect teeth
- Inspect roof (hard palate) and floor of the mouth
- Test hypoglossal nerve, or CN XII (symmetry of tongue protrusion)
- Inspect tongue
- Palpate tongue (if indicated)
- Inspect soft palate, anterior and posterior pillars, uvula, tonsils, and pharynx
- Test vagus nerve, or CN X (symmetry of uvula)

⚕ Mouth

Inspect the:

- Lips

  Cyanosis, pallor, cheilosis; see Table 14-1, Abnormalities of the Lips, pp. 216–217

- Oral mucosa

  Aphthous ulcers (canker sores)

- Gums

  Gingivitis, periodontal disease

- Teeth

  Dental caries, tooth loss

- Roof of the mouth

  Torus palatinus (benign)

- Tongue, including:

  - Papillae

    Glossitis

  - Symmetry

    Deviation to one side from paralysis of CN XII from CVA

TECHNIQUES OF EXAMINATION	POSSIBLE FINDINGS

■ Any lesions

Erythroplakia, leukoplakia (precancerous); squamous cell or other carcinomas; see Table 14-2, Abnormalities of the Tongue, pp. 218–219

■ Floor of the mouth

Lesions suspicious for cancer

Pharynx

Inspect for:

■ Color or any exudate

Pharyngitis

■ Presence and size of tonsils

Exudates, tonsillitis, peritonsillar abscess

■ Symmetry of the soft palate as patient says "ah"

Soft palate fails to rise, uvula deviates to opposite side in CN X paralysis from CVA. See Table 14-3, Abnormalities of the Pharynx, p. 220.

RECORDING YOUR FINDINGS

Recording the Head, Eyes, Ears, Nose, and Throat (HEENT) Examination

Head—The skull is normocephalic/atraumatic. Frontal balding. *Eyes*—Visual acuity 20/100 bilaterally. Sclera white; conjunctiva injected. Pupils constrict from 3 to 2 mm, equally round and reactive to light and accommodation. Disc margins sharp; no hemorrhages or exudates. Arteriolar-to-venous ratio (AV ratio) 2:4; no AV nicking. *Ears*—Acuity diminished to whispered voice; intact to spoken voice. TMs clear. *Nose*—Mucosa swollen with erythema and clear drainage. Septum midline. Tender over maxillary sinuses. **Throat— Oral mucosa pink, dental caries in lower molars, pharynx erythematous, no exudates.**
Neck—Trachea midline. Neck supple; thyroid isthmus midline, lobes palpable but not enlarged.
Lymph Nodes—Submandibular and anterior cervical lymph nodes tender, 1×1 cm, rubbery and mobile; no posterior cervical, epitrochlear, axillary, or inguinal lymphadenopathy.

These findings suggest a possible upper respiratory infection.

HEALTH PROMOTION AND COUNSELING: EVIDENCE AND RECOMMENDATIONS

Important Topics for Health Promotion and Counseling

- Oral health
- Oral and pharyngeal cancer

Oral Health

Be sure to promote oral health: 19% of children age 2 to 19 years have untreated cavities, and about 5% of adults age 40 to 59 years and 25% of those older than age 60 years have no teeth at all. Inspect the oral cavity for decayed or loose teeth, inflammation of the gingiva, signs of periodontal disease (bleeding, pus, receding gums, and bad breath), and oral cancers. Counsel patients to use fluoride-containing toothpastes, brush, floss, and seek dental care at least annually.

Oral and Pharyngeal Cancer

Tobacco and alcohol account for about 75% of oral cavity cancers. Human papillomavirus (HPV) infection is an increasingly important cause of oropharyngeal cancers (lesions of the tonsils, oropharynx, and base of tongue), accounting for about 70% of cases.

The primary screening test for these cancers is a thorough examination of the oral cavity. Although the U.S. Preventive Services Task Force concluded in 2014 that evidence was insufficient to recommend routinely screening asymptomatic adults for oral cancer (I statement), the American Dental Association (ADA) does recommend that patients with a suspicious oral mucosal lesion be promptly referred to a specialist for biopsy evaluation.

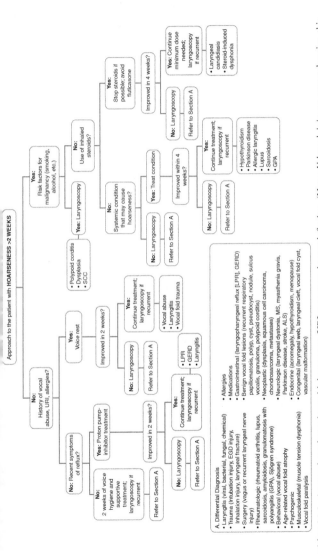

Approach to the patient with HOARSENESS >2 WEEKS

No: History of vocal abuse, URI, allergies?

No: Recent symptoms of reflux?

No: 2 weeks of voice hygiene and supportive treatment; laryngoscopy if recurrent

Yes: Proton pump-inhibitor treatment

Improved in 2 weeks?

No: Laryngoscopy
Refer to Section A

Yes: Continue treatment; laryngoscopy if recurrent
• LPR
• GERD
• Laryngitis

Yes: Voice rest

Improved in 2 weeks?

No: Laryngoscopy
Refer to Section A

Yes: Continue treatment; laryngoscopy if recurrent
• Vocal abuse
• Laryngitis
• Vocal fold trauma

Yes: Risk factors for malignancy (smoking, alcohol, etc.)

Yes: Laryngoscopy
• Polypoid corditis
• Dysplasia
• SCC

No: Systemic condition that may cause hoarseness?

Yes: Treat condition

Improved within 4 weeks?

No: Laryngoscopy
Refer to Section A

Yes: Continue treatment; laryngoscopy if recurrent
• Hypothyroidism
• Parkinson disease
• Allergic laryngitis
• Lupus
• Sarcoidosis
• GPA

Yes: Use of inhaled steroids?

Stop steroids if possible; avoid fluticasone

Improved in 4 weeks?

No: Laryngoscopy
Refer to Section A

Yes: Continue minimum dose needed; laryngoscopy if recurrent
• Laryngeal candidiasis
• Steroid-induced dysphonia

A. Differential Diagnosis
• Laryngitis (viral, bacterial, fungal, chemical)
• Trauma (intubation injury, EGD injury, Inhalation injury, laryngeal fracture)
• Surgery (vagus or recurrent laryngeal nerve injury)
• Rheumatologic (rheumatoid arthritis, lupus, sarcoidosis, amyloidosis, granulomatosis with polyangiitis (GPA), Sjögren syndrome)
• Behavioral (vocal abuse)
• Age-related vocal fold atrophy
• Psychogenic
• Musculoskeletal (muscle tension dysphonia)
• Vocal fold paralysis
• Allergies
• Medications
• Gastrointestinal (laryngopharyngeal reflux [LPR], GERD)
• Benign vocal fold lesions (recurrent respiratory papillomatosis, polyp, cyst, pseudocyst, nodule, sulcus vocalis, granuloma, polypoid corditis)
• Neoplastic (dysplasia, squamous cell carcinoma, chondrosarcoma, metastases)
• Neurologic (laryngeal dystonia, MS, myasthenia gravis, Parkinson disease, stroke, ALS)
• Endocrine (acromegaly, hypothyroidism, menopause)
• Congenital (laryngeal web, laryngeal cleft, vocal fold cyst, vascular malformation)

Algorithm 14-1. Approach to the patient with hoarseness. URI, upper respiratory infection. (Note: Although it is not comprehensive, this algorithm may be a helpful starting approach.)

INTERPRETATION AIDS

TABLE 14-1. Abnormalities of the Lips

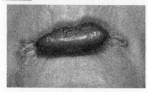

Angular cheilitis. Softening and cracking of the angles of the mouth

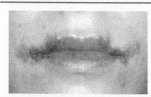

Herpes simplex. Painful vesicles, followed by crusting; also called *cold sore* or *fever blister*

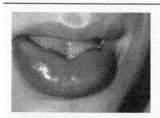

Angioedema. Diffuse, tense, subcutaneous swelling, usually allergic in cause

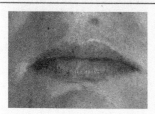

Hereditary hemorrhagic telangiectasia. Small red spots. Autosomal dominant disorder causing vascular fragility and arteriovascular malformations (AVMs), including in the brain and lungs. Associated bleeding in nose and GI tract

TABLE 14-1. Abnormalities of the Lips (continued)

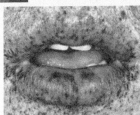

Peutz–Jeghers syndrome. Brown spots of the lips and buccal mucosa, significant because of associated intestinal polyposis and high risk of GI cancer

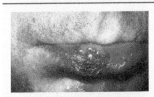

Syphilitic chancre. A firm lesion that ulcerates and may crust

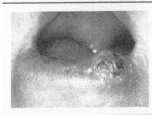

Carcinoma of the lip. A thickened plaque or irregular nodule that may ulcerate or crust; malignant

Sources of photos: Angular Cheilitis, Herpes Simplex, Angioedema—Neville B, et al. *Color Atlas of Clinical Oral Pathology.* Philadelphia: Lea & Febiger, 1991. Hereditary Hemorrhagic Telangiectasia—Mansoor AM. *Frameworks for Internal Medicine.* Wolters Kluwer; 2019. Figure 40-2. Peutz-Jeghers Syndrome—Robinson HBG, et al. *Colby, Kerr, and Robinson's Color Atlas of Oral Pathology.* 5th ed. JB Lippincott; 1990. Chancre of Syphilis—Reprinted from Wisdom A. *A Colour Atlas of Sexually Transmitted Diseases.* 2nd ed. Wolfe Medical Publications; 1989. Copyright © 1989 Elsevier. With permission. Carcinoma of the Lip—Reprinted from Tyldesley WR. *A Colour Atlas of Orofacial Diseases.* 2nd ed. Wolfe Medical Publications; 1991. Copyright © 1991 Elsevier. With permission.

TABLE 14-2. Abnormalities of the Tongue

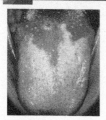

Geographic tongue. Scattered areas in which the papillae are lost, giving a map-like appearance; benign

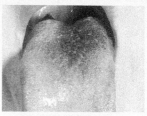

Hairy tongue. Results from elongated papillae that may look yellowish, brown, or black; benign

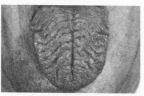

Fissured tongue. May appear with aging; benign

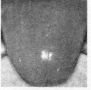

Smooth tongue. Results from loss of papillae; seen in deficiency of riboflavin, niacin, folic acid, vitamin B12, pyridoxine, or iron, and treatment with chemotherapy

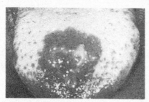

Candidiasis. May show a thick, white coat, which, when scraped off, leaves a raw red surface; tongue may also be red; antibiotics, corticosteroids, AIDS may predispose

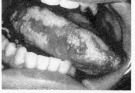

Hairy leukoplakia. White raised, feathery areas, usually on sides of tongue. Seen in HIV/AIDS

TABLE 14-2. Abnormalities of the Tongue *(continued)*

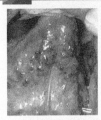

Varicose veins. Dark round spots in the undersurface of the tongue, associated with aging; also called *caviar lesions*

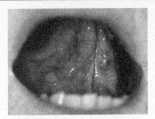

Aphthous ulcer (canker sore). Painful, small, whitish ulcer with a red halo; heals in 7–10 days

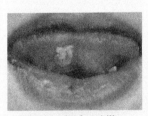

Mucous patch of syphilis. Slightly raised, oval lesion, covered by a grayish membrane

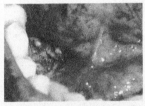

Carcinoma of the tongue or floor of the mouth. Malignancy should be considered in any nodule or nonhealing ulcer at the base or edges of the mouth

Sources of photos: Fissured Tongue, Candidiasis, Mucous Patch, Leukoplakia, Carcinoma—Robinson HBG, et al. *Colby, Kerr, and Robinson's Color Atlas of Oral Pathology.* 5th ed. JB Lippincott; 1990. Smooth Tongue—Jensen S. *Nursing Health Assessment: A Best Practice Approach.* 3rd ed. Wolters Kluwer; 2019. Figure 15-25. Geographic Tongue—From the Centers for Disease Control Public Health Image Library; ID #16520. Hairy Leukoplakia—From the Centers for Disease Control Public Health Image Library, photo credit Sol Silverman, Jr., DDS; ID #6061. Varicose Veins—Neville B, et al. *Color Atlas of Clinical Oral Pathology.* Lea & Febiger, 1991.

TABLE 14-3. Abnormalities of the Pharynx

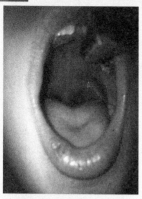

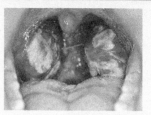

Exudative tonsillitis. A sore red throat with patches of white exudate on the tonsils is associated with streptococcal pharyngitis and some viral illnesses

Pharyngitis, mild to moderate. Note redness and vascularity of the pillars and uvula

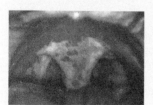

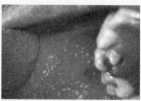

Diphtheria. An acute infection caused by *Corynebacterium diphtheriae*. The throat is dull red, and a gray exudate appears on the uvula, pharynx, and tongue

Koplik spots. These small white specks that resemble grains of salt on a red background are an early sign of measles

Thorax and Lungs

HEALTH HISTORY

Common or Concerning Symptoms

- Shortness of breath (dyspnea)
- Wheezing
- Cough and hemoptysis
- Daytime sleepiness, snoring, and disordered sleep
- Chest pain (also see Chapter 16, Cardiovascular System)

Shortness of Breath (Dyspnea)

Shortness of breath, or *dyspnea,* is a painless but uncomfortable awareness of breathing that is inappropriate to the level of exertion. For patients who are short of breath, focus on possible pulmonary or cardiovascular complaints.

Because of variations in age, body weight, and physical fitness, there is no absolute scale for quantifying shortness of breath. Instead, make every effort to determine its severity based on the patient's daily activities.

See Table 15-1, Dyspnea, pp. 234–235 and Algorithm 15-1, Approach to the patient with dyspnea, p. 231.

Wheezing

Wheezes are musical respiratory sounds that may be audible to the patient and to others.

Occurs in partial lower airway obstruction from secretions and tissue inflammation in asthma, or a foreign body

Cough and Hemoptysis

For complaints of cough, pursue a thorough assessment. Duration: *acute* (<3 weeks), *subacute* (3 to 8 weeks), or *chronic* (>8 weeks)? Dry or productive of sputum? With blood streaks

See Table 15-2, Cough and Hemoptysis, pp. 236–238, Algorithm 15-2, Approach to the patient with cough, p. 232, and Algorithm 15-3, Approach to the patient with hemoptysis, p. 233.

or frank blood coughed up, known as
hemoptysis?

Daytime Sleepiness, Snoring, and Disordered Sleep

Patients may report excessive daytime sleepiness and fatigue. Ask the
patient or bed partner about problems with snoring.

Snoring, witnessed apneas ≥10 seconds,
awakening with a choking sensation, or
morning headache point to obstructive
sleep apnea.

Chest Pain

Complaints of *chest pain* or *chest discomfort* raise concerns about the heart
but often arise from conditions in the
thorax and lungs. For this important
symptom, keep in mind the possible
causes shown in Box 15-1.

Also see Table 16-1, Chest Pain,
pp. 262–263 in Chapter 16, Cardiovascular System.

BOX 15-1. Sources of Chest Pain and Related Causes	
Source	**Possible Causes**
Myocardium	Angina pectoris, myocardial infarction, myocarditis
Pericardium	Pericarditis
Aorta	Aortic dissection
Trachea and large bronchi	Bronchitis
Parietal pleura	Pericarditis, pneumonia, pneumothorax, pleural effusion, pulmonary embolus, connective tissue disease
The chest wall, including the skin, musculoskeletal and neurologic systems	Costochondritis, herpes zoster
Esophagus	Gastroesophageal reflux disease, esophageal spasm, esophageal tear
Extrathoracic structures such as the neck, gallbladder, and stomach	Cervical arthritis, biliary colic, gastritis

For further discussion of exertional chest pain possibly related to cardiovascular causes, see
Chapter 16, Cardiovascular System (see pp. 262–263).

TECHNIQUES OF EXAMINATION

Key Components of the Thorax and Lung Examination

- Survey respiration (rate, rhythm, depth, effort of breathing)
- Examine the anterior and posterior chest:
  - Inspect chest
  - Palpate chest
  - Percuss chest
  - Auscultate chest

Thorax

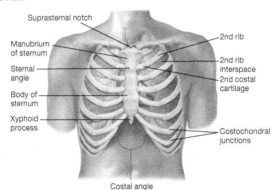

FIGURE 15-1. Chest wall anatomy.

Inspect the thorax (Fig. 15-1) and its respiratory movements.

Theoretical vertical lines used to describe anatomical locations on the chest are shown in Figs. 15-2 and 15-3.

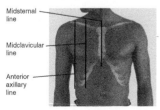

FIGURE 15-2. Midsternal and midclavicular lines.

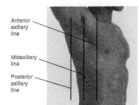

FIGURE 15-3. Anterior axillary, midaxillary, and posterior axillary lines.

TECHNIQUES OF EXAMINATION	POSSIBLE FINDINGS

Note:

- Facial color

  Cyanosis and pallor in lips and oral mucosa signal hypoxia

- Rate, rhythm, depth, and effort of breathing. Normally 14 to 20 breaths/min in adults

  Tachypnea, hyperpnea, Cheyne–Stokes breathing. See Table 15-3, Abnormalities in Rate and Rhythm of Breathing, p. 239.

- Inspiratory retraction of the supraclavicular areas

  Occurs in chronic obstructive pulmonary disease (COPD), asthma, upper airway obstruction

- Inspiratory contraction of the sternocleidomastoids

  Indicates severe breathing difficulty

Observe shape of patient's chest.

Normal or barrel chest (see Table 15-4, Deformities of the Thorax, pp. 240–241)

Posterior Chest

Inspect the posterior chest for:

- Asymmetry in chest expansion

  Asymmetric expansion occurs in large pleural effusions.

- Abnormal inspiratory retraction of the interspaces

  Retraction in asthma, COPD, upper airway obstruction

- Impairment or unilateral *lag* in respiratory movement

  Disease of the underlying lung or pleura, phrenic nerve palsy

Palpate the chest for:

- Tender areas

  Fractured ribs

- Assessment of visible abnormalities

  Masses, sinus tracts

- Chest expansion (Fig. 15-4)

  Impairment, both sides in COPD and restrictive lung disease; unilateral decrease or delay in chronic fibrosis of the underlying lung or pleura, pleural effusion, lobar pneumonia, pleural pain with associated splinting, unilateral bronchial obstruction, and paralysis of the hemidiaphragm

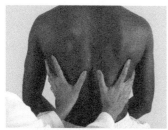

FIGURE 15-4. Assessing lung expansion.

- Tactile fremitus—ask the patient to repeat the words "*ninety-nine*" or "*one-one-one.*" Identify and locate any areas of *increased*, *decreased*, or *absent* fremitus.

Decreased or absent fremitus when transmission of vibrations to the chest is impeded by a thick chest wall, obstructed bronchus, COPD, or pleural effusion, fibrosis, air (*pneumothorax*), or an infiltrating tumor

Asymmetric decreased fremitus in unilateral pleural effusion, pneumothorax, or neoplasm; asymmetric increased fremitus occurs in unilateral pneumonia, which increases transmission through consolidated tissue

Percuss the chest, comparing one side with the other at each level (Box 15-2), using the side-to-side "ladder pattern," as shown in Figures 15-5 and 15-6.

Dullness when fluid or solid tissue replaces normally air-filled lung; hyperresonance in emphysema or pneumothorax

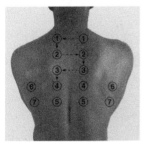

FIGURE 15-5. "Ladder" pattern for percussion and auscultation.

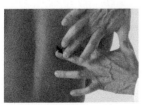

FIGURE 15-6. Striking the pleximeter finger with the right middle finger.

BOX 15-2. Percussion Notes and Their Characteristics

	Relative Intensity, Pitch, and Duration	Examples
Flat	Soft/high/short	Large pleural effusion
Dull	Medium/medium/medium	Lobar pneumonia
Resonant	Loud/low/long	Healthy lung, simple chronic bronchitis
Hyperresonant	Louder/lower/longer	COPD, pneumothorax
Tympanitic	Loud/high (timbre is musical)	Large pneumothorax

Percuss level of diaphragmatic dullness on each side and estimate diaphragmatic descent after patient takes full inspiration (Fig. 15-7).

Pleural effusion or a paralyzed diaphragm raises level of dullness.

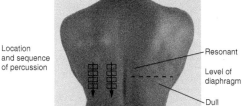

Location and sequence of percussion

Resonant

Level of diaphragm

Dull

FIGURE 15-7. Identify the extent of diaphragmatic excursion.

Auscultate the chest with stethoscope in the "ladder" pattern, again comparing sides.

See Table 15-5, Physical Findings in Selected Chest Disorders, p. 242.

- Evaluate the breath sounds (Box 15-3).

Vesicular, bronchovesicular, or bronchial breath sounds; decreased breath sounds from decreased airflow

- Note any *adventitious* (added) sounds (Box 15-4).

Crackles (fine and coarse) and continuous sounds (wheezes and rhonchi)

BOX 15-3. Characteristics of Breath Sounds

	Duration	Intensity and Pitch of Expiratory Sound	Example Locations
Vesicular	Insp > Exp	Soft/low	Most of the lungs
Bronchovesicular	Insp = Exp	Medium/medium	1st and 2nd interspaces, interscapular area
Bronchial	Insp < Exp	Loud/high	Over the manubrium
Tracheal	Insp = Exp	Very loud/high	Over the trachea

Duration is indicated by the length of the line, intensity by the width of the line, and pitch by the slope of the line.

BOX 15-4. Adventitious or Added Breath Sounds

Crackles (or Rales)

Discontinuous
- Intermittent, nonmusical, and brief
- Like dots in time
- *Fine crackles:* soft, high-pitched (~650 Hz), very brief (5–10 ms)

  • • • • •

- *Coarse crackles:* somewhat louder, lower in pitch (~350 Hz), brief (15–30 ms)

  • • • • • •

Wheezes and Rhonchi

Continuous
- Sinusoidal, musical, prolonged (but not necessarily persisting throughout respiratory cycle)
- Like dashes in time
- *Wheezes:* relatively high-pitched (≥400 Hz) with hissing or shrill quality (>80 ms)

  〰〰〰〰

- *Rhonchi:* relatively low-pitched (150–200 Hz) with snoring quality (>80 ms)

  〜〰

Source: Loudon R, et al. Lung sounds. *Am Rev Respir Dis.* 1994;130:663; Bohadana A, et al. Fundamentals of lung auscultation. *N Engl J Med.* 2014;370:744.

TECHNIQUES OF EXAMINATION	POSSIBLE FINDINGS

Observe qualities of breath sound, timing in the respiratory cycle, and location on the chest wall. Do they clear with deep breathing or coughing?

Clearing after cough suggests atelectasis.

If distress, auscultate the neck and lungs for:

- Audible high-pitched inspiratory whistling (*stridor*)

Stridor may occur in upper airway obstruction from foreign body or epiglottitis and requires prompt evaluation.

Assess transmitted voice sounds (Box 15-5) and bronchial breath sounds heard in abnormal places. Ask patient to:

- Say "ninety-nine" and "ee."

Bronchophony if sounds become louder; *egophony* if "ee" to "A" change from lobar consolidation

- Whisper "ninety-nine" or "one-two-three."

Whispered pectoriloquy if whispered sounds transmit louder and more clearly

BOX 15-5. Transmitted Voice Sounds

Through Normally Air-Filled Lung	Through Airless Lung[a]
Usually accompanied by vesicular breath sounds and normal tactile fremitus	Usually accompanied by bronchial or bronchovesicular breath sounds and increased tactile fremitus
Spoken words muffled and indistinct	Spoken words louder, clearer (*bronchophony*)
Spoken "ee" heard as "ee"	Spoken "ee" heard as "ay" (*egophony*)
Whispered words faint and indistinct, if heard at all	Whispered words louder, clearer (*whispered pectoriloquy*)

[a]As in lobar pneumonia and toward the top of a large pleural effusion.

Anterior Chest

Inspect the anterior chest for:

- Deformities or asymmetry

Pectus excavatum

- Intercostal retraction

From obstructed airways

- Impaired or lagging respiratory movement

Disease of the underlying lung or pleura, phrenic nerve palsy

| TECHNIQUES OF EXAMINATION | POSSIBLE FINDINGS |

Palpate the chest for:

- Tender areas
- Assessment of visible abnormalities
- Respiratory expansion
- Tactile fremitus

Tender pectoral muscles, costochondritis

Flail chest

Percuss the chest in the areas illustrated in Figure 15-8.

Normal cardiac dullness may disappear in emphysema.

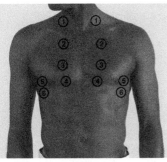

FIGURE 15-8. Locations for percussing anterior chest in ladder pattern.

Auscultate the chest. Assess breath sounds, adventitious sounds, and if indicated transmitted voice sounds as previously discussed.

RECORDING YOUR FINDINGS

Recording the Thorax and Lungs Examination

"Thorax is symmetric with good expansion. Lungs resonant. Breath sounds vesicular; no rales, wheezes, or rhonchi. Diaphragms descend 4 cm bilaterally."

OR

"Thorax symmetric with moderate kyphosis and increased anteroposterior (AP) diameter, decreased expansion. Lungs are hyperresonant. Breath sounds distant with delayed expiratory phase and scattered expiratory wheezes. Fremitus decreased; no bronchophony, egophony, or whispered pectoriloquy. Diaphragms descend 2 cm bilaterally."

These findings suggest COPD.

HEALTH PROMOTION AND COUNSELING: EVIDENCE AND RECOMMENDATIONS

> ### Important Topics for Health Promotion and Counseling
>
> - Lung cancer screening
> - Latent tuberculosis
> - Screening for obstructive sleep apnea
> - Tobacco cessation (see Chapter 6, Health Maintenance and Screening, pp. 92–93)
> - Immunizations—influenza and streptococcal pneumonia vaccines (see Chapter 6, Health Maintenance and Screening, pp. 95–97)

Lung Cancer

Lung cancer is the second most frequently diagnosed cancer in the United States and the leading cause of cancer death for both men and women. Cigarette smoking is far and away the leading risk factor for lung cancer, accounting for about 90% of lung cancer deaths. Annual low-dose computed tomography (LDCT) screening is recommended by the U.S. Preventive Services Task Force (USPSTF) for current smokers (or those who have quit within the last 15 years) if they have smoked an average of one pack of cigarettes for 30 years and are age 55 to 80 years (grade B recommendation).

Latent Tuberculosis

As opposed to those with active tuberculosis, people with latent tuberculosis have no symptoms and are not contagious. However, they may develop active tuberculosis if they do not receive treatment. The USPSTF favors screening in asymptomatic adults with the tuberculin skin test (TST) or interferon-gamma release assay (IGRA) blood tests (grade B recommendation).

Screening for Obstructive Sleep Apnea

In 2017, the USPSTF concluded that the evidence was insufficient to assess the balance of benefits and harms of screening asymptomatic adults for obstructive sleep apnea (OSA).

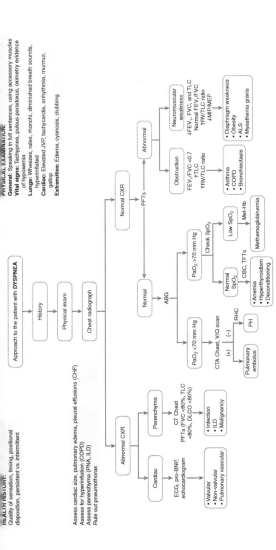

HEALTH HISTORY:
Quality of sensation, timing, positional disposition, persistent vs. intermittent

PHYSICAL EXAMINATION:
General: Speaking in full sentences, using accessory muscles of hypoxemia
Vital signs: Tachypnea, pulsus paradoxus, oximetry evidence of hypoxemia
Lungs: Wheezes, rales, rhonchi, diminished breath sounds, hyperinflated
Cardiac: Elevated JVP, tachycardia, arrhythmia, murmur, gallop
Extremities: Edema, cyanosis, clubbing

Approach to the patient with **DYSPNEA**

History

Physical exam

Chest radiograph

Assess cardiac size, pulmonary edema, pleural effusions (CHF)
Assess for hyperinflation (COPD)
Assess parenchyma (PNA, ILD)
Rule out pneumothorax

Abnormal CXR

Cardiac
ECG, pro-BNP, echocardiogram
• Valvular
• Non-valvular
• Pulmonary vascular

Parenchyma
CT Chest
PFTs (FVC <80%, TLC <80%, DLCO <80%)
• Infection
• ILD
• Malignancy

Normal CXR

Normal

ABG

PaO$_2$ <70 mm Hg
CTA Chest, V/Q scan
(+) → Pulmonary embolism
(−) → PH → RHC

PaO$_2$ >70 mm Hg
Check SpO$_2$
Low SpO$_2$ → Methemoglobinemia → Met-Hb
Normal SpO$_2$ → CBC, TFTs
• Anemia
• Hyperthyroidism
• Deconditioning

PFTs

Abnormal

Obstruction
FEV$_1$/FVC <0.7
↑TLC
↑RV/TLC ratio
• Asthma
• COPD
• Bronchiectasis

Neuromuscular weakness
↓FEV$_1$, FVC, and TLC
Normal FEV$_1$/FVC
↓MIP/MEP
• Diaphragm weakness
• Obesity
• ALS
• Myasthenia gravis

Algorithm 15-1. Approach to the patient with dyspnea. (Note: Although it is not comprehensive, this algorithm may be a helpful starting approach for synthesizing information gathered from the history and physical.) ALS, amyotrophic lateral sclerosis; pro-BNP, brain natriuretic peptide; CHF, congestive heart failure; COPD, chronic obstructive pulmonary disease; CT, computed tomography; CTA, computed tomography angiography; CXR, chest x-ray; ECG, electrocardiogram; FEV, forced expiratory volume; FVC, forced vital capacity; HPI, history of present illness; ILD, interstitial lung disease; JVP, jugular venous pressure; MEP, maximal expiratory pressure; MIP, maximal inspiratory pressure; PH, pulmonary hypertension; PFTs, pulmonary function tests; PNA, pulmonary nodular amyloidosis; RHC, right heart catheterization; RV, residual volume; TFTs, thyroid function tests; TLC, total lung capacity.

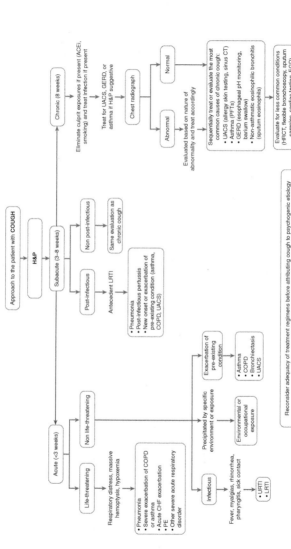

Algorithm 15-2. Approach to the patient with cough. (Note: Although it is not comprehensive, this algorithm may be a helpful starting approach for synthesizing information gathered from the history and physical.) CHF, congestive heart failure; COPD, chronic obstructive pulmonary disease; CT, computed tomography; EGD, esophagogastroduodenoscopy; GERD, gastroesophageal reflux disease; H&P, history and physical examination; HRCT, high-resolution computed tomography; LRTI, lower respiratory tract infection; PE, pulmonary embolism; PFTs, pulmonary

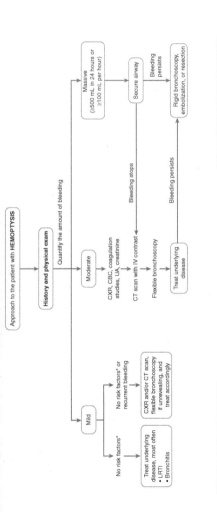

Algorithm 15-3. Approach to the patient with hemoptysis. (Note: Although it is not comprehensive, this algorithm may be a helpful starting approach for synthesizing information gathered from the history and physical.) *Risk factors: tobacco use, age >40, high risk for tuberculosis or malignancy. AVM, arteriovenous malformation; CBC, complete blood count; CHF, congestive heart failure; CT, computed tomography; CXR = chest x-ray; DIC = disseminated intravascular coagulation; H&P = history and physical examination; LRTI = lower respiratory tract infection; PE = pulmonary embolism; UA = urinalysis.

Approach to the patient with **HEMOPTYSIS**

History and physical exam

Quantify the amount of bleeding

Mild

No risk factors*

Treat underlying disease, most often
• LRTI
• Bronchitis

No risk factors* or recurrent bleeding

CXR and/or CT scan, flexible bronchoscopy if unrevealing, and treat accordingly

Moderate

CXR, CBC, coagulation studies, UA, creatinine

CT scan with IV contrast

Flexible bronchoscopy

Treat underlying disease

Bleeding stops

Bleeding persists

Massive
(≥500 mL in 24 hours or ≥100 mL per hour)

Secure airway

Bleeding persists

Rigid bronchoscopy, embolization, or resection

Rule out other sources (pseudohemoptysis):
• Nasal (epistaxis)
• Oropharynx
• Gastrointestinal tract (hematemesis)

Airway: foreign body, bronchitis, bronchiectasis, cancer, Dieulafoy vessel
Parenchyma: infection, rheumatic
Vascular: CHF, mitral stenosis, endocarditis, AVM, PE, pulmonary artery aneurysm, vasculitis
Coagulopathy: DIC, systemic anticoagulation
Miscellaneous: drugs, trauma, idiopathic

INTERPRETATION AIDS

TABLE 15-1. Dyspnea

Problem	Timing	Provoking/Relieving Factors; Associated Symptoms
Left-Sided Heart Failure (*Left ventricular failure or mitral stenosis*)	Dyspnea may progress slowly or suddenly, as in acute pulmonary edema	↑ by exertion, lying down ↓ by rest, sitting up, though dyspnea may become persistent *Associated Symptoms:* Often cough, orthopnea, paroxysmal nocturnal dyspnea; sometimes wheezing
Chronic Bronchitis (*may be seen with COPD*)	Chronic productive cough followed by slowly progressive dyspnea	↑ by exertion, inhaled irritants, respiratory infections ↓ by expectoration, rest though dyspnea may become persistent *Associated Symptoms:* Chronic productive cough, recurrent respiratory infections; wheezing possible
Chronic Obstructive Pulmonary Disease (COPD)	Slowly progressive; relatively mild cough later	↑ by exertion ↓ by rest, though dyspnea may become persistent *Associated Symptoms:* Cough with scant mucoid sputum

Asthma	Acute episodes, then symptom-free periods; nocturnal episodes common	↑ by allergens, irritants, respiratory infections, exercise, emotion ↓ by separation from aggravating factors *Associated Symptoms:* Wheezing, cough, tightness in chest
Diffuse Interstitial Lung Diseases (*Sarcoidosis, neoplasms, asbestosis, idiopathic pulmonary fibrosis*)	Progressive; varies in rate of development depending on cause	↑ by exertion ↓ by rest, though dyspnea may become persistent *Associated Symptoms:* Often weakness, fatigue; cough less common than in other lung diseases
Pneumonia	Acute illness; timing varies with causative agent	*Associated Symptoms:* Pleuritic pain, cough, sputum, fever, though not necessarily present
Spontaneous Pneumothorax	Sudden onset of dyspnea	*Associated Symptoms:* Pleuritic pain, cough
Acute Pulmonary Embolism	Sudden onset of dyspnea	*Associated Symptoms:* Often none; retrosternal oppressive pain if massive occlusion; pleuritic pain, cough, syncope, hemoptysis, and/or unilateral leg swelling and pain from instigating deep vein thrombosis; anxiety

TABLE 15-2. Cough and Hemoptysis

Problem	Cough, Sputum, Associated Symptoms, and Setting
Acute Inflammation	
Laryngitis	*Cough and sputum:* Dry, or with variable amounts of sputum
	Associated Symptoms and Setting: Acute, fairly minor illness with hoarseness. Associated with viral nasopharyngitis
Acute bronchitis	*Cough and Sputum:* Dry or productive of sputum
	Associated Symptoms and Setting: An acute, often viral illness, with burning retrosternal discomfort
Mycoplasma and viral pneumonias	*Cough and Sputum:* Dry and hacking often with mucoid sputum
	Associated Symptoms and Setting: Acute febrile illness, often with malaise, headache, and possibly dyspnea
Bacterial pneumonias	*Cough and Sputum:* Sputum is mucoid or purulent; may be blood streaked, diffusely pinkish, or rusty
	Associated Symptoms and Setting: Acute illness with chills, often high fever, dyspnea, and chest pain. Commonly from *Streptococcus pneumonia, Haemophilus influenzae, Moraxella catarrhalis; Klebsiella* in alcoholism
Chronic Inflammation	
Postnasal drip	*Cough and Sputum:* Chronic cough with mucoid or mucopurulent sputum
	Associated Symptoms and Setting: Repeated attempts to clear the throat. Postnasal drip, discharge in posterior pharynx. Associated with chronic rhinitis, with or without sinusitis

TABLE 15-2. Cough and Hemoptysis *(continued)*

Problem	Cough, Sputum, Associated Symptoms, and Setting
Chronic bronchitis	*Cough:* Chronic
	Sputum: Mucoid to purulent; may be blood streaked or even bloody
	Associated Symptoms and Setting: Often long history of cigarette smoking. Recurrent superimposed infections; often wheezing and dyspnea
Bronchiectasis	*Cough and Sputum:* Chronic cough; sputum mucoid to purulent, may be blood streaked or even bloody
	Associated Symptoms and Setting: Recurrent bronchopulmonary infections common; sinusitis may coexist
Pulmonary tuberculosis	*Cough and Sputum:* Dry, mucoid or purulent; may be blood streaked or bloody
	Associated Symptoms and Setting: Early, no symptoms. Later, anorexia, weight loss, fatigue, fever, and night sweats
Lung abscess	*Cough and Sputum:* Sputum purulent and foul smelling; may be bloody
	Associated Symptoms and Setting: Often from aspiration pneumonia from oral anaerobes and poor dental hygiene; often with dysphagia, impaired consciousness
Asthma	*Cough and Sputum:* Thick and mucoid, especially near end of an attack
	Associated Symptoms and Setting: Episodic wheezing and dyspnea, but cough may occur alone. Often a history of allergy
Gastroesophageal reflux	*Cough and Sputum:* Chronic cough, especially at night or early morning
	Associated Symptoms and Setting: Wheezing, especially at night (often mistaken for asthma), early morning hoarseness, repeated attempts to clear throat. Often with history of heartburn and regurgitation

continued

TABLE 15-2. Cough and Hemoptysis *(continued)*

Problem	Cough, Sputum, Associated Symptoms, and Setting
Neoplasm *Lung cancer*	*Cough:* Dry to productive *Sputum and Cough:* Cough, dry to productive; sputum may be blood-streaked or bloody *Associated symptoms and setting:* Commonly with dyspnea, weight loss, and history of tobacco abuse

Cardiovascular Disorders

Left ventricular failure or mitral stenosis	*Cough and Sputum:* Cough often dry, especially on exertion or at night. Sputum may progress to pink and frothy, as in pulmonary edema, or to frank hemoptysis *Associated Symptoms and Setting:* Dyspnea, orthopnea, paroxysmal nocturnal dyspnea
Pulmonary embolism	*Cough and Sputum:* Dry cough, at times with hemoptysis *Associated Symptoms and Setting:* Tachypnea, chest or pleuritic pain, dyspnea, fever, syncope, anxiety; factors that predispose to deep venous thrombosis
Irritating Particles, Chemicals, or Gases	*Cough and Sputum:* Variable. May be a latent period between exposure and symptoms *Associated Symptoms and Setting:* Exposure to irritants; eye, nose, and throat symptoms

Sources: Irwin RS, Madison JM. The diagnosis and treatment of cough. *N Engl J Med.* 2000;343:1715; Metlay JP, Kapoor WN, Fine MJ. Does this patient have community-acquired pneumonia? Diagnosing pneumonia by history and physical examination. *JAMA.* 1997;378:1440; Neiderman M. In the clinic: community-acquired pneumonia. *Ann Intern Med.* 2009;151:ITC4–1; Barker A. Bronchiectasis. *N Engl J Med.* 2002;346:1383; Wenzel RP, Fowler AA. Acute bronchitis. *N Engl J Med.* 2006;355:2125; Kerlin MP. In the clinic. Asthma. *Ann Intern Med.* 2014;160:ITC3–1; Escalante P. In the clinic: tuberculosis. *Ann Intern Med.* 2009;150:ITC6–1; Agnelli G, Becattini C. Acute pulmonary embolism. *N Engl J Med.* 2010;363:266.

TABLE 15-3. Abnormalities in Rate and Rhythm of Breathing

Inspiration Expiration

Normal. In adults, 14–20 per min; in infants, up to 44 per min.

Rapid Shallow Breathing (*Tachypnea*). Many causes, including salicylate intoxication, restrictive lung disease, pleuritic chest pain, and an elevated diaphragm.

Rapid Deep Breathing (*Hyperpnea, Hyperventilation*). Many causes, including exercise, anxiety, metabolic acidosis, brainstem injury. Kussmaul breathing, due to metabolic acidosis, is deep, but rate may be fast, slow, or normal.

Slow Breathing (*Bradypnea*). May be secondary to diabetic coma, drug-induced respiratory depression.

Hyperpnea Apnea

Cheyne–Stokes Breathing. Rhythmically alternating periods of hyperpnea and apnea. In infants and the aged, may be normal during sleep; also accompanies brain damage, heart failure, uremia, drug-induced respiratory depression.

Ataxic (*Biot*) Breathing. Unpredictable irregularity of depth and rate. Causes include meningitis, respiratory depression, and brain injury.

Sighs

Sighing Breathing. Breathing punctuated by frequent sighs. When associated with other symptoms, it suggests the hyperventilation syndrome. Occasional sighs are normal.

Prolonged expiration

Obstructive Breathing. In obstructive lung disease, expiration is prolonged due to narrowed airways that increase the resistance to air flow. Causes include asthma, chronic bronchitis, and COPD.

TABLE 15-4. Deformities of the Thorax

Normal Adult

The thorax is wider than it is deep; lateral diameter is greater than anteroposterior (AP) diameter.

Barrel Chest

Has increased AP diameter, seen in normal infants and normal aging; also in COPD.

 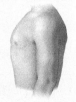

Traumatic Flail Chest

If multiple ribs are fractured, can see paradoxical movements of the thorax. Descent of the diaphragm decreases intrathoracic pressure on inspiration. The injured area may cave inward; on expiration, it moves outward.

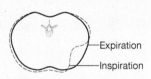

—Expiration

—Inspiration

Funnel Chest (Pectus Excavatum)

Depression in the lower portion of the sternum. Related compression of the heart and great vessels may cause murmurs.

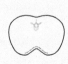

TABLE 15-4. Deformities of the Thorax *(continued)*

Pigeon Chest (Pectus Carinatum)

Sternum is displaced anteriorly, increasing the AP diameter; costal cartilages adjacent to the protruding sternum are depressed.

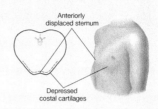

Anteriorly displaced sternum

Depressed costal cartilages

Thoracic Kyphoscoliosis

Abnormal spinal curvatures and vertebral rotation deform the chest, making interpretation of lung findings difficult.

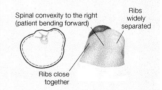

Spinal convexity to the right (patient bending forward)

Ribs widely separated

Ribs close together

TABLE 15-5. Physical Findings in Selected Chest Disorders

	Trachea	Percussion Note	Breath Sounds	Transmitted Voice Sounds	Adventitious Sounds
Chronic Bronchitis	Midline	Resonant	Normal	Normal	None, or wheezes, rhonchi, crackles
Left Heart Failure (Early)	Midline	Resonant	Normal	Normal	Late inspiratory crackles in lower lungs; possible wheezes
Consolidation[a]	Midline	Dull	Bronchial	Increased[b]	Late inspiratory crackles
Atelectasis (Lobar Obstruction)	May be shifted *toward* involved side	Dull	Usually absent	Usually absent	None
Pleural Effusion	May be shifted *away*	Dull	Decreased to absent	Decreased to absent	Usually none, possible pleural rub
Pneumothorax	May be shifted *away*	Hyperresonant or tympanitic	Decreased to absent	Decreased to absent	Possible pleural rub
COPD	Midline	Hyperresonant	Decreased to absent	Decreased	None or the wheezes and rhonchi of chronic bronchitis
Asthma	Midline	Resonant to hyperresonant	May be obscured by wheezes	Decreased	Wheezes, perhaps crackles

[a]As in lobar pneumonia, pulmonary edema, or pulmonary hemorrhage.

[b]With increased tactile fremitus, bronchophony, egophony, whispered pectoriloquy.

Cardiovascular System

HEALTH HISTORY

Common or Concerning Symptoms

- Chest pain (also see Chapter 15, Thorax and Lungs)
- Shortness of breath: dyspnea, orthopnea, or paroxysmal nocturnal dyspnea
- Palpitations
- Swelling (*edema*) and fainting (*syncope*)

Chest Pain

Be systematic as you think through the range of possible cardiac, pulmonary, and extrathoracic etiologies. Classic exertional pain, pressure, or discomfort in the chest, shoulder, back, neck, or arm is seen in angina pectoris or myocardial infarction. Atypical descriptors also are common, such as cramping, grinding, pricking or, rarely, tooth or jaw pain.

Anterior chest pain, often tearing or ripping and radiating into the back or neck, occurs in acute aortic dissection.

See Table 16-1, Chest Pain, pp. 262–263 and Algorithm 16-1, Approach to the patient with chest pain, p. 259.

Shortness of Breath

Ask about any shortness of breath or *dyspnea* (an uncomfortable awareness of breathing that is inappropriate for a given level of exertion); also ask about *orthopnea* (dyspnea that occurs when the patient is supine and improves when the patient sits up) or *paroxysmal nocturnal dyspnea* (nighttime episodes of sudden dyspnea that awakens one from sleep).

Orthopnea and PND occur in left ventricular heart failure and mitral stenosis and also in obstructive lung disease.

See Algorithm 15-1, Approach to the patient with dyspnea, p. 231 in Chapter 15, Thorax and Lungs.

Remember that symptoms such as dyspnea, wheezing, cough, and even hemoptysis can be cardiac as well as pulmonary in origin.

Palpitations

Ask about any unpleasant awareness of the heartbeat, *palpitations*. Other descriptive terms include skipping, racing, fluttering, pounding, or stopping of the heart. Palpitations do not necessarily indicate heart disease, however.

If there are symptoms or signs of irregular heart action, obtain an ECG. Atrial fibrillation, which causes an "irregularly irregular" pulse, is often identified at the bedside.

Anxious and hyperthyroid patients may report palpitations; see Algorithm 16-2, Approach to the patient with palpitations, p. 260.

Swelling and Fainting

Also ask about any swelling (*edema*) especially in the legs and feet; or any episodes of fainting (*syncope*).

Causes of edema are frequently cardiac (right or left ventricular dysfunction; pulmonary hypertension) or pulmonary (obstructive lung disease).

Syncope occurs in end-stage heart failure and arrhythmias.

Also, when assessing cardiac symptoms, it is important to quantify the patient's baseline level of activity compared to the symptomatic episode.

TECHNIQUES OF EXAMINATION

Key Components of the Cardiovascular Examination

- Note general appearance and measure blood pressure and heart rate
- Estimate level of jugular venous pressure
- Auscultate carotids (bruit) one at a time
- Palpate carotid pulse including carotid upstroke (amplitude, contour, timing) and presence of a thrill
- Inspect anterior chest wall (apical impulse, precordial movements)
- Palpate precordium for any heaves, thrills, or palpable heart sounds
- Palpate and locate PMI or apical impulse
- Palpate for systolic impulse of the right ventricle, pulmonary artery, and aortic outflow tract areas on chest wall

- Auscultate S_1 and S_2 in six positions from the base to apex
- Identify physiologic and paradoxical splitting of S_2
- Auscultate and recognize abnormal sounds in early diastole, including S_3 and OS of mitral stenosis and S_4 later in diastole
- Distinguish systolic and diastolic murmurs, using maneuvers when needed; if present, identify timing, shape, grade, location, radiation, pitch, and quality

Heart Rate and Blood Pressure

Count the radial or apical pulse.

Estimate systolic blood pressure by palpation and *add* 30 mm Hg. Use this sum as the target for further cuff inflations.

This step helps you to detect an auscultatory gap and avoid recording an inappropriately low systolic blood pressure.

Measure blood pressure with a sphygmomanometer. If indicated, *recheck* it.

Orthostatic (postural) hypotension within 3 minutes of position change from supine to standing is SBP↓ ≥20 mm Hg; HR↑ ≥20 beats/min.

Jugular Veins

Jugular Venous Pulsations. In the right internal jugular vein identify their highest point in the neck. Start with head of the bed at 30°; adjust the head of the bed as necessary, giving consideration to volume status.

Jugular Venous Pressure (JVP). Measure the vertical distance between this highest point and the sternal angle, normally <3 to 4 cm (Fig. 16-1).

Elevated JVP in right-sided heart failure; decreased JVP in hypovolemia from dehydration or gastrointestinal bleeding.

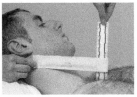

FIGURE 16-1. Measuring the height of the JVP.

Study the waves of venous pulsation. Note the *a* wave of atrial contraction and the *v* wave of venous filling.

Abnormally *prominent a waves* in tricuspid stenosis, pulmonary hypertension, and pulmonic stenosis; *absent a waves* in atrial fibrillation. *Increased v waves* in tricuspid regurgitation, atrial septal defects, and constrictive pericarditis.

Carotid Pulse

Palpate the amplitude and contour of the carotid upstroke. The normal upstroke is brisk.

A delayed upstroke in aortic stenosis; a bounding upstroke in aortic insufficiency.

Pulsus Alternans. Palpate for alteration in carotid pulse amplitude. Lower pressure of blood pressure cuff slowly to systolic level while you listen with your stethoscope over the brachial artery.

Alternating amplitude of pulse or sudden doubling of Korotkoff sounds indicates *pulsus alternans*—a sign of left ventricular heart failure.

Pulsus Paradoxus (Paradoxical Pulse). Lower pressure of BP cuff slowly and note two pressure levels: (1) where Korotkoff sounds are first heard and (2) where they first persist through the respiratory cycle. These levels are normally not more than 3 to 4 mm Hg apart.

A drop of >10 mm Hg during inspiration signifies pulsus paradoxus. Consider obstructive pulmonary disease, asthma, pericardial tamponade, or constrictive pericarditis.

Auscultate for Bruits. *Bruits* are murmur-like sounds arising from turbulent arterial blood flow. Ask the patient to stop breathing for ~10 seconds, then listen with the diaphragm of the stethoscope.

Although usually caused by atherosclerotic luminal stenosis, bruits are also caused by a tortuous carotid artery, external carotid arterial disease, aortic stenosis, hypervascularity of hyperthyroidism, and external compression from thoracic outlet syndrome. Bruits do not correlate with clinically significant underlying disease.

Heart

See Box 16-1 for the patient positions and a suggested sequence for the cardiac examination.

BOX 16-1. Sequence of the Cardiac Examination

Patient Position	Examination
Supine, with the head elevated 30°	After examining the JVP and carotid pulse, inspect and palpate the precordium: the second right and left intercostal spaces; the RV; and the LV, including the apical impulse (diameter, location).
Left lateral decubitus	Palpate the apical impulse to assess its diameter. Listen at the apex with the *bell* of the stethoscope for low-pitched extra sounds such as an S_3, opening snap, diastolic rumble of mitral stenosis.
Supine, with the head elevated 30°	Listen at the six areas with the *diaphragm* then *bell*: the 2nd right and left interspaces, down the left sternal border to the 4th and 5th interspaces, and across to the apex (see p. 252). As indicated, listen at the lower right sternal border for right-sided murmurs and sounds, often accentuated with inspiration, with the *diaphragm* and *bell*.
Sitting, leaning forward, after full exhalation	Listen down the left sternal border and at the apex with the *diaphragm* for the soft decrescendo murmur of aortic insufficiency.

Inspection and Palpation. Inspect and palpate the anterior chest for heaves, lifts, and thrills.

Inspect and palpate the *apical impulse* (Fig. 16-2).

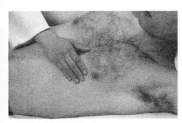

FIGURE 16-2. Palpating the apical impulse.

Turn patient to left as necessary. Note:

- Location of impulse

Displaced in heart failure, cardiomyopathy, and ischemic heart disease.

TECHNIQUES OF EXAMINATION	POSSIBLE FINDINGS

- Diameter or area (usually measures <2.5 cm in a supine patient)

Increased diameter, amplitude, and duration in left ventricular dilatation from heart failure or ischemic cardiomyopathy.

- Amplitude—usually *tapping*

Sustained in left ventricular hypertrophy; *diffuse* in CHF.

- Duration—feel for a right ventricular impulse in left parasternal and epigastric areas.

Prominent impulses suggest right ventricular enlargement.

Palpate left and right second interspaces close to sternum. Note any thrills in these areas.

Pulsations of great vessels; accentuated S_2; thrills of aortic or pulmonic stenosis.

Auscultation. Listen to the heart by "inching" your stethoscope from the base to the apex (or apex to base) in the areas illustrated in Figure 16-3.

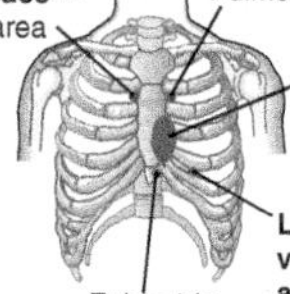

Right 2nd interspace— Aortic area

Left 2nd interspace— Pulmonic area

Right ventricular area— Left sternal border

Left ventricular area— Apex

Epigastric (subxiphoid)

FIGURE 16-3. Auscultate the heart from the base to the apex.

Use the *diaphragm* to detect the relatively *high-pitched sounds* like S_1, S_2.

Also murmurs of aortic and mitral regurgitation, pericardial friction rubs.

Use the *bell* for *low-pitched sounds* at the lower left sternal border and apex.

S_3, S_4, murmur of mitral stenosis

Listen at each area for:

- S_1

See Table 16-2, Heart Sounds, p. 264; Table 16-3, Variations in the First Heart Sound—S_1, p. 265; and Table 16-4, Variations in the Second Heart Sound—S_2 During Inspiration and Expiration, pp. 266–267.

- S_2. Is splitting normal in left 2nd and 3rd interspaces?

Physiologic (inspiratory) or pathologic (expiratory) splitting.

TECHNIQUES OF EXAMINATION	POSSIBLE FINDINGS
■ Extra sounds in systole	Systolic clicks.
■ Extra sounds in diastole	S_3, S_4.
■ Systolic murmurs	Midsystolic, pansystolic, late systolic murmurs.
■ Diastolic murmurs	Early, mid-, or late diastolic murmurs.

Use two maneuvers as needed to help identify the murmurs of mitral stenosis and aortic regurgitation.

Listen at the apex with patient turned toward left side for low-pitched sounds (Fig. 16-4).

Left-sided S_3, and diastolic murmur of mitral stenosis.

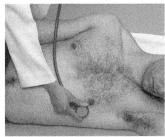

FIGURE 16-4. Listening at the apex for low-pitched sounds.

Listen down the left sternal border to the apex as patient sits, leaning forward, with breath held after exhalation (Fig. 16-5).

Diastolic decrescendo murmur of aortic regurgitation.

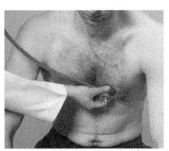

FIGURE 16-5. Listening at the lower left sternal border for aortic insufficiency.

Assessing and Describing Murmurs. If murmurs are present, identify their:

- Timing in the cardiac cycle (systole, diastole). It is helpful to palpate the carotid upstroke while listening to any murmur—murmurs occurring simultaneously with the upstroke are systolic.

See Table 16-5, Heart Murmurs, p. 268 and Algorithm 16-3, Approach to the patient with a murmur, p. 261.

- Shape

Plateau, crescendo, decrescendo

S₁   S₂

A *crescendo–decrescendo* murmur first rises in intensity, then falls (e.g., aortic stenosis).

S₁   S₂

A *plateau* murmur has the same intensity throughout (e.g., mitral regurgitation).

S₂   S₁

A *crescendo* murmur grows louder (e.g., mitral stenosis).

S₂   S₁

A *decrescendo* murmur grows softer (e.g., aortic regurgitation).

- Location of maximal intensity

Murmurs loudest at the *base* are often aortic; at the *apex*, they are often mitral.

- Radiation

- Pitch

High, medium, low

- Quality

Blowing, harsh, musical, rumbling

- Intensity of murmurs (Boxes 16-2 and 16-3).

Special Techniques

Aids to Identify Systolic Murmurs

Valsalva Maneuver. Ask patient to strain down.

BOX 16-2. Gradations of Systolic Murmurs

Grade	Description
Grade 1	Softer in volume than S_1 and S_2, very faint
Grade 2	Equal in volume to S_1 and S_2, quiet, but heard immediately
Grade 3	Louder in volume than S_1 and S_2, moderately loud
Grade 4	Louder in volume than S_1 and S_2, with *palpable thrill*
Grade 5	Louder in volume than S_1 and S_2, with *thrill*; may be heard when the stethoscope is partly off the chest
Grade 6	Louder in volume than S_1 and S_2, with *thrill*; may be heard with stethoscope entirely off the chest

BOX 16-3. Gradations of Diastolic Murmurs

Grade	Description
Grade 1	Softer in volume than S_1 and S_2, very faint
Grade 2	Equal in volume to S_1 and S_2, quiet, but heard immediately
Grade 3	Louder in volume than S_1 and S_2; moderately loud
Grade 4	Louder in volume than S_1 and S_2; may be heard with stethoscope off the chest

In suspected mitral valve prolapse (MVP), listen to the timing of click and murmur.

Ventricular filling decreases, the systolic click of MVP is earlier, and the murmur lengthens.

To distinguish aortic stenosis (AS) from hypertrophic cardiomyopathy (HCM), listen to the intensity of the murmur.

In AS, the murmur decreases; in HCM, it often increases.

Squatting and Standing. In suspected MVP, listen for the click and murmur in both positions.

Squatting increases ventricular filling and delays the click and murmur. Standing reverses the changes.

Try to distinguish AS from HCM by listening to the murmur in both positions.

Squatting increases murmur of AS and decreases murmur of HCM. Standing reverses the changes.

RECORDING YOUR FINDINGS

Recording the Cardiovascular Examination

"The jugular venous pulse is 3 cm above the sternal angle with the head of the bed elevated to 30°. Carotid upstrokes are brisk, without bruits. The point of maximal impulse (PMI) is tapping, 1 cm lateral to the midclavicular line in the 5th intercostal space. Crisp S_1 and S_2. At the base, S_2 is louder than S_1 and physiologically split, with $A_2 > P_2$. At the apex, S_1 is greater than S_2 and constant. No murmurs or extra sounds."

OR

"The JVP is 5 cm above the sternal angle with the head of the bed elevated to 50°. Carotid upstrokes are brisk; a bruit is heard over the left carotid artery. The PMI is diffuse, 3 cm in diameter, palpated at the anterior axillary line in the 5th and 6th intercostal spaces. S_1 and S_2 are soft. S_3 present at the apex. High-pitched, harsh 2/6 holosystolic murmur best heard at the apex, radiating to the axilla. No S_4 or diastolic murmurs."

These findings suggest CHF with possible left carotid stenosis and mitral regurgitation.

HEALTH PROMOTION AND COUNSELING: EVIDENCE AND RECOMMENDATIONS

Important Topics for Health Promotion and Counseling

- Screening for cardiovascular risk factors
    - *Step 1:* Screen for global risk factors
    - *Step 2:* Calculate 10-year and lifetime global CVD risk using a web-based calculator
    - *Step 3:* Address individual risk factors—hypertension, diabetes, dyslipidemias, metabolic syndrome, smoking, family history, and obesity
- Promoting lifestyle changes and risk factor modification

Cardiovascular disease (CVD), which consists primarily of hypertension (the vast majority of diagnoses), coronary heart disease (CHD), heart failure, and stroke, is the leading cause of death for both men and women in the United States. *Primary prevention,* in those without evidence of CVD, and *secondary prevention,* in those with known cardiovascular events, remain important clinical priorities.

Provide education and counseling to promote optimal levels of blood pressure, cholesterol, weight, exercise, and smoking cessation and to reduce risk factors for CVD and stroke.

Screening for Cardiovascular Risk Factors

Step 1: Screen for Global Risk Factors. Begin routine screening at age 20 for combined individual risk factors or "global" risk of CVD and any family history or premature heart disease, defined as onset at age <55 years in first-degree male relatives and <65 years in first-degree female relatives. Recommended screening intervals are listed in Box 16-4.

BOX 16-4. Major Cardiovascular Risk Factors and Screening Frequency

Risk Factor	Screening Frequency	Goal
Family history of premature CVD	Update regularly	Estimate CVD risk
Cigarette smoking	At each visit	Cessation or continued abstinence
Unhealthy diet	At each visit	Improved overall eating pattern
Physical inactivity	At each visit	30 minutes moderate intensity exercise five times weekly
Obesity, especially central adiposity	At each visit	BMI ≤25 kg/m²; waist circumference: ≤40 in for men, ≤35 in for women
Hypertension	At each visit	<130/80 mm Hg for adults
Dyslipidemias	Every 5 years in average-risk adults from ages 40 to 75	Initiate statin therapy if meeting ACC/AHA guidelines

continued

Risk Factor	Screening Frequency	Goal
Diabetes	Every 3 years (if normal) beginning at age 45 years; more frequently at any age if with risk factors	Prevent/delay diabetes for those with HbA$_{1c}$ of 5.7%–6.4%
Pulse	At each visit	Identify and treat atrial fibrillation

Sources: Arnett DK, Blumenthal RS, Albert MA, et al. 2019 ACC/AHA guideline on the primary prevention of cardiovascular disease: executive summary: a report of the American College of Cardiology/American Heart Association Task Force on Clinical Practice Guidelines. *J Am Coll Cardiol*. 2019;74(10):1376–1414; Grundy SM, Stone NJ, Bailey AL, et al. 2018 AHA/ACC/AACVPR/AAPA/ABC/ACPM/ADA/AGS/APhA/ASPC/NLA/PCNA guideline on the management of blood cholesterol: executive summary: a report of the American College of Cardiology/American Heart Association Task Force on Clinical Practice Guidelines. *Circulation*. 2019;139(25):e1046–e1081; James PA, Oparil S, Carter BL, et al. 2014 evidence-based guideline for the management of high blood pressure in adults: report from the panel members appointed to the Eighth Joint National Committee (JNC 8). *JAMA*. 2014;311:507; Meschia JF, Bushnell C, Boden-Albala B, et al. Guidelines for the primary prevention of stroke: a statement for healthcare professionals from the American Heart Association/American Stroke Association. *Stroke*. 2014;45:3754; Flack JM, Sica DA, Bakris G, et al. Management of high blood pressure in Blacks: an update of the International Society on Hypertension in Blacks consensus statement. *Hypertension*. 2010;56:780; and American Diabetes Association. Standards of medical care in diabetes. *Diabetes Care* 2004;27(suppl 1):s15–s35.

Step 2: Calculate 10-Year and Lifetime Global CVD Risk Using a Web-Based Calculator. Use the CVD risk calculators to establish 10-year and lifetime risk for ages 40 to 79 years (Box 16-5). The primary use of these risk estimates is to support and facilitate the important discussion regarding risk reduction between the clinician and patient.

BOX 16-5. Selected Web-Based Global CVD Risk Calculators

American College of Cardiology/American Heart Association	http://www.cvriskcalculator.com
American College of Cardiology	http://tools.acc.org/ASCVD-Risk-Estimator-Plus/#!/calculate/estimate

Step 3: Address Individual Risk Factors—Hypertension, Diabetes, Dyslipidemias, Metabolic Syndrome, Smoking, Family History, and Obesity.

Hypertension. The U.S. Preventive Services Task Force (USPSTF) recommends *screening all people age ≥18 years for high blood pressure.* Use the blood pressure classification of the Eighth Report of the Joint National Committee on Prevention, Detection, Evaluation, and Treatment of High Blood Pressure (JNC 8) based on rigorous scientific review of clinical trial data (Box 16-6).

BOX 16-6. Blood Pressure Categories for Adults (JNC 8)

Category[a]	Systolic (mm Hg)		Diastolic (mm Hg)
Normal	<120	and	<80
Elevated	120–129	and	<80
Stage 1 hypertension	130–139	or	80–89
Stage 2 hypertension	≥140	or	≥90

Patients with SBP and DBP in 2 categories should be designated to the higher BP category.

[a]BP indicates blood pressure (based on an average of 2 careful readings obtained on 2 occasions.

Source: James PA, Oparil S, Carter BL, et al. 2014 evidence-based guideline for the management of high blood pressure in adults: report from the panel members appointed to the Eighth Joint National Committee (JNC 8). *JAMA*. 2014;311(5):507–520.

Diabetes. Use the screening and diagnostic criteria shown in Boxes 16-7 and 16-8, respectively.

BOX 16-7. American Diabetes Association 2017: Classification and Diagnosis of Diabetes—Screening

Screening Criteria

For healthy adults with no risk factors: begin at age 45 years, repeat at 3-year intervals.

For adults with BMI ≥25 kg/m² and additional risk factors:

- HbA$_{1c}$ ≥5.7%, impaired glucose tolerance, or impaired fasting glucose on previous testing
- First-degree relative with diabetes
- High-risk ethnic population—African American, Native American, Latino American, Asian American, Pacific Islander
- Mothers of infants ≥4.08 kg (9 lb) at birth or diagnosed with gestational DM
- History of CVD
- Hypertension ≥140/90 mm Hg or on therapy for hypertension
- HDL cholesterol <35 mg/dL and/or triglycerides >250 mg/dL
- Women with polycystic ovary syndrome
- Physical inactivity
- Other conditions associated with insulin resistance such as severe obesity, acanthosis nigricans

Source: American Diabetes Association. Classification and diagnosis of diabetes. *Diabetes Care*. Jan 2017;40 (Supplement 1):S11–S24.

BOX 16-8. American Diabetes Association 2017: Classification and Diagnosis of Diabetes—Diagnosis

Diagnostic Criteria	Diabetes[a]	Prediabetes
HbA$_{1c}$	≥6.5%	5.7–6.4%
Fasting plasma glucose (on at least 2 occasions)	≥126 mg/dL	100–125 mg/dL
2-Hour plasma glucose (oral glucose tolerance test)	≥200 mg/dL	140–199 mg/dL
Random glucose if classic symptoms	≥200 mg/dL	

[a]In the absence of classic symptoms, an abnormal test must be repeated to confirm the diagnosis. However, if two different tests are both abnormal then no additional testing is necessary.

Source: American Diabetes Association. Classification and diagnosis of diabetes. *Diabetes Care.* 2017;40(Suppl 1):S11–S24.

Dyslipidemias. LDL is the primary target of cholesterol-lowering therapy. The USPSTF has issued a grade A recommendation for routine lipid screening for all men of age >35 years and women >45 years who are at increased risk for CHD; and a grade B recommendation to screen for lipid disorders beginning at age 20 years for men and women who have diabetes, hypertension, obesity, tobacco use, noncoronary atherosclerosis, or family history of early CVD. The most recent ACC/AHA Cholesterol Guideline provides evidence-based recommendations for initiating statin therapy based on high-, moderately high-, and low-risk level (Fig. 16-6).

Metabolic Syndrome. The *metabolic syndrome* consists of a cluster of risk factors which confer and increased risk of both CVD and diabetes. In 2009, the International Diabetes Association and other societies harmonized diagnostic criteria as the presence of any three of the following five risk factors: (1) an elevated waist circumference (population- and country-specific), (2) elevated triglycerides, (3) reduced HDL cholesterol, (4) elevated blood pressure, and (5) elevated fasting plasma glucose.

Other Risk Factors: Smoking, Family History, and Obesity. *Smoking* increases the risk of CHD and stroke by two- to fourfold compared to nonsmokers or past smokers who quit >10 years previously; about a third of the annual coronary heart disease deaths in the population, or over 120,000 deaths, are attributed to smoking. Among adults, 12% report a *family history* of heart attack or angina before age 50 years. Along with a family history of premature revascularization, this risk factor is associated with about a 50%

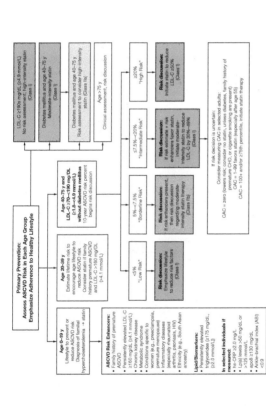

FIGURE 16-6. American College of Cardiology/American Heart Association Cholesterol Guideline. (Reprinted with permission from Grundy SM, et al. 2018 AHA/ACC/AACVPR/AAPA/ABC/ACPM/ADA/AGS/APhA/ASPC/NLA/PCNA Guideline on the Management of Blood Cholesterol: A Report of the American College of Cardiology/American Heart Association Task Force on Clinical Practice Guidelines. *Circulation.* 139(25):e1082-e1143. Copyright ©2018 American Heart Association, Inc.)

increased lifetime risk for CHD and for CVD mortality. *Obesity*, or BMI over 30 kg/m², contributed to 112,000 excess adult deaths compared to those of normal weight.

Promoting Lifestyle Change and Risk Factor Modification

Motivating behavior change is challenging, but it is an essential clinical skill for promoting risk factor reduction. Encourage the ACC/AHA recommendations (Box 16-9).

BOX 16-9. Lifestyle Modifications for Cardiovascular Health

- Optimal weight, or BMI of 18.5–24.9 kg/m²
- Intake of <6 g of sodium chloride or 2.3 g of sodium per day
- Regular aerobic exercise such as brisk walking three to four times a week, averaging 40 minutes per session
- Moderate alcohol consumption per day of ≤2 drinks for men and ≤1 drink for women (2 drinks = 1 oz ethanol, 24 oz beer, 10 oz wine, or 2–3 oz whiskey). Diet rich in fruits, vegetables, whole grains, and low-fat dairy products with reduced intake of saturated and total fat, sweets, and red meats.

Source: Eckel RH, Jakicic JM, Ard JD, et al. 2013 AHA/ACC guideline on lifestyle management to reduce cardiovascular risk: a report of the American College of Cardiology/American Heart Association Task Force on Practice Guidelines. *Circulation*. 2014;129:S76.

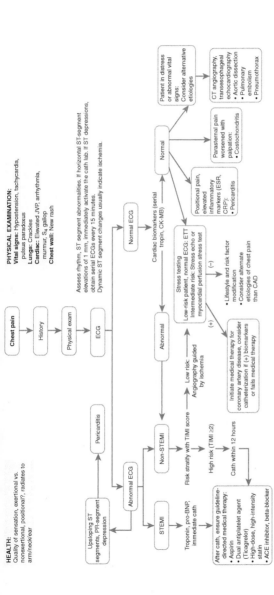

Algorithm 16-1. Approach to the patient with chest pain. (Note: Although it is not comprehensive, this algorithm may be a helpful starting approach for synthesizing information gathered from the history and physical.) *Risk factors: tobacco use, diabetes, hyperlipidemia, male age >55, female age >65, family history of CAD. BNP, brain natriuretic peptide; CAD, coronary artery disease; Cath, coronary angiography; CK-MB, creatine kinase-myocardial fraction; CRP, C-reactive protein; ECG, electrocardiogram; ESR, erythrocyte sedimentation rate; ETT, exercise treadmill test; HPI, history of present illness; TIMI, thrombolysis in myocardial infarction score. (One point for each: Known CAD ≥50% stenosis, + biomarkers, age ≥65, ≥three risk factors for CAD, ≥two anginal episodes in 24 hours, ST deviation by 0.5 mm, aspirin use in the last 7 days.)

HEALTH:
Quality of sensation, exertional vs.
nonexertional, positional?, radiates to
arm/neck/ear

PHYSICAL EXAMINATION:
Vital signs: Hypotension, tachycardia,
pulsus paradoxus
Lungs: Crackles
Cardiac: Elevated JVP, arrhythmia,
murmur, S₄ gallop
Chest wall: New rash

Chest pain

History

Physical exam

ECG

Assess rhythm, ST segment abnormalities. If horizontal ST-segment
elevations of 1 mm, immediately activate the cath lab. If ST depressions,
obtain serial ECGs every 15 minutes.
Dynamic ST segment changes usually indicate ischemia.

Pericarditis

Abnormal ECG

Upsloping ST
segments, PR-segment
depression

STEMI

Troponin, pro-BNP,
immediate cath

After cath, ensure guideline-
directed medical therapy:
• Aspirin
• Dual antiplatelet agent
  (Ticagrelor)
• High-dose, high-intensity
  statin
• ACE inhibitor, beta-blocker

Non-STEMI

Risk stratify with TIMI score

High risk (TIMI ≥2)

Cath within 12 hours

Low risk:
Angiography guided
by ischemia

Initiate medical therapy for
coronary artery disease, consider
catheterization if (+) biomarkers
or fails medical therapy

Normal ECG

Cardiac biomarkers (serial
tropin, CK-MB)

Abnormal

Stress testing
Low-risk patient, normal ECG: ETT
intermediate risk: Stress echo or
myocardial perfusion stress test

(+)

(−)
• Lifestyle and risk factor
  modification
• Consider alternate
  etiologies of chest pain
  than CAD

Normal

Positional pain,
elevated
inflammatory
markers (ESR,
CRP):
• Pericarditis

Parasternal pain
worsened with
palpation:
• Costochondritis

Patient in distress
or abnormal vital
signs:
Consider alternative
etiologies

CT angiography,
transesophageal
echocardiography
• Aortic dissection
• Pulmonary
  embolism
• Pneumothorax

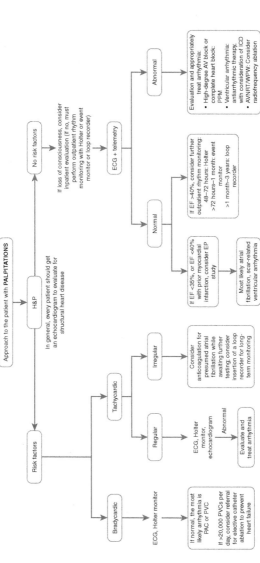

Algorithm 16-2. Approach to the patient with palpitations. (Note: Although it is not comprehensive, this algorithm may be a helpful starting approach for synthesizing information gathered from the history and physical.) *Risk factors: prior myocardial infarction, syncope, unexplained fracture, known reduced ejection fraction, palpitations >two times weekly. AVNRT, atrioventricular nodal reentry tachycardia; ECG, electrocardiogram; EF, ejection fraction; EP study, electrophysiologic study; H&P, history and physical examination; ICD, implantable cardiodefibrillator; PAC, premature atrial contraction; PPM, permanent pacemaker; PVC, premature ventricular contraction; WPW, Wolff–Parkinson–White syndrome.

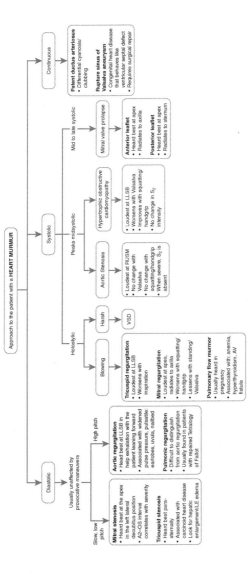

Algorithm 16-3. Approach to the patient with a murmur. (Note: Although it is not comprehensive, this algorithm may be a helpful starting approach for synthesizing information gathered from the history and physical.) AV, arteriovenous; LE, lower extremity; LLSB, left lower sternal border; RUSB, right upper sternal border; VSD, ventricular septal defect.

INTERPRETATION AIDS

TABLE 16-1. Chest Pain

Problem and Location	Quality, Severity, Timing, and Associated Symptoms
Pulmonary *Pleuritic Pain* Chest wall overlying the process	■ Sharp, knifelike quality ■ Often severe ■ Persistent timing ■ Associated symptoms of the underlying illness (often pneumonia, pulmonary embolism)
Cardiovascular *Angina Pectoris* Retrosternal or across the anterior chest, sometimes radiating to the shoulders, arms, neck, lower jaw, or upper abdomen	■ Pressing, squeezing, tight, heavy, occasionally burning ■ Mild to moderate severity, sometimes perceived as discomfort rather than pain ■ Usually 1–3 min but up to 10 min; prolonged episodes up to 20 min ■ Sometimes with dyspnea, nausea, swelling
Myocardial Infarction Same as in angina	■ Same as in angina ■ Often but not always a severe pain ■ 20 min to several hours ■ Associated with nausea, vomiting, sweating, weakness
Pericarditis *Retrosternal or Precordial:* May radiate to the tip of the shoulder and to the neck	■ Sharp, knifelike quality ■ Often severe ■ Persistent timing ■ Relieved by leaning forward ■ Seen in autoimmune disorders, postmyocardial infarction, viral infection, chest irradiation

TABLE 16-1. Chest Pain *(continued)*

Problem and Location	Quality, Severity, Timing, and Associated Symptoms
Dissecting Aortic Aneurysm Anterior chest, radiating to the neck, back, or abdomen	■ Ripping, tearing quality ■ Very severe ■ Abrupt onset, early peak, persistent for hours or more ■ Associated syncope, hemiplegia, paraplegia
Gastrointestinal *Gastrointestinal Reflux Disease* Retrosternal, may radiate to the back	■ Burning quality, may be squeezing ■ Mild to severe ■ Variable timing ■ Associated with regurgitation, dysphagia; also cough, laryngitis, asthma
Diffuse Esophageal Spasm Retrosternal, may radiate to the back, arms, and jaw	■ Usually squeezing quality ■ Mild to severe ■ Variable timing ■ Associated dysphagia
Others *Chest Wall Pain, Costochondritis* Often below the left breast or along the costal cartilages	■ Stabbing, sticking, or dull aching quality ■ Variable severity ■ Fleeting timing, hours or days ■ Often with local tenderness
Anxiety, Panic Disorder	■ Pain may be stabbing, sticking, or dull, aching ■ Can mimic angina ■ Associated with breathlessness, palpitations, weakness, anxiety

TABLE 16-2. Heart Sounds

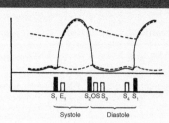

Finding	Possible Causes
S₁ accentuated	Tachycardia, states of high cardiac output; mitral stenosis
S₁ diminished	First-degree heart block; reduced left ventricular contractility; immobile mitral valve, as in mitral regurgitation
Systolic click(s)	Mitral valve prolapse
S₂ accentuated in right 2nd interspace	Systemic hypertension, dilated aortic root
S₂ diminished or absent in right 2nd interspace	Immobile aortic valve, as in calcific aortic stenosis
P₂ accentuated	Pulmonary hypertension, dilated pulmonary artery, atrial septal defect
P₂ diminished or absent	Aging, pulmonic stenosis
Opening snap	Mitral stenosis
S₃	Physiologic (usually in children and young adults); volume overload of ventricle, as in mitral regurgitation or heart failure
S₄	Excellent physical conditioning (trained athletes); resistance to ventricular filling because of decreased compliance, left ventricular hypertrophy from pressure overload, as in hypertensive heart disease or aortic stenosis

TABLE 16-3. Variations in the First Heart Sound—S_1

Normal Variations

S_1 is softer than S_2 at the *base* (right and left 2nd interspaces).

S_1 S_2

S_1 is often but not always louder than S_2 at the *apex*.

S_1 S_2

Accentuated S_1

S_1 S_2

Occurs in (1) tachycardia, rhythms with a short PR interval, and high cardiac output states (e.g., exercise, anemia, hyperthyroidism), and (2) mitral stenosis.

Diminished S_1

S_1 S_2

Occurs in first-degree heart block, calcified mitral valve of mitral regurgitation, and ↓ left ventricular contractility in heart failure or coronary heart disease.

Varying S_1

S_1 S_2 S_1 S_2

S_1 varies in complete heart block and any totally irregular rhythm (e.g., atrial fibrillation).

Split S_1

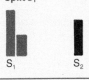

S_1 S_2

Normally heard along the **lower left sternal border** if audible tricuspid component. If S_1 sounds split at apex, consider an S_4, an aortic ejection sound, an early systolic click, right bundle branch block, and premature ventricular contractions.

TABLE 16-4. Variations in the Second Heart Sound—S₂ During Inspiration and Expiration

Physiologic Splitting

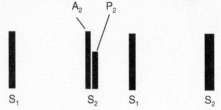

Heard in the 2nd or 3rd left interspace: the pulmonic component of S₂ is usually too faint to be heard at the apex or aortic area, where S₂ is single and derived from aortic valve closure alone. Accentuated by inspiration; usually disappears on exertion.

Pathologic Splitting

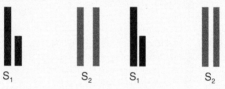

Wide splitting of S₂ persists throughout respiration; arises from delayed closure of the pulmonic valve (e.g., by pulmonic stenosis or right bundle branch block); also from early closure of the aortic valve, as in mitral regurgitation.

Fixed Splitting

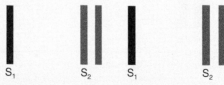

Does not vary with respiration, as in atrial septal defect, right ventricular failure.

**TABLE 16-4. Variations in the Second Heart Sound—
S₂ During Inspiration and Expiration** *(continued)*

Paradoxical or Reversed Splitting

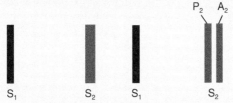

Appears on expiration and disappears on inspiration. Closure of the aortic valve is abnormally delayed, so A_2 follows P_2 on expiration, as in left bundle branch block.

More on A_2 and P_2

Increased Intensity of A_2, 2nd Right Interspace (where only A_2 can usually be heard) occurs in systemic hypertension because of the increased ejection pressure. It also occurs when the aortic root is dilated, probably because the aortic valve is then closer to the chest wall.

Decreased or Absent A_2, 2nd Right Interspace is noted in calcific aortic stenosis because of immobility of the valve. If A_2 is inaudible, no splitting is heard.

Increased Intensity of P_2. When P_2 is equal to or louder than A_2, pulmonary hypertension may be suspected. Other causes include a dilated pulmonary artery and an atrial septal defect. When a split S_2 is heard widely, even at the apex and the right base, P_2 is accentuated.

Decreased or Absent P_2 is most commonly due to the increased anteroposterior diameter of the chest associated with aging. It can also result from pulmonic stenosis. If P_2 is inaudible, no splitting is heard.

TABLE 16-5. Heart Murmurs

	Likely Causes
Midsystolic	Innocent murmurs (no valve abnormality)
	Physiologic murmurs (from ↑ flow across a semilunar valve, as in pregnancy, fever, anemia)
	Aortic stenosis
	Murmurs that mimic aortic stenosis—aortic sclerosis, bicuspid aortic valve, dilated aorta, and pathologically ↑ systolic flow across aortic valve
	Hypertrophic cardiomyopathy
	Pulmonic stenosis
Pansystolic	Mitral regurgitation
	Tricuspid regurgitation
	Ventricular septal defect
Late Systolic	Mitral valve prolapse, often with click (C)
Early Diastolic	Aortic regurgitation
Middiastolic and Presystolic	Mitral stenosis—note opening snap (OS)
Continuous Murmurs and Sounds	Patent ductus arteriosus—harsh, machinery-like
	Pericardial friction rub—a scratchy sound with 1–3 components
	Venous hum—continuous, above midclavicles, loudest in diastole

Peripheral Vascular System

HEALTH HISTORY

Common or Concerning Symptoms

- Pain and swelling of legs and arms
- Cramping in legs on exertion with relief with rest (*intermittent claudication*)
- Cold, numbness, pallor, or discoloration in legs; hair loss
- Abdominal, flank, or back pain

Pain and Swelling in Arms and Legs

Ask about any pain in the arms and legs.

Cold-induced digital ischemic change with blanching then cyanosis then rubor in Raynaud phenomenon or disease. See Algorithm 17-1, Approach to the patient with leg pain, p. 280.

Ask about *swelling of feet and legs*, or any ulcers on lower legs, often near the ankles from peripheral vascular disease.

Calf swelling in deep venous thrombosis (DVT); hyperpigmentation, edema, and possible cyanosis, especially when legs are dependent, in *venous stasis ulcers;* swelling with redness and tenderness in *cellulitis.* See Algorithm 17-2, Approach to the patient with leg swelling, p. 281.

Cramping in Legs on Exertion and Relief with Rest (Intermittent Claudication)

Is there *intermittent claudication,* exercise-induced pain that is absent at rest, makes the patient stop exertion, and abates within about 10 minutes? Ask "Have you ever had any pain or cramping in your legs when you walk or exercise?" "How far can you walk

Peripheral arterial disease (PAD) can cause symptomatic limb ischemia with exertion; distinguish this from the neurogenic pain of spinal stenosis, which produces leg pain with exertion, often reduced by leaning forward (stretching the spinal cord in the narrowed vertebral canal) and less readily relieved by rest.

without stopping to rest?" and "Does pain improve with rest?"

Because patients have few symptoms, identify risk factors—tobacco abuse, hypertension, diabetes, hyperlipidemia, and coronary artery disease—and PAD warning signs (Box 17-1).

Only 10% to 30% of affected patients have the classic symptoms of exertional calf pain relieved by rest.

BOX 17-1. Peripheral Arterial Disease Warning Signs

- Fatigue, aching, numbness, or pain that limits walking or exertion in the legs; if present, identify the location. Ask also about erectile dysfunction.
- Any poorly healing or nonhealing wounds of the legs or feet
- Any pain present when at rest in the lower leg or foot and changes when standing or supine

- Abdominal pain after meals and associated *food fear* (patients do not want to eat because they experience the pain) and weight loss

- Any first-degree relatives with an AAA

Symptom location suggests the site of arterial ischemia:

- Buttock, hip: *aortoiliac*
- Erectile dysfunction: *iliac–pudenda*
- Thigh: *common femoral* or *aortoiliac*
- Upper calf: *superficial femoral*
- Lower calf: *popliteal*
- Foot: *tibial* or *peroneal*

These symptoms suggest intestinal ischemia of the *celiac* or *superior* or *inferior mesenteric arteries.*

Prevalence of AAAs in first-degree relatives is 15% to 28%.

Cold, Numbness, Pallor, or Discoloration in Legs; Hair Loss

Ask also about *coldness, numbness,* or *pallor* in legs or feet or *hair loss* over the anterior tibial surfaces.

Hair loss over the anterior tibiae in PAD. "Dry" or brown–black ulcers from gangrene may ensue. See Algorithm 17-3, Approach to the patient with leg discoloration, p. 282.

Abdominal, Flank, or Back Pain

Ask about abdominal, flank, or back pain, especially in older male smokers.

An expanding abdominal aortic aneurysm (AAA) may compress arteries or ureters.

TECHNIQUES OF EXAMINATION

Key Components of the Peripheral Vascular System Examination

Arms:
- Inspect upper extremities
- Palpate upper extremities (radial pulse, brachial pulse, epitrochlear lymph nodes)

Abdomen:
- Palpate inguinal lymph nodes
- Palpate abdomen (aortic width and pulsation)
- Auscultate abdomen (aortic, renal, and femoral bruits)

Legs:
- Inspect lower extremities
- Palpate lower extremities (femoral pulse, popliteal pulse, dorsalis pedis pulse, posterior tibial pulse, temperature, swelling)

In addition, review the techniques for assessing blood pressure, carotid artery, aorta, renal and femoral arteries:
- Measure blood pressure in both arms (see Chapter 8, General Survey, Vital Signs, and Pain, pp. 116–121)
- Palpate carotid upstroke, auscultate for bruits (see Chapter 16, Cardiovascular System, pp. 244–246)
- Auscultate for aortic, renal, and femoral bruits; palpate aorta and assess its maximal diameter (see Chapter 19, Abdomen, pp. 304–307)

♀ Arms

Inspect for:

Size and symmetry, any swelling	Lymphedema, venous obstruction.
Venous pattern	Visible venous collaterals, swelling, edema, and discoloration signal upper extremity DVT.
Color and texture of skin and nails	Sharply demarcated pallor of the fingers in Raynaud disease.

Palpate and grade the pulses (Box 17-2):

BOX 17-2. Recommended Grading of Arterial Pulses

3+	Bounding
2+	Brisk, expected (normal)
1+	Diminished, weaker than expected
0	Absent, unable to palpate

■ Radial (Fig. 17-1)

Bounding radial, carotid, and femoral pulses in aortic regurgitation.

Lost in thromboangiitis obliterans or acute arterial occlusion.

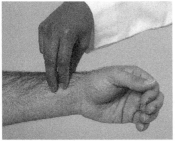

FIGURE 17-1. Palpating the radial pulse.

■ Brachial (Fig. 17-2)

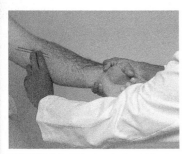

FIGURE 17-2. Palpating the brachial pulse.

Feel for the epitrochlear nodes.

Lymphadenopathy from local or distal infection, lymphoma, or human immunodeficiency virus (HIV).

๐ Abdomen

Auscultate for aortic, renal, and femoral bruits.

Palpate gently and estimate the width of the abdominal aorta between your two fingers (see p. 545).

Pulsatile mass, AAA if width ≥4 cm.

Palpate the superficial inguinal nodes (Fig. 17-3). Note size, consistency, discreteness, and any tenderness.

Lymphadenopathy in genital infections, lymphoma, AIDS.

- Horizontal group

- Vertical group

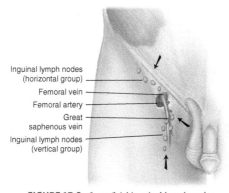

Inguinal lymph nodes
(horizontal group)
Femoral vein
Femoral artery
Great
saphenous vein
Inguinal lymph nodes
(vertical group)

FIGURE 17-3. Superficial inguinal lymph nodes.

๐ Legs

Inspect for:

See Table 17-1, Chronic Insufficiency of Arteries and Veins, p. 283, and Table 17-2, Common Ulcers of the Feet and Ankles, p. 284.

- Size and symmetry, any swelling in thigh or calf

Venous insufficiency, lymphedema; DVT. Calf asymmetry >3 cm (measure 10 cm below tibial tuberosity) doubles the risk of DVT.

- Venous pattern

Varicose veins

- Color and texture of skin

Pallor, rubor, cyanosis; erythema, warmth in *cellulitis, thrombophlebitis*; pigmentation, ulcers of the feet in PAD

- Hair distribution, temperature

Palpate and grade the pulses:

- Femoral

- Popliteal (Fig. 17-4)

Atrophic hairless cool skin in PAD

Loss of pulses in acute arterial occlusion and arteriosclerosis obliterans

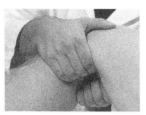

FIGURE 17-4. Palpating the popliteal pulse.

- Dorsalis pedis and posterior tibial (Figs. 17-5 and 17-6)

Absent pedal pulses with normal femoral and popliteal pulses make PAD highly likely. Confirm with the ABI (see Box 17-3, Using the Ankle–Brachial Index, pp. 275–276).

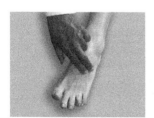

FIGURE 17-5. Palpating the dorsalis pedis pulse.

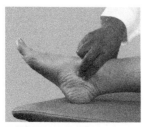

FIGURE 17-6. Palpating the posterior tibial pulse.

Palpate for pitting edema.	Dependent edema, heart failure, hypo-albuminemia, nephrotic syndrome.
Palpate the calves.	Possible cord and tenderness in DVT (not always present).
Ask patient to stand and reinspect the venous pattern.	Varicose veins.

Special Techniques

Assessing for Peripheral Arterial Disease. To screen for PAD, use the *ankle–brachial index (ABI)*, which is the ratio of blood pressure measurements in the foot and arm (Box 17-3); values <0.9 are considered abnormal.

BOX 17-3. Measuring the Ankle–Brachial Index

Instructions for Measuring the Ankle–Brachial Index (ABI)

1. Patient should rest supine in a warm room for at least 10 minutes before testing.

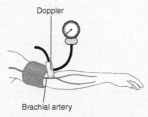

2. Place blood pressure cuffs on both arms and ankles as illustrated, then apply ultrasound gel over brachial, dorsalis pedis, and posterior tibial arteries.
3. Measure systolic pressures in the arms (brachial pressure)
   - Use vascular Doppler to locate brachial pulse
   - Inflate cuff 20 mm Hg above last audible pulse
   - Deflate cuff slowly and record pressure at which pulse becomes audible
   - Obtain 2 measures in each arm and record the average as the brachial pressure in that arm

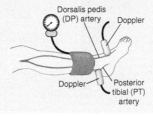

continued

4. Measure systolic pressures in ankles (ankle pressure)
   - Use vascular Doppler to locate dorsalis pedis pulse
   - Inflate cuff 20 mm Hg above last audible pulse
   - Deflate cuff slowly and record pressure at which pulse becomes audible
   - Obtain 2 measures in each ankle and record the average as the dorsalis pedis pressure in that leg
   - Repeat above steps for posterior tibial arteries
5. Calculate ABI for each leg.
   - Calculated ABI values should be recorded to 2 decimal places.

$$\text{Right ABI} = \frac{\text{highest right average ankle pressure (DP or PT)}}{\text{highest average arm pressure (right or left)}}$$

$$\text{Left ABI} = \frac{\text{highest left average ankle pressure (DP or PT)}}{\text{highest average arm pressure (right or left)}}$$

Interpretation of Ankle–Brachial Index

Ankle–Brachial Index Result	Clinical Interpretation
>0.90 (with a range of 0.90 to 1.30)	Normal lower extremity blood flow
>0.60 to <0.89	Mild PAD
>0.40 to <0.59	Moderate PAD
<0.39	Severe PAD

⚕ Evaluating Arterial Supply to the Hand. Feel ulnar pulse, if possible. Perform an *Allen test.*

1. Ask the patient to make a tight fist, palm up. Occlude both radial and ulnar arteries with your thumb (Fig. 17-7).

2. Ask the patient to open hand into a relaxed, slightly flexed position (Fig. 17-8).

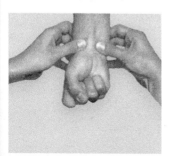

FIGURE 17-7. Compress the radial and ulnar arteries.

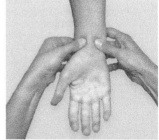

FIGURE 17-8. Pallor when hand relaxed.

3. Release your pressure over one artery. Palm should flush within 3 to 5 seconds (Fig. 17-9).

4. Repeat, releasing other artery. Persisting pallor of palm indicates occlusion of the released artery or its distal branches (Fig. 17-10).

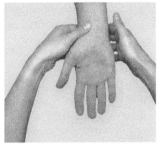

FIGURE 17-9. Palmar flushing—Allen test negative showing patent arterial circulation.

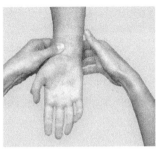

FIGURE 17-10. Palmar pallor—Allen test positive showing possible occlusive disease.

RECORDING YOUR FINDINGS

Recording the Peripheral Vascular System Examination

"Extremities are warm and without edema. No varicosities or stasis changes. Calves are supple and nontender. No femoral or abdominal bruits. Brachial, radial, femoral, popliteal, dorsalis pedis (DP), and posterior tibial (PT) pulses are 2+ and symmetric."

OR

"Extremities are pale below the midcalf, with notable hair loss. Redness noted when legs dependent but no edema or ulceration. Bilateral femoral bruits; no abdominal bruits heard. Brachial and radial pulses 2+; femoral, popliteal, DP, and PT pulses 1+." Alternatively, pulses can be recorded as below.

	Radial	Brachial	Femoral	Popliteal	Dorsalis Pedis	Posterior Tibial
RT	2+	2+	1+	1+	1+	1+
LT	2+	2+	1+	1+	1+	1+

These findings suggest atherosclerotic PAD.

HEALTH PROMOTION AND COUNSELING: EVIDENCE AND RECOMMENDATIONS

Important Topics for Health Promotion and Counseling

- Screening for lower extremity peripheral artery disease
- Screening for abdominal aortic aneurysm

Screening for Peripheral Arterial Disease

PAD prevalence increases with age, ranging from around 8% of adults age 65 to 75 years to 18% in persons aged 75 years and older. Cardiovascular risk factors, particularly smoking and diabetes, increase risk: An estimated 40% to 60% of PAD patients have coexisting coronary artery disease and/or cerebral artery disease, and the presence of PAD significantly increases risk of cardiovascular events. Most patients with PAD have either no symptoms or a range of nonspecific leg symptoms, such as aching, cramping, numbness, or fatigue. The USPSTF does not advocate PAD screening due to insufficient available evidence to estimate the relative benefits and harms of ankle–brachial index (ABI) testing (I statement). However, the American Heart Association/American College of Cardiology practice guideline suggests that it is reasonable to use ABI to screen for PAD in patients with risk factors (Box 17-4).

BOX 17-4. Risk Factors for Lower Extremity Peripheral Arterial Disease

- Age ≥65 years
- Age ≥50 years with a history of diabetes or smoking
- Leg symptoms with exertion
- Nonhealing wounds

Screening for Abdominal Aortic Aneurysm

AAA is present when the infrarenal aortic diameter exceeds 3 cm. Rupture and mortality rates dramatically increase for AAAs exceeding 5.5 cm in diameter. Additional risk factors are smoking, age older than 65 years, family history, coronary artery disease, PAD, hypertension, and elevated cholesterol level. Because symptoms are rare, and screening has been shown to reduce mortality by 50% over 13 to 15 years, the U.S. Preventive Services Task Force (USPSTF) recommends one-time screening by ultrasound in men between 65 and 75 years of age with a history of "ever smoking," defined as more than 100 cigarettes in a lifetime; evidence is insufficient regarding screening women in this age range who have ever smoked (I statement); and the USPSTF recommends against screening women who have never smoked (grade D).

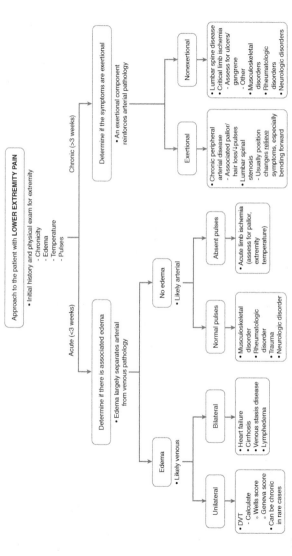

Algorithm 17-1. Approach to the patient with leg pain. (Note: Although it is not comprehensive, this algorithm may be a helpful starting approach for synthesizing information gathered from the history and physical.) DVT, deep vein thrombosis.

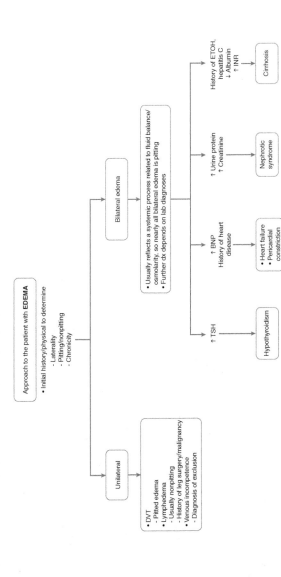

Algorithm 17-2. Approach to the patient with leg swelling. (Note: Although it is not comprehensive, this algorithm may be a helpful starting approach for synthesizing information gathered from the history and physical.) BNP, brain natriuretic peptide; DVT, deep vein thrombosis; EtOH, ethanol; INR, international normalized ratio; TSH, thyroid-stimulating hormone.

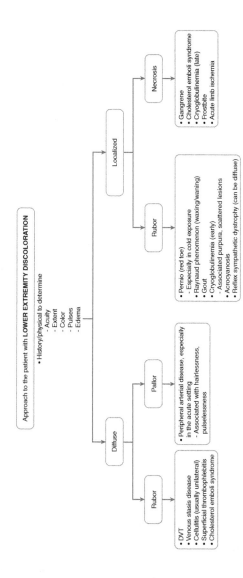

Algorithm 17-3. Approach to the patient with leg discoloration. (Note: Although it is not comprehensive, this algorithm may be a helpful starting approach for synthesizing information gathered from the history and physical.) DVT, deep vein thrombosis.

INTERPRETATION AIDS

TABLE 17-1. Chronic Insufficiency of Arteries and Veins

Condition	Characteristics
Chronic Arterial Insufficiency 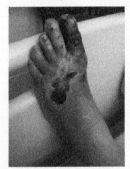	Intermittent claudication progressing to pain at rest. Decreased or absent pulses. Pale, especially on elevation; dusky red on dependency. Cool. Absent or mild edema, which may develop on lowering the leg to relieve pain. Thin, shiny, atrophic skin; hair loss over foot and toes; thickened, ridged nails. Possible ulceration on toes or points of trauma on feet. Potential for gangrene.
Chronic Venous Insufficiency 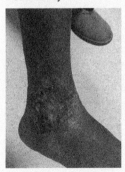	No pain to aching pain on dependency. Normal pulses, though may be hard to feel because of edema. Color normal or cyanotic on dependency; petechiae or brown pigment may develop. Often marked edema. Stasis dermatitis, possible thickening of skin, and narrowing of leg as scarring develops. Potential ulceration at sides of ankles. No gangrene.

Source of photos: Courtesy of Daniel Han, MD.

TABLE 17-2. Common Ulcers of the Feet and Ankles

Ulcer	Characteristics
Arterial Insufficiency 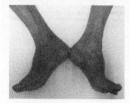	Located on toes, feet, or possible areas of trauma. No callus or excess pigment. May be atrophic. Pain often severe, unless masked by neuropathy. Possible gangrene. Decreased pulses, trophic changes, pallor of foot on elevation, dusky rubor on dependency.
Chronic Venous Insufficiency 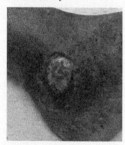	Located on inner or outer ankle. Pigmented, sometimes fibrotic. Pain not severe. No gangrene. Edema, pigmentation, stasis dermatitis, and possibly cyanosis of feet on dependency.
Neuropathic Ulcer 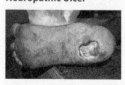	Located on pressure points in areas with diminished sensation, as in diabetic neuropathy. Skin calloused. No pain (which may cause ulcer to go unnoticed). Usually no gangrene. Decreased sensation, absent ankle jerks.

Breasts and Axillae

HEALTH HISTORY

Common or Concerning Symptoms

- Breast lump or mass
- Breast discomfort or pain
- Nipple discharge

Breast Lump or Mass

Ask, "Do you examine your breasts?", "How often?" Ask about any masses or lumps in the breasts. Identify precise location, how long it has been present, any history of trauma, tender, and any change in size or variation with menstrual cycle. All breast masses warrant careful evaluation, and definitive diagnostic measures should be pursued.

Lumps may be physiologic or pathologic, ranging from cysts and fibroadenomas to breast cancer. See Algorithm 18-1, Approach to the patient with a breast lump or mass, p. 293.

See Table 18-1, Palpable Masses of the Breast, p. 296.

Breast Discomfort or Pain

Ask about any discomfort, or pain in the breasts.

Medications associated with breast pain include selective serotonin-reuptake inhibitors, haloperiodol, spironolactone, and digoxin. See Algorithm 18-2, Approach to the patient with breast discomfort or pain, p. 294.

Nipple Discharge

Also ask about any discharge from the nipples, change in breast contour, dimpling, swelling, or puckering of the skin over the breasts (see Algorithm 18-3, Approach to the patient with nipple discharge, p. 295).

TECHNIQUES OF EXAMINATION

Key Components of the Breasts and Axillae Examination

In women:
- Inspect breasts in four views: arms at sides, arms over head, arms pressed against hips, and leaning forward (skin appearance, size, symmetry, contour, nipple characteristics)
- Palpate breasts
- Inspect axillae
- Palpate axillary nodes

In men:
- Inspect nipple and areola
- Palpate areola and breast tissue

Female Breast

Inspect the breasts in four positions, identifying the quadrant where changes appear (Figs. 18-1 through 18-5).

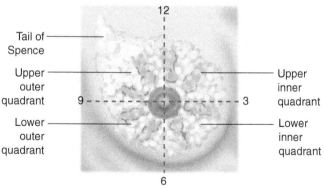

FIGURE 18-1. Breast quadrants.

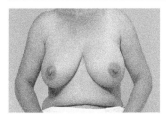

FIGURE 18-2. Inspection with arms at sides.

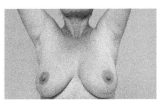

FIGURE 18-3. Inspection with arms overhead.

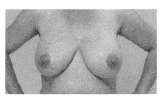

FIGURE 18-4. Inspection with hands pressed against hips.

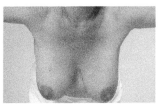

FIGURE 18-5. Inspection while leaning forward.

Note:

- Size and symmetry

  See Table 18-2, Visible Signs of Breast Cancer, p. 297.

- Contour

  Flattening, dimpling suspicious for malignancy

- Appearance of the skin

  Edema (peau d'orange) in breast cancer

Inspect the nipples.

- Compare their size, shape, and direction of pointing.

  Inversion, retraction, deviation

- Note any rashes, ulcerations, or discharge.

  Paget disease of the nipple, galactorrhea

Palpate the breasts, including augmented breasts. Breast tissue should be flattened and the patient supine.

Use a *vertical strip pattern* (currently the best validated technique) or a circular or wedge pattern. Palpate in *small, concentric circles.*

- For *the lateral portion of the breast,* ask the patient to roll onto the opposite hip, place her hand on her forehead, but keep shoulders pressed against the bed or examining table (Fig. 18-6).

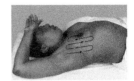

FIGURE 18-6. Vertical strip pattern—lateral breast.

- For *the medial portion of the breast,* ask the patient to lie with her shoulders flat against the bed or examining table, place her hand at her neck, and lift up her elbow until it is even with her shoulder (Fig. 18-7).

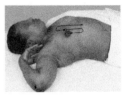

FIGURE 18-7. Vertical strip pattern—medial breast.

Palpate a rectangular area extending from the clavicle to the inframammary fold, and from the midsternal line to the posterior axillary line and well into the axilla for the tail of Spence.

Note:

- Consistency   Physiologic nodularity

- Tenderness   Infection, premenstrual tenderness

- Nodules. If present, note location,   Cyst, fibroadenoma, cancer
  size, shape, consistency, delimitation,
  tenderness, and mobility.

Palpate each nipple.   Thickening in cancer

Compress the areola in a spoke-like   Type and source of discharge may be
pattern around the nipple. Watch for   identified.
discharge.

Palpate and inspect along the incision Local recurrences of breast cancer
lines of mastectomy.

Male Breast

Inspect and palpate the nipple and areola.

Gynecomastia, mass suspicious for cancer, fat

Axillae

Inspect for rashes, infection, and pigmentation.

Hidradenitis suppurativa, acanthosis nigricans

Palpate the axillary nodes, including the central, pectoral, lateral, and subscapular groups (Fig. 18-8).

Lymphadenopathy

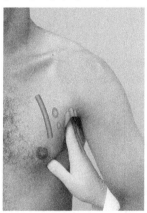

FIGURE 18-8. Palpating the left axilla.

RECORDING YOUR FINDINGS

Recording the Breasts and Axillae Examination

"Breasts symmetric and smooth, without masses. Nipples without discharge." (Axillary adenopathy usually included after neck in section on lymph nodes.)

OR

"Breasts pendulous with diffuse fibrocystic changes. Single firm 1×1 cm mass, mobile and nontender, with overlying peau d'orange appearance in right breast, upper outer quadrant at 11 o'clock, 2 cm from the nipple."

These findings suggest possible breast cancer.

HEALTH PROMOTION AND COUNSELING: EVIDENCE AND RECOMMENDATIONS

Important Topics for Health Promotion and Counseling

- Breast cancer risk assessment
- Breast cancer screening

Breast Cancer Risk Assessment

About 50% of affected women have no known predisposing risk factors; however, selected risk factors are well established (Box 18-1).

BOX 18-1. Breast Cancer Risk Factors

Nonmodifiable risk factors:
- Age (most important)
- Family history of breast and ovarian cancers
- Inherited genetic mutations
- Personal history of breast cancer or lobular carcinoma in situ
- High levels of endogenous hormones
- Breast tissue density
- Proliferative lesions with atypia on breast biopsy
- Duration of unopposed estrogen exposure related to early menarche
- Age of first full-term pregnancy
- Late menopause
- Breast density on mammograms (commands increasing importance as a strong independent risk factor)
- History of radiation to the chest
- History of diethylstilbestrol (DES) exposure

Modifiable risk factors:
- Breastfeeding for <1 year
- Postmenopausal obesity
- Use of hormone replacement therapy (HRT)
- Cigarette smoking
- Alcohol ingestion
- Physical inactivity
- Type of contraception

See Table 18-3, Breast Cancer in Women: Factors that Increase Relative Risk for Breast Cancer in Women, p. 298.

A number of breast cancer risk assessment calculators and tools can be used to help women determine their personal risk of developing breast cancer (Box 18-2).

BOX 18-2. Calculators for Assessing Risk of Breast Cancer

- Gail model: http://www.cancer.gov/bcrisktool/
- Centers for Disease Control and Prevention Division of Cancer Prevention and Control—Know BRCA Tool: https://www.knowbrca.org/

Breast Cancer Screening

Mammography combined with the clinical breast exam (CBE) are the most common screening modalities; however, recommendations from professional groups vary about how to screen, when to start screening, and screening intervals, as shown in Box 18-3. Clinicians should be well informed as they counsel individual patients, particularly as more evidence emerges to guide risk-based screening.

BOX 18-3. Recommendations for Breast Cancer Screening in Average-Risk Women

Organization	Mammography	Clinical Breast Examination	Breast Self-Examination
U.S. Preventative Services Task Force—average-risk women	50–74 years—biennially <50 years—individualize screening based on patient specific factors ≥75 years—insufficient evidence to assess the balance of benefits and harms	Insufficient evidence to assess the additional benefits and harms beyond screening mammography	Recommends against teaching breast self-examination, supports breast self-awareness

continued

Organization	Mammography	Clinical Breast Examination	Breast Self-Examination
American Cancer Society—average-risk women (2015)	40–45 years—optional annual screening 45–54 years—annual screening ≥55 years—biennial screening with option to continue annual screens Continue screening if good health and life expectancy ≥10 years	Not recommended	Not recommended
American College of Obstetricians and Gynecologists	Offer screening starting at age 40 years Screening should be every 1 or 2 years based on a shared decision-making process Continue screening until at least age 75	May be offered in context of a shared decision-making process every 1–3 years for women aged 25–39 years and annually for women 40 years and older	Not recommended, but women should be counseled about breast self-awareness

Sources: Siu AL, U.S. Preventive Services Task Force. Screening for breast cancer: U.S. Preventive services task force recommendation statement. *Ann Intern Med*. 2016;164:279–296; Oeffinger KC, Fontham ET, Etzioni R, et al. Breast cancer screening for women at average risk: 2015 guideline update from the American cancer society. *JAMA*. 2015;314:1599–1614; Practice bulletin No. 179 Summary: Breast cancer risk assessment and screening in average-risk women. *Obstet Gynecol*. 2017;130:241–243.

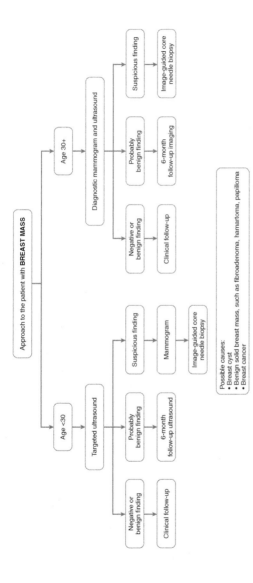

Algorithm 18-1. Approach to the patient with a breast lump or mass. (Note: Although it is not comprehensive, this algorithm may be a helpful starting approach for synthesizing information gathered from the history and physical.)

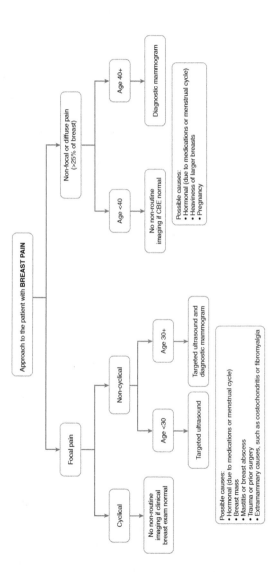

Algorithm 18-2. Approach to the patient with breast discomfort or pain. (Note: Although it is not comprehensive, this algorithm may be a helpful starting approach for synthesizing information gathered from the history and physical.) CBE, clinical breast exam.

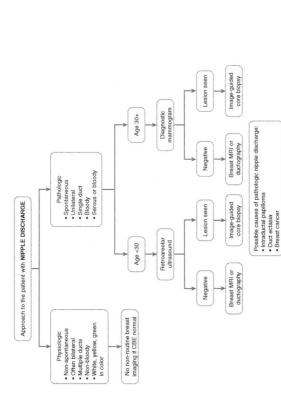

Algorithm 18-3. Approach to the patient with nipple discharge. (Note: Although it is not comprehensive, this algorithm may be a helpful starting approach for synthesizing information gathered from the history and physical.) CBE, clinical breast exam; MRI, magnetic resonance imaging.

INTERPRETATION AIDS

TABLE 18-1. Palpable Masses of the Breast

Age	Common Lesion	Characteristics
15–25	Fibroadenoma	Usually smooth, rubbery, round, mobile, nontender
25–50	Cysts	Usually soft to firm, round, mobile; often tender
	Fibrocystic changes	Nodular, rope-like
	Cancer	Irregular, firm, may be mobile or fixed to surrounding tissue
Over 50	Cancer until proven otherwise	Irregular, firm, may be mobile or fixed to surrounding tissue
Pregnancy/lactation	Lactating adenomas, cysts, mastitis, and cancer	Irregular, firm, may be mobile or fixed to surrounding tissue

Adapted from Schultz MZ, Ward BA, Reiss M. Breast diseases. In: Noble J, Greene HL, Levinson W, et al. eds. *Primary Care Medicine*. 3rd ed. St. Louis, MO; 2000; Pruthi S. Detection and evaluation of a palpable breast mass. *Mayo Clin Proc*. 2001;76(6):641–647.

TABLE 18-2. Visible Signs of Breast Cancer

Retraction Signs

Fibrosis from breast cancer, fat necrosis, and mammary duct ectasia can produce the three retraction signs illustrated here.

Skin Dimpling

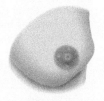

Abnormal Contours
Look for any variation in the normal convexity of each breast, and compare one side with the other.

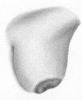

Nipple Retraction and Deviation
A retracted nipple is flattened or pulled inward and may be broadened and thickened. Typically, the nipple deviates toward the underlying cancer.

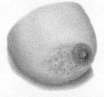

Edema of the Skin
From lymphatic blockade, appearing as thickened skin with enlarged pores—the so-called *peau d'orange* (orange peel) *sign.*

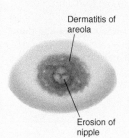

Dermatitis of areola

Erosion of nipple

Paget Disease of the Nipple
An uncommon form of breast cancer that usually starts as a scaly, eczema-like lesion that may weep, crust, or erode. A breast mass may be present. Suspect Paget disease in any persisting dermatitis of the nipple and areola.

TABLE 18-3. Factors that Increase Relative Risk for Breast Cancer in Women

Relative Risk	Factor
>4.0	■ Age (65+ versus <65 years, although risk increases across all ages until age 80) ■ Atypical hyperplasia ■ Lobular carcinoma in situ ■ Pathogenic genetic variations (e.g., *BRCA1*, *BRCA2*, *PALB2*, *TP53*)
2.1–4.0	■ Ductal carcinoma in situ ■ High endogenous hormone levels (postmenopausal) ■ High-dose radiation to chest (e.g., Hodgkin lymphoma treatment) ■ Mammographically dense breasts ■ Two or more first-degree relatives with breast cancer
1.1–2.0	■ Alcohol consumption ■ Early menarche (<11 years) ■ Excess body weight ■ High endogenous estrogen or testosterone levels (premenopausal) ■ Late age at first full-term pregnancy (>30 years) ■ Late menopause (≥55 years) ■ Never breastfed a child ■ No full-term pregnancies ■ One first-degree relative with breast cancer ■ Obesity (postmenopausal) ■ Personal history of ovarian or endometrial cancer ■ Physical inactivity ■ Proliferative breast disease without atypia (usual ductal hyperplasia, fibroadenoma) ■ Recent and long-term use of menopausal hormone therapy containing estrogen and progestin ■ Recent hormonal contraceptive use ■ Weight gain in adulthood ■ Tall height

Note: Relative risks for some factors vary by breast cancer molecular subtype.

Source: Reprinted with permission from American Cancer Society. *Breast Cancer Facts and Figures 2019–2020*. Atlanta: American Cancer Society, Inc.; 2019. Available at https://www.cancer.org/content/dam/cancer-org/research/cancer-facts-and-statistics/breast-cancer-facts-and-figures/breast-cancer-facts-and-figures-2019-2020.pdf. Accessed July 21, 2020.

Abdomen

HEALTH HISTORY

Common or Concerning Symptoms

Gastrointestinal Disorders	Urinary and Renal Disorders
<ul><li>Abdominal pain, acute and chronic</li><li>Indigestion, nausea, vomiting including blood (*hematemesis*), loss of appetite (*anorexia*), early satiety</li><li>Difficulty swallowing (*dysphagia*) and/or painful swallowing (*odynophagia*)</li><li>Change in bowel function</li><li>Diarrhea, constipation</li><li>Jaundice</li></ul>	<ul><li>Suprapubic pain</li><li>Difficulty urinating (*dysuria*), urgency, or frequency</li><li>Excessive urination (*polyuria*) or excess urination at night (*nocturia*)</li><li>Urinary incontinence</li><li>Blood in the urine (*hematuria*)</li><li>Flank pain and ureteral colic</li></ul>

Mechanisms of Abdominal Pain

Be familiar with three broad categories (Box 19-1):

BOX 19-1. Categories of Abdominal Pain

Visceral pain	<ul><li>Occurs when hollow abdominal organs such as the intestine or biliary tree contract unusually forcefully or are distended or stretched.</li></ul>	<ul><li>May be difficult to localize</li><li>Varies in quality; may be gnawing, burning, cramping, or aching</li><li>When severe, may be associated with sweating, pallor, nausea, vomiting, restlessness.</li></ul>

Visceral pain in the right upper quadrant (RUQ) from liver distention against its capsule from the various causes of hepatitis, including alcoholic hepatitis

continued

Somatic or Parietal pain	■ From inflammation of the parietal peritoneum.	■ Steady, aching ■ Usually more severe ■ Usually more precisely localized over the involved structure than visceral pain	Visceral periumbilical pain in early acute appendicitis from distention of inflamed appendix gradually changes to parietal pain in the right lower quadrant (RLQ) from inflammation of the adjacent parietal peritoneum.
Referred pain	■ Occurs in more distant sites innervated at approximately the same spinal levels as the disordered structure.	■ Pain from the chest, spine, or pelvis may be referred to the abdomen. ■ Palpation at the site of referred pain often does not result in tenderness.	Pain from pleurisy or acute myocardial infarction may be referred to the epigastric area. Pain of duodenal or pancreatic origin may be referred to the back; pain from the biliary tree—to the right shoulder or right posterior chest.

Gastrointestinal Tract

Ask patients to *describe the pain in their own words*, especially timing of the pain (acute or chronic); then ask them to *point to the pain*.

See Algorithm 19-1, Approach to the patient with abdominal pain, based on location, p. 314.

Pursue important details:

"Where does the pain start?"
"What is the pain like?"
"How severe is it on a scale of 1 to 10?"
"What makes it better or worse?"
"Does it radiate or travel?"

Doubling over with cramping colicky pain signals a renal stone. Sudden knife-like epigastric pain often radiating to the back is typical of pancreatitis.

Epigastric pain occurs with gastroesophageal reflux disease (GERD), pancreatitis, and perforated ulcers. RUQ and upper abdominal pain are common in cholecystitis and cholangitis.

Elicit any *symptoms associated with the pain*, such as fever or chills; ask about their sequence.

Upper Abdominal Pain, Discomfort, or Heartburn. Ask about chronic or recurrent upper abdominal discomfort, or *dyspepsia*. Related symptoms include bloating, nausea, upper abdominal fullness, and heartburn. Note any:

- Bloating from excessive gas, especially with frequent belching, abdominal distention, or flatus, the passage of gas by rectum

Bloating may occur with lactose intolerance, inflammatory bowel disease, or ovarian cancer; belching results from *aerophagia*, or swallowing air. See Algorithm 19-2, Approach to the patient with right upper quadrant pain, p. 315.

- Unpleasant *abdominal fullness* after normal meals or *early satiety*, the inability to eat a full meal

Consider diabetic gastroparesis, anticholinergic drugs, gastric outlet obstruction, gastric cancer. Early satiety may signify hepatitis.

- *Heartburn, dysphagia, or regurgitation?*

Suggests GERD. Up to 90% of patients with asthma have GERD-like symptoms.

Lower Abdominal Pain or Discomfort—Acute and Chronic. If acute, is the pain sharp and continuous or intermittent and cramping?

RLQ pain, or pain migrating from periumbilical region in appendicitis; in women with RLQ pain, possible pelvic inflammatory disease, ectopic pregnancy, ruptured ovarian follicle; see Algorithm 19-3, Approach to the patient with right lower quadrant pain, p. 316.

Left lower quadrant (LLQ) pain in diverticulitis, diffuse abdominal pain with abdominal distention, hyperactive bowel sounds, and tenderness on palpation in small or large bowel obstruction; pain with absent bowel sounds, rigidity, percussion tenderness, and guarding in peritonitis; see Algorithm 19-4, Approach to the patient with left lower quadrant pain, p. 317.

If chronic, is there a change in bowel habits? Alternating diarrhea and constipation?

Colon cancer; irritable bowel syndrome (IBS)

Abdominal Pain with Associated GI Symptoms

■ Nausea, vomiting, loss of appetite (*anorexia*)	Pregnancy, diabetic ketoacidosis, adrenal insufficiency, hypercalcemia, uremia, liver disease. Induced vomiting without nausea in anorexia/bulimia.
■ Regurgitation	GERD, esophageal stricture, and esophageal cancer
■ Coffee-ground emesis (*hematemesis*)	Esophageal or gastric varices, Mallory–Weiss tears, peptic ulcer disease
■ Difficulty swallowing (*dysphagia*)	If solids and liquids, neuromuscular disorders affecting motility (e.g., achalasia). If only solids, consider structural conditions like Zenker diverticulum, Schatzki ring, stricture, neoplasm.
■ Painful swallowing (*odynophagia*)	Radiation; caustic ingestion, infection from cytomegalovirus, herpes simplex, HIV, esophageal ulceration from aspirin or NSAIDs
■ Diarrhea, acute (<14 days), persistent (14 to 30 days) and chronic (>30 days)	Acute infection (viral, salmonella, shigella, etc.); chronic in Crohn disease, ulcerative colitis; oily diarrhea (*steatorrhea*)—in pancreatic insufficiency. See Table 19-1, Diarrhea, pp. 319–320.
■ Constipation	Medications, especially anticholinergic agents and opioids; colon cancer, diabetes, hypothyroidism, hypercalcemia, multiple sclerosis, Parkinson disease
■ Black, tarry stools (*melena*)	Upper GI bleed
■ Jaundice from increased levels of bilirubin; apparent when plasma bilirubin is >3 mg/dL	Impaired excretion of conjugated bilirubin in viral hepatitis, cirrhosis, primary biliary cirrhosis, drug-induced cholestasis
	Common bile duct obstruction from gallstones or pancreatic, cholangio-, or duodenal carcinoma
Ask about the color of *the urine and stool*.	Dark urine from increased conjugated bilirubin excreted in urine (hepatitis); acholic clay-colored stool when bilirubin excretion into intestine is obstructed
Does the skin itch without other obvious explanation?	Itching or pruritus occurs in cholestatic or obstructive jaundice when bilirubin levels are markedly elevated.

Ask about risk factors for liver diseases (Box 19-2).

BOX 19-2. Risk Factors for Liver Disease

- *Hepatitis:* Travel or meals in areas of poor sanitation, ingestion of contaminated water or foodstuffs (*hepatitis A*); parenteral or mucous membrane exposure to infectious body fluids such as blood, serum, semen, and saliva, especially through sexual contact with an infected partner or use of shared needles for injection drug use (*hepatitis B*); illicit injection drug use or blood transfusion (*hepatitis C*)
- *Alcoholic hepatitis* or *alcoholic cirrhosis* (screen patients carefully about alcohol use)
- *Toxic liver damage* from medications, industrial solvents, environmental toxins, or some anesthetic agents
- *Gallbladder disease* or *surgery* that may result in extrahepatic biliary obstruction
- *Hereditary disorders* in the Family History

Urinary Tract

Ask about *pain on urination,* usually a burning sensation, sometimes termed *dysuria* (also refers to difficulty voiding).

Bladder infection (*cystitis*)

Also seen in urethritis, urinary tract infections, bladder stones, tumors, and, in men, acute prostatitis. In women, internal burning in urethritis, external burning in vulvovaginitis

Note any:

- *Urgency,* an unusually intense and immediate desire to void

May lead to urge incontinence

- *Urinary frequency,* or abnormally frequent voiding

Urinary tract infection

- Fever or chills; blood in the urine

Urinary tract infection

- Any pain in the abdomen, flank, or back

Dull, steady pain in pyelonephritis; severe colicky pain in ureteral obstruction from renal stone

- In those with prostates, *hesitancy* in starting the urine stream, *straining to void, reduced caliber and force of the urine stream,* or *dribbling* as they complete voiding.

Prostatitis, urethritis

Assess any:

- *Polyuria,* a significant increase in 24-hour urine volume

  Diabetes mellitus, diabetes insipidus

- *Nocturia,* urinary frequency at night

  Bladder obstruction

- *Urinary incontinence,* involuntary loss of urine (Algorithm 19-5):

  See Table 19-2, Urinary Incontinence, p. 321.

  - From coughing, sneezing, lifting

    Stress incontinence (poor urethral sphincter tone)

  - From urge to void

    Urge incontinence (detrusor overactivity or overactive bladder)

  - From bladder fullness with leaking but incomplete emptying

    Overflow incontinence (anatomic obstruction, impaired neural innervation to bladder); see Algorithm 19-5, Approach to the patient with urinary incontinence, p. 318.

TECHNIQUES OF EXAMINATION

Key Components of the Abdominal Examination

Abdomen
- Note patient's general appearance (demeanor, distress, color, mental status)
- Inspect surface, contours, and movements of the abdomen
- Prior to palpation or percussion, place the diaphragm of your stethoscope in one abdominal region and listen for bowel sounds
- Percuss abdomen lightly in all four quadrants
- Palpate lightly with one hand in all four quadrants
- Palpate deeply with two hands in all four quadrants
- Check for signs of peritonitis

Liver
- Estimate liver size along right midclavicular line
- Palpate and characterize liver edge

Spleen
- Percuss for splenic enlargement along the Traube space
- Palpate for splenic edge with patient supine and in the right lateral decubitus position

Kidneys
- Check for costovertebral angle (CVA) tenderness using fist percussion

Urinary Bladder
- Percuss the urinary bladder

Special Techniques
- Perform special techniques if indicated

Abdomen

Inspect the abdomen, including:

- Skin

  Scars, striae, veins, ecchymoses (in intra- or retroperitoneal hemorrhages)

- Umbilicus

  Hernia, inflammation

- Contours for shape, symmetry, enlarged organs or masses

  Bulging flanks of ascites, suprapubic bulge, large liver or spleen, tumors

- Any peristaltic waves

  Increased in GI obstruction

- Any pulsations

  Increased in aortic aneurysm

Auscultate the abdomen for:

- Bowel sounds

  Increased or decreased motility

  Changes in bowel sounds heard are typically nonspecific and nondiagnostic.

- Bruits (Fig. 19-1)

  Hepatic bruit in carcinoma of the liver and alcoholic hepatitis

  Arterial bruits in partial obstruction of the aorta or renal, iliac, or femoral arteries.

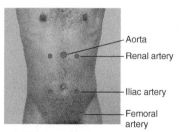

— Aorta
— Renal artery
— Iliac artery
— Femoral artery

FIGURE 19-1. Abdominal auscultatory areas for bruits.

- Friction rubs

  Liver tumor, splenic infarct

Percuss the abdomen for patterns of tympany and dullness.

  Ascites, GI obstruction, pregnant uterus, ovarian tumor

Palpate all quadrants of the abdomen:

- Lightly for guarding, rebound, and tenderness (Fig. 19-2)

See Table 19-3, Abdominal Tenderness, p. 322. "Acute abdomen" or peritonitis:

Guarding if patient voluntary tenses abdominal wall due to pain.

Rebound tenderness from peritoneal inflammation; pain is greater when you withdraw your hand than when you press down. Press slowly on a tender area, then quickly release.

Firm and rigid abdominal wall suggests peritoneal inflammation.

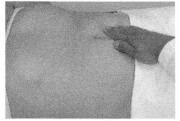

FIGURE 19-2. Using one hand to lightly palpate the abdomen in all four quadrants.

- Deeply for masses or tenderness (Fig. 19-3)

Tumors, a distended viscus

Abdominal masses may be physiologic (pregnant uterus), inflammatory (diverticulitis), vascular (AAA), neoplastic (colon cancer), or obstructive (distended bladder or dilated loop of bowel).

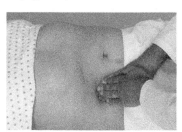

FIGURE 19-3. Using two hands to deeply palpate the abdomen in all four quadrants.

⚬ Liver

Percuss span of liver dullness in the midclavicular line (MCL), Figure 19-4.

Increased dullness in hepatomegaly from acute hepatitis, heart failure; decreased dullness in cirrhosis

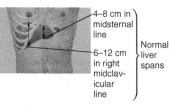

4–8 cm in midsternal line
6–12 cm in right midclavicular line
} Normal liver spans

FIGURE 19-4. Area of percussion for estimating liver size along midclavicular line.

TECHNIQUES OF EXAMINATION	POSSIBLE FINDINGS

Feel the liver edge, if possible, as patient breathes in.

Firm edge of cirrhosis

Starting well below the costal margin, measure distance of the liver edge from the costal margin in the MCL (Fig. 19-5).

Increased distance in hepatomegaly—may be missed (as in Fig. 19-6) by starting palpation too high in the RUQ

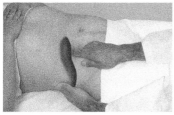

FIGURE 19-5. Palpating for the liver edge.

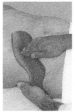

FIGURE 19-6. Palpating first at the costal margin may miss the liver edge.

Note any tenderness or masses.

Tender liver of hepatitis or heart failure; tumor mass

Spleen

Percuss across left lower anterior chest (*Traube space*), noting change from tympany to dullness.

⟳ Palpate the spleen with the patient supine then lying on the right side with legs flexed at hips and knees (Fig. 19-7).

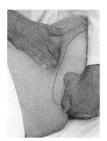

FIGURE 19-7. Spleen tip (purple) palpable below costal margin.

ᴏ— Kidneys

The kidneys are retroperitoneal and usually not palpable unless markedly enlarged.

᭏ Check for costovertebral angle (CVA) tenderness (Fig. 19-8).

Tender in pyelonephritis

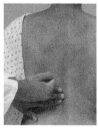

FIGURE 19-8. Fist percussion to detect costovertebral angle (CVA) tenderness.

ᴏ— Aorta

Gently palpate the aorta's pulsations (Fig. 19-9). In older people, estimate its width.

Periumbilical mass with expansile pulsations ≥3 cm in diameter in abdominal aortic aneurysm. Assess further due to risk of rupture.

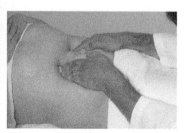

FIGURE 19-9. Palpating the epigastrium on both sides of the aorta.

Special Techniques

- Ascites
- Appendicitis
- Acute cholecystitis

Assessing Ascites

○—/○— Palpate for shifting dullness. Map areas of tympany and dullness with patient supine, then lying on side (Fig. 19-10).

Ascitic fluid usually shifts to dependent side, changing the margin of dullness (Fig. 19-11).

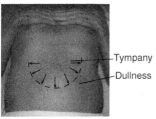

FIGURE 19-10. Area and direction outward to map percussion dullness from ascites.

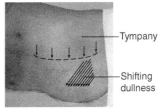

FIGURE 19-11. Area of percussion for shifting dullness with the patient turned to right side.

Results of fluid wave test are not specific.

Ballotte an organ or mass in an ascitic abdomen. Place your stiffened and straightened fingers on the abdomen, briefly jab them toward the structure, and try to touch its surface.

Your hand, quickly displacing the fluid, stops abruptly as it touches the solid surface (Fig. 19-12).

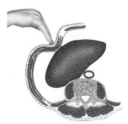

FIGURE 19-12. Displacement of ascitic fluid by ballottement allowing palpation of liver.

Assessing Possible Appendicitis. Palpate for local tenderness; often at the McBurney point (Fig. 19-13).

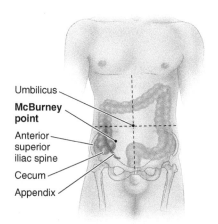

FIGURE 19-13. Surface projection of pelvis, cecum, and appendix showing McBurney point. (From Honan L. *Focus on Adult Health: Medical-Surgical Nursing.* 2nd ed. Wolters Kluwer; 2019. Figure 24-2.)

Palpate for muscular rigidity.

Perform a rectal examination and, in women, a pelvic examination.

Local tenderness, especially if appendix is retrocecal

Special Maneuvers for Appendicitis

- *Rovsing sign:* Press deeply and evenly in the *left* lower quadrant. Then quickly withdraw your fingers.

  Pain in the *right* lower quadrant during *left*-sided pressure suggests appendicitis (a *positive* Rovsing sign).

- *Psoas sign:* Place your hand just above the patient's right knee. Ask the patient to raise that thigh against your hand. Or, ask the patient to turn onto the left side. Then extend the patient's right leg at the hip to stretch the psoas muscle.

  Pain from irritation of the psoas muscle suggests an inflamed appendix (a *positive* psoas sign).

- *Obturator sign:* Flex the patient's right thigh at the hip, with the knee bent, and rotate the leg internally at

  Right hypogastric pain in a *positive* obturator sign, suggesting irritation of the obturator muscle by an inflamed appendix.

the hip, which stretches the internal obturator muscle.

Appendicitis is twice as likely in the presence of RLQ tenderness, Rovsing sign (indirect tenderness), and the psoas sign; it is three times more likely with McBurney point tenderness (McBurney sign).

Assessing Possible Acute Cholecystitis. Auscultate, percuss, and palpate the abdomen for tenderness.

Bowel sounds may be active or decreased; tympany may increase with an ileus; assess any RUQ tenderness.

Assess for the *Murphy sign*. Hook your thumb under the right costal margin at edge of rectus muscle, and ask patient to take a deep breath.

Sharp tenderness and a sudden stop in inspiratory effort constitute a *positive* Murphy sign.

RECORDING YOUR FINDINGS

Recording the Abdominal Examination

"Abdomen is protuberant with active bowel sounds. It is soft and nontender; no palpable masses or hepatosplenomegaly. Liver span is 7 cm and in the right MCL; edge is smooth and palpable 1 cm below the right costal margin. Spleen not felt. No CVA tenderness."

OR

"Abdomen is flat. No bowel sounds heard. It is firm and board-like, with increased tenderness, guarding, and rebound in the right lower quadrant. Liver percusses to 7 cm in the MCL; edge not felt. Spleen not felt. No palpable mass. No CVA tenderness. Psoas sign positive."

These findings suggest possible peritonitis from possible appendicitis.

HEALTH PROMOTION AND COUNSELING: EVIDENCE AND RECOMMENDATIONS

Important Topics for Health Promotion and Counseling

- Viral hepatitis: risk factors, screening, and vaccination
- Screening for colorectal cancer

Viral Hepatitis: Risk Factors, Screening, and Vaccination

Protective measures against *infectious hepatitis* include counseling about transmission (Box 19-3).

- *Hepatitis A:* Transmission is fecal–oral. Illness occurs approximately 30 days after exposure. Advise hand washing with soap and water after bathroom use or changing diapers and before preparing or eating food. Diluted bleach can be used to clean environmental surfaces.

BOX 19-3. Centers for Disease Control and Prevention Recommendations for Hepatitis A Vaccination

- All children at age 1 year
- Individuals with chronic liver disease
- Groups at increased risk of acquiring hepatitis A virus: travelers to areas with high endemic rates of infection, men who have sex with men, injection and illicit drug users, individuals working with nonhuman primates, and persons who have clotting-factor disorders
- The vaccine alone may be administered at any time before traveling to endemic areas.

- *Hepatitis B:* Transmission occurs during contact with infected body fluids, such as blood, semen, saliva, and vaginal secretions. Infection increases risk of fulminant hepatitis, chronic infection, and subsequent cirrhosis and hepatocellular carcinoma. Provide counseling and serologic screening for patients at risk (Box 19-4).

BOX 19-4. Centers for Disease Control and Prevention Recommendations for Hepatitis B Vaccination: High-Risk Groups and Settings

- *All adults in high-risk settings,* such as sexually transmitted infection (STI) clinics, HIV testing and treatment programs, drug-abuse treatment programs and programs for persons who inject drugs, correctional facilities, programs for men having sex with men, chronic hemodialysis facilities and end-stage renal disease programs, and facilities for people with developmental disabilities
- *People with percutaneous or mucosal exposure to blood,* including injection drug users, household contacts of antigen-positive

persons, residents and staff of facilities for the developmentally disabled, health care workers, and people on dialysis

- *Sexual contacts,* including sex partners of hepatitis B surface antigen-positive persons, people with more than one sex partner in the prior 6 months, people seeking evaluation and treatment for sexually transmitted infections, and men who have sex with men

- *Others,* including travelers to endemic areas, people with chronic liver disease and HIV infection, and people seeking protection from hepatitis B infection

- *Hepatitis C:* Hepatitis C, now the most common form of hepatitis, is spread by blood exposure and injection drug use. There is no vaccine for hepatitis C, so prevention targets counseling to avoid risk factors. Serologic screening should be recommended for high-risk groups.

Screening for Colorectal Cancer

Adopt the 2016 recommendations of the U.S. Preventive Services Task Force (Box 19-5).

BOX 19-5. Screening for Colorectal Cancer–U.S. Preventive Services Task Force 2016

- Adults age 50 to 75 years—options (grade A recommendation)
  - Stool-based tests
  - Fecal immunochemical test (FIT) annually
  - High-sensitivity guaiac-based fecal occult blood testing annually
  - FIT-DNA testing every 1 or 3 years
  - Direct visualization tests
  - Colonoscopy every 10 years
  - Sigmoidoscopy every 5 years
  - Flexible sigmoidoscopy every 10 years with FIT every 3 years
  - CT colonography every 5 years
- Adults age 76 to 85 years—individualized decision making (grade C recommendation), decisions should take into consideration life expectancy and previous screening. Previously unscreened adults might benefit from screening.
- Adults older than age 85—do not screen (grade D recommendation), because "competing causes of mortality preclude a mortality benefit that would outweigh the harms"

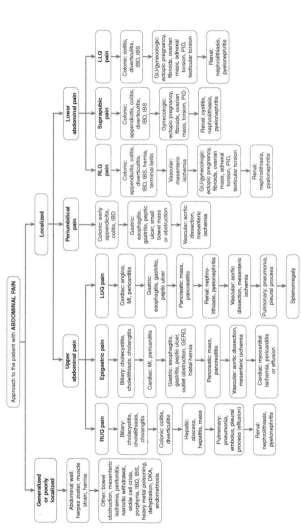

Algorithm 19-1. Approach to the patient with abdominal pain, based on location. (Note: Although it is not comprehensive, this algorithm may be a helpful starting approach for synthesizing information gathered from the history and physical.) DKA, diabetic ketoacidosis; GERD, gastroesophageal reflux disease; IBD, inflammatory bowel disease; IBS, irritable bowel syndrome; LLQ, left lower quadrant; LUQ, left upper quadrant; MI, myocardial infarction; PID, pelvic inflammatory disease; RLQ, right lower quadrant; RUQ, right upper quadrant.

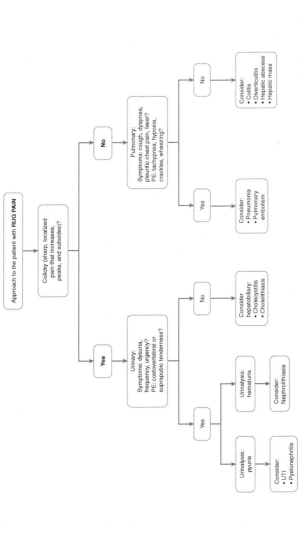

Algorithm 19-2. Approach to the patient with right upper quadrant pain. (Note: Although it is not comprehensive, this algorithm may be a helpful starting approach for synthesizing information gathered from the history and physical.) PE, physical examination; RUQ, right upper quadrant; UTI, urinary tract infection.

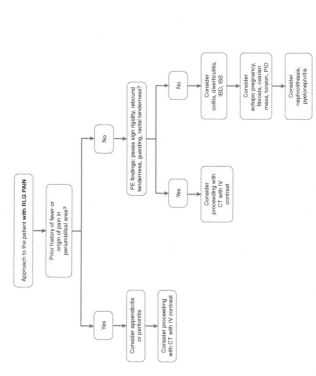

Algorithm 19-3. Approach to the patient with right lower quadrant pain. (Note: Although it is not comprehensive, this algorithm may be a helpful starting approach for synthesizing information gathered from the history and physical.) CT, computed tomography; IBD, inflammatory bowel disease; IBS, irritable bowel syndrome; IV, intravenous; PE, physical examination; PID, pelvic inflammatory disease; RLQ, right lower quadrant.

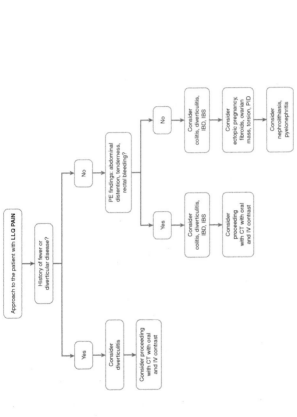

Algorithm 19-4. Approach to the patient with left lower quadrant pain. (Note: Although it is not comprehensive, this algorithm may be a helpful starting approach for synthesizing information gathered from the history and physical.) CT, computed tomography; IBD, inflammatory bowel disease; IBS, irritable bowel syndrome; IV, intravenous; LLQ, left lower quadrant; PE, physical examination; PID, pelvic inflammatory disease.

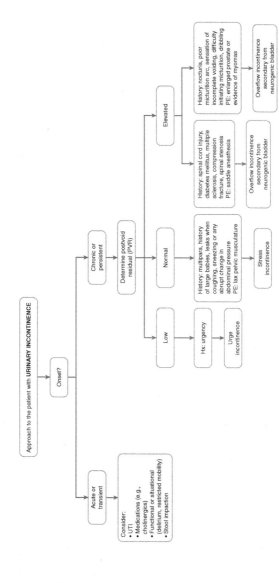

Algorithm 19-5. Approach to the patient with urinary incontinence. (Note: Although it is not comprehensive, this algorithm may be a helpful starting approach for synthesizing information gathered from the history and physical.) Hx, history; PE, physical exam; UTI, urinary tract infection.

INTERPRETATION AIDS

TABLE 19-1. Diarrhea

Problem/Process	Characteristics of Stool
Acute Diarrhea	
Secretory Infection (noninflammatory)	
Infection by viruses; preformed bacterial toxins such as *Staphylococcus aureus, Clostridium perfringens*, toxigenic *Escherichia coli; Vibrio cholerae, Cryptosporidium, Giardia lamblia*, rotavirus	Watery, without blood, pus, or mucus
Inflammatory Infection	
Colonization or invasion of intestinal mucosa as in nontyphoid *Salmonella, Shigella, Yersinia, Campylobacter*, enteropathic *E. coli, Entamoeba histolytica, Clostridium difficile*	Loose to watery, often with blood, pus, or mucus
Drug-Induced Diarrhea	
Action of many drugs, such as magnesium-containing antacids, antibiotics, antineoplastic agents, and laxatives	Loose to watery
Chronic Diarrhea (≥30 days)	
Diarrheal Syndromes	
Irritable bowel syndrome: A disorder of bowel motility with alternating diarrhea and constipation	Loose; may show mucus but no blood. Small, hard stools with constipation
Cancer of the sigmoid colon: Partial obstruction by a malignant neoplasm	May be blood-streaked

continued

TABLE 19-1. Diarrhea *(continued)*

Problem/Process	Characteristics of Stool
Inflammatory Bowel Disease	
Ulcerative colitis: inflammation and ulceration of the mucosa and submucosa of the rectum and colon	Soft to watery, often containing blood
Crohn disease of the small bowel (regional enteritis) or colon (granulomatous colitis): chronic inflammation of the bowel wall, typically involving the terminal ileum, proximal colon, or both	Small, soft to loose or watery, usually free of gross blood (enteritis) or with less bleeding than ulcerative colitis (colitis)
Voluminous Diarrhea	
Malabsorption syndrome: Defective absorption of fat, including fat-soluble vitamins, with steatorrhea (excessive excretion of fat) as in pancreatic insufficiency, bile salt deficiency, bacterial overgrowth	Typically, bulky, soft, light yellow to gray, greasy or oily; foul smelling; usually floats in the toilet (*steatorrhea*)
Osmotic Diarrheas	
■ Lactose intolerance: Deficiency in intestinal lactase	Watery diarrhea
■ Abuse of osmotic purgatives: Laxative habit, often surreptitious	Watery diarrhea
Secretory diarrheas from bacterial infection, secreting villous adenoma, fat or bile salt malabsorption, hormone-mediated conditions (gastrin in Zollinger–Ellison syndrome, vasoactive intestinal peptide): Process is variable.	Watery diarrhea

TABLE 19-2. Urinary Incontinence*

Problem	Mechanisms
Stress Incontinence: Urethral sphincter weakened. Transient increases in intra-abdominal pressure raise bladder pressure to levels exceeding urethral resistance. Leads to voiding *small amounts* during laughing, coughing, and sneezing.	■ In women, weakness of the pelvic floor with inadequate muscular support of the bladder and proximal urethra and a change in the angle between the bladder and the urethra from childbirth, surgery, and local conditions affecting the internal urethral sphincter, such as postmenopausal atrophy of the mucosa and urethral infection ■ In men, prostatic surgery
Urge Incontinence: Detrusor contractions are stronger than normal and overcome normal urethral resistance. Bladder is typically small. Results in voiding *moderate amounts*, urgency, frequency, and nocturia.	■ Decreased cortical inhibition of detrusor contractions, as in stroke, brain tumor, dementia, and lesions of the spinal cord above the sacral level ■ Hyperexcitability of sensory pathways, as in bladder infection, tumor, and fecal impaction ■ Deconditioning of voiding reflexes, caused by frequent voluntary voiding at low bladder volumes
Overflow Incontinence: Detrusor contractions are insufficient to overcome urethral resistance. Bladder is typically large, even after an effort to void, leading to *continuous dribbling*.	■ Obstruction of the bladder outlet, as by benign prostatic hyperplasia or tumor ■ Weakness of detrusor muscle associated with peripheral nerve disease at the sacral level ■ Impaired bladder sensation that interrupts the reflex arc, as in diabetic neuropathy
Functional Incontinence: Inability to get to the toilet in time because of impaired health or environmental conditions	■ Problems in mobility from weakness, arthritis, poor vision, other conditions; environmental factors such as unfamiliar setting, distant bathroom facilities, bed rails, physical restraints
Incontinence Secondary to Medications: Drugs may contribute to any type of incontinence listed.	■ Sedatives, tranquilizers, anticholinergics, sympathetic blockers, potent diuretics

*Patients may have more than one kind of incontinence.

TABLE 19-3. Abdominal Tenderness

Visceral Tenderness

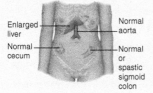

Enlarged liver

Normal aorta

Normal cecum

Normal or spastic sigmoid colon

Peritoneal Tenderness

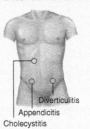

Diverticulitis

Appendicitis

Cholecystitis

Tenderness from Disease in the Chest and Pelvis

Acute Pleurisy

Unilateral or bilateral, upper or lower abdomen

Acute Salpingitis

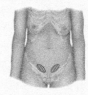

Male Genitalia

HEALTH HISTORY

Common Concerns

- Penile discharge or lesions
- Scrotal or testicular swelling or pain

Penile Discharge or Lesions

To assess possible infection from sexually transmitted infections (STIs), ask about any discharge from the penis, dripping, or staining of underwear. If penile discharge is present, clarify the amount; color; and any fever, chills, rash, or associated symptoms.

Penile discharge in gonococcal (usually yellow) and nongonococcal (clear or white) urethritis

Inquire about sores or growths on the penis.

STIs may involve other parts of the body. Ask about practices of oral and anal sex and any related sore throat, oral itching or pain, diarrhea, or rectal bleeding.

Rash in disseminated gonococcal infection.

See Table 20-1, Sexually Transmitted Infections of Male Genitalia, pp. 330–331 and Algorithm 20-1, Approach to the patient with a penile mass or lesion, p. 328.

Scrotal or Testicular Swelling or Pain

Ask about swelling or pain in the scrotum or on the testicles.

Look for scrotal swelling in mumps orchitis, scrotal edema, and testicular cancer, and pain in testicular torsion, epididymitis, and orchitis. See Algorithm 20-2, Approach to the patient with a scrotal mass or pain, p. 329.

TECHNIQUES OF EXAMINATION

Key Components of the Male Genitalia Examination

- Inspect skin, prepuce, and glans
- Inspect urethral meatus, and, if indicated, strip or "milk" penile shaft
- Palpate shaft of the penis
- Inspect scrotum including skin, hair, and contour
- Palpate each testis including epididymis and spermatic cord
- Perform special techniques as indicated:
  - Evaluate for groin hernias
  - Evaluate for scrotal mass

Male Genitalia

Wear gloves to examine the male genitalia (Fig. 20-1). The patient may be standing or supine.

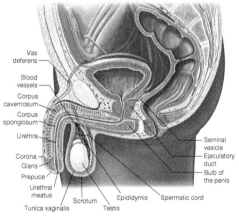

Vas deferens
Blood vessels
Corpus cavernosum
Corpus spongiosum
Urethra
Corona
Glans
Prepuce
Urethral meatus
Tunica vaginalis
Scrotum
Epididymis
Testis
Spermatic cord
Seminal vesicle
Ejaculatory duct
Bulb of the penis

FIGURE 20-1. Anatomy of male genitalia.

Penis. Inspect the:

- Development of the penis and the skin and pubic hair at its base

Sexual maturation, lice, scabies

See Table 25-7, Sex Maturity Ratings in Boys (Tanner Stages), Chapter 25, Children: Infancy through Adolescence, p. 497.

TECHNIQUES OF EXAMINATION	POSSIBLE FINDINGS
■ Prepuce (if present, retract the fore-skin)	Phimosis, cancer
■ Glans	Balanitis, chancre, herpes, warts, cancer
■ Urethral meatus (compress the glans to inspect the meatus for discharge)	Hypospadias, discharge of urethritis

Palpate:

■ Any visible lesions	Peyronie disease, chancre, cancer
■ Penile shaft	Urethral stricture or cancer
	See Table 20-2, Abnormalities of the Penis and Scrotum, p. 332.

Scrotum and Its Contents. Inspect:

■ Skin of scrotum	Rashes
■ Contours of scrotum	Hernia, hydrocele, cryptorchidism
■ Inguinal areas	Fungal infection

Palpate each:

■ Testis (Fig. 20-2), assess size, shape, consistency noting any:	See Table 20-3, Abnormalities of the Testis, p. 333.

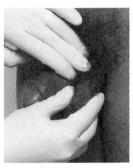

FIGURE 20-2. Palpating the testis and epididymis.

■ Lumps or nodules	Testicular carcinoma
■ Tenderness	Acute epididymitis, acute orchitis, torsion of the spermatic cord, strangu-lated inguinal hernia
■ Epididymis	Epididymitis, cyst

- Spermatic cord and adjacent areas (Fig. 20-3)

Varicocele if multiple tortuous veins; cystic structure may be a hydrocele

See Table 20-4, Abnormalities of the Epididymis and Spermatic Cord, p. 334.

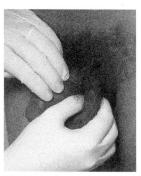

FIGURE 20-3. Palpating the spermatic cord.

Special Technique

Evaluating Groin Hernias. Patient is usually standing.

See Table 20-5, Hernias in the Groin, p. 335.

Inspect inguinal and femoral areas as patient strains down (*Valsalva*).

Inguinal and femoral hernias

Palpate external inguinal ring through scrotal skin and ask patient to strain down (Fig. 20-4).

Indirect and direct inguinal hernias

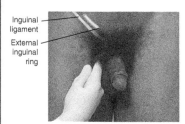

Inguinal ligament

External inguinal ring

FIGURE 20-4. Invaginating redundant scrotal skin.

Scrotal Transillumination. Hold a strong light source behind scrotal mass. Cystic (light shines through as a red glow) or solid (light blocked).

Hydrocoele

RECORDING YOUR FINDINGS

Recording the Male Genitalia Examination

"Circumcised male. No penile discharge or lesions. No scrotal swelling or discoloration. Testes descended bilaterally, smooth, without masses. Epididymis nontender. No inguinal or femoral hernias."

OR

"Uncircumcised male; prepuce easily retractable. No penile discharge or lesions. No scrotal swelling or discoloration. Testes descended bilaterally; right testicle smooth; 1 × 1 cm firm nodule on left lateral testicle. It is fixed and nontender. Epididymis nontender. No inguinal or femoral hernias."

These findings are suspicious for testicular carcinoma.

HEALTH PROMOTION AND COUNSELING: EVIDENCE AND RECOMMENDATIONS

Important Topics for Health Promotion and Counseling

- Screening for testicular cancer
- Sexually transmitted infections (See Chapter 6, Health Maintenance and Screening, pp. 93–95.)

Screening for Testicular Cancer

Testicular cancer is rare but highly treatable when detected early. It is the most commonly diagnosed cancer in white men ages 20 to 34 years. Risk factors are white ethnicity, family history, human immunodeficiency virus (HIV) infection, and a history of cryptorchidism. In 2011, the U.S. Preventive Services Task Force (USPSTF) concluded that meaningful health benefits from screening are unlikely, either by clinical examination or testicular self-examination (TSE), and advised against screening for testicular cancer in asymptomatic adolescent and adult males (grade D recommendation). In contrast, the American Cancer Society (ACS) supports testicular examination as part of a general physical examination. The ACS does not have a recommendation for regular TSE but does advise men to seek medical attention for any of the following: painless lump, swelling, or enlargement in either testicle; pain or discomfort in testicle or scrotum; breast growth or soreness; or dull ache in the lower abdomen or groin.

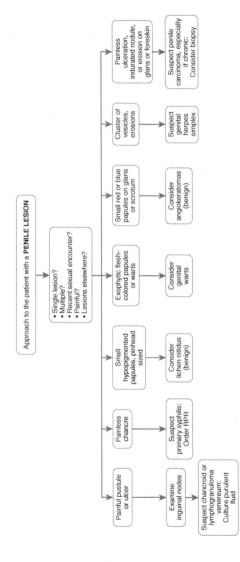

Algorithm 20-1. Approach to the patient with a penile mass or lesion. (Note: Although it is not comprehensive, this algorithm may be a helpful starting approach for synthesizing information gathered from the history and physical.) RPR, rapid plasma regain test.

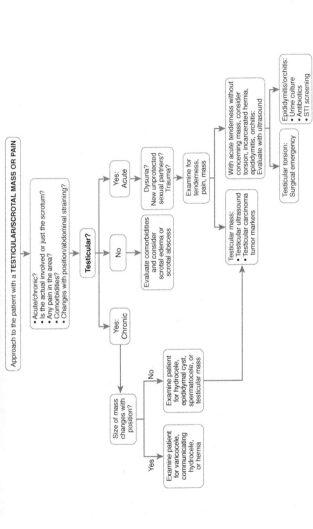

Algorithm 20-2. Approach to the patient with a scrotal mass or pain. (Note: Although it is not comprehensive, this algorithm may be a helpful starting approach for synthesizing information gathered from the history and physical.) STI, sexually transmitted infection.

INTERPRETATION AIDS

TABLE 20-1. Sexually Transmitted Infections of Male Genitalia

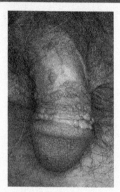

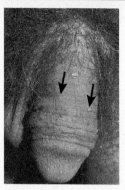

Genital Warts (Condylomata Acuminata)

- *Appearance:* Single or multiple papules or plaques of variable shapes; may be round, acuminate (or pointed), or thin and slender. May be raised, flat, or cauliflower-like (verrucous).
- *Causative organism:* Human papillomavirus (HPV), usually from subtypes 6, 11; carcinogenic subtypes rare, approximately 5–10% of all anogenital warts.
- *Incubation:* Weeks to months; infected contact may have no visible warts.
- Can arise on penis, scrotum, groin, thighs, anus; usually asymptomatic, occasionally cause itching and pain.
- May disappear without treatment.

Genital Herpes Simplex

- *Appearance:* Small scattered or grouped vesicles, 1–3 mm in size, on glans or shaft of penis. Appear as erosions if vesicular membrane breaks.
- *Causative organism:* Usually *Herpes simplex virus 2* (90%), a double-stranded DNA virus. *Incubation:* 2–7 days after exposure.
- Primary episode may be asymptomatic; recurrence usually less painful, of shorter duration.
- Associated with fever, malaise, headache, arthralgias; local pain and edema, lymphadenopathy.
- Need to distinguish from genital herpes zoster (usually in older patients with dermatomal distribution); candidiasis.

TABLE 20-1. Sexually Transmitted Infections of Male Genitalia *(continued)*

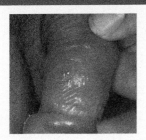

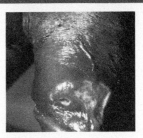

Primary Syphilis

- *Appearance:* Small red papule that becomes a chancre, or painless erosion up to 2 cm in diameter. Base of chancre is clean, red, smooth, and glistening; borders are raised and indurated. Chancre heals within 3–8 wks.
- *Causative organism: Treponema pallidum,* a spirochete.
- *Incubation:* 9–90 days after exposure.
- May develop inguinal lymphadenopathy within 7 days; lymph nodes are rubbery, nontender, mobile.
- 20–30% of patients develop secondary syphilis while chancre still present (suggests coinfection with HIV).
- Distinguish from: genital herpes simplex, chancroid, granuloma inguinale from *Klebsiella granulomatis* (rare in the United States; four variants, so difficult to identify).

Chancroid

- *Appearance:* Red papule or pustule initially, then forms a painful deep ulcer with ragged nonindurated margins; contains necrotic exudate, has a friable base.
- *Causative organism: Haemophilus ducreyi,* an anaerobic bacillus.
- *Incubation:* 3–7 days after exposure.
- Painful inguinal adenopathy; suppurative bobos in 25% of patients.
- Need to distinguish from: primary syphilis; genital herpes simplex; lymphogranuloma venereum, granuloma inguinale from *Klebsiella granulomatis* (both rare in the United States).

TABLE 20-2. Abnormalities of the Penis and Scrotum

Hypospadias
A congenital displacement of the urethral meatus to the inferior surface of the penis. A groove extends from the actual urethral meatus to its normal location on the tip of the glans.

Fingers can get above mass

Scrotal Edema
Pitting edema may make the scrotal skin taut; seen in heart failure or nephrotic syndrome.

Peyronie Disease
Palpable, nontender, hard plaques are found just beneath the skin, usually along the dorsum of the penis. The patient complains of crooked, painful erections.

Fingers can get above mass

Hydrocele
A nontender, fluid-filled mass within the tunica vaginalis. It transilluminates, and the examining fingers can get above the mass within the scrotum.

Carcinoma of the Penis
An indurated nodule or ulcer that is usually nontender. Limited almost completely to men who are not circumcised, it may be masked by the prepuce. Any persistent penile sore is suspicious.

Fingers cannot get above mass

Scrotal Hernia
Usually an *indirect inguinal hernia* that comes through the external inguinal ring, so the examining fingers cannot get above it within the scrotum.

TABLE 20-3. Abnormalities of the Testis

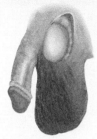

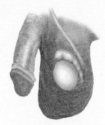

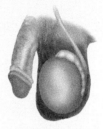

Cryptorchidism
Testis is atrophied and may lie in the inguinal canal or the abdomen, resulting in an unfilled scrotum. As above, there is no palpable left testis or epididymis. Cryptorchidism markedly raises the risk for testicular cancer.

Small Testis
In adults, testicular length is usually ≤3.5 cm. Small, firm testes seen in *Klinefelter syndrome*, usually ≤2 cm. Small, soft testes suggesting atrophy seen in cirrhosis, myotonic dystrophy, use of estrogens, and hypopituitarism; may also follow orchitis.

Acute Orchitis
The testis is acutely inflamed, painful, tender, and swollen. It may be difficult to distinguish from the epididymis. The scrotum may be reddened. Seen in mumps and other viral infections; usually unilateral.

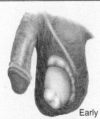
Early

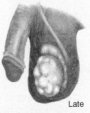
Late

Tumor of the Testis
Usually appears as a painless nodule. Any nodule within the testis warrants investigation for malignancy.

As a testicular neoplasm grows and spreads, it may seem to replace the entire organ. The testicle characteristically feels heavier than normal.

TABLE 20-4. Abnormalities of the Epididymis and Spermatic Cord

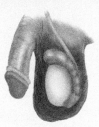

Acute Epididymitis
An acutely inflamed epididymis is tender and swollen and may be difficult to distinguish from the testis. The scrotum may be reddened and the vas deferens inflamed. It occurs chiefly in adults. Coexisting urinary tract infection or prostatitis supports the diagnosis.

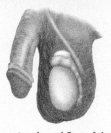

Spermatocele and Cyst of the Epididymis
A painless, movable cystic mass just above the testis suggests a spermatocele or an epididymal cyst. Both transilluminate. The former contains sperm, and the latter does not, but they are clinically indistinguishable.

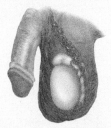

Varicocele of the Spermatic Cord
Varicocele refers to varicose veins of the spermatic cord, usually found on the left. It feels like a soft "bag of worms" separate from the testis, and slowly collapses when the scrotum is elevated in the supine patient.

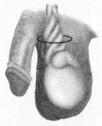

Torsion of the Spermatic Cord
Twisting of the testicle on its spermatic cord produces an acutely painful and swollen organ that is retracted upward in the scrotum, which becomes red and edematous. There is no associated urinary infection. It is a surgical emergency because of obstructed circulation.

TABLE 20-5. Hernias in the Groin

Indirect Inguinal

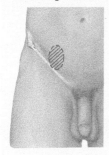

Most common hernia at all ages, both sexes. Originates above inguinal ligament and often passes into scrotum. *May touch examiner's fingertip in inguinal canal.*

Direct Inguinal

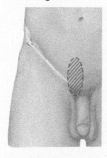

Less common than indirect hernia, usually occurs in men older than 40 yrs. Originates above inguinal ligament near external inguinal ring and *rarely enters scrotum. May bulge anteriorly, touching side of examiner's finger.*

Femoral

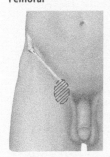

Least common hernia, more common in women than in men. Originates below inguinal ligament, more lateral than inguinal hernia. *Never enters scrotum.*

21

Female Genitalia

HEALTH HISTORY

Common Concerns

- Menarche, menstruation
- Menopause, postmenopausal bleeding
- Vulvovaginal symptoms
- Pelvic pain—acute and chronic
- Sexually transmitted infections
- Pregnancy

Menarche, Menstruation

For the *menstrual history*, ask when menstrual periods began (age at *menarche*).

When did her last menstrual period (LMP) start, and the one prior menstrual period (PMP)? What is the interval between periods, from the first day of one to the first day of the next? Are menses regular or irregular? How long do they last? How heavy is the flow?

Changes in the interval between periods can signal possible pregnancy or menstrual irregularities.

Amenorrhea is the absence of periods. Failure to begin periods is *primary amenorrhea*, whereas cessation of established periods is *secondary amenorrhea*.

Secondary amenorrhea from pregnancy, lactation, menopause; low body weight from conditions of malnutrition, anorexia nervosa, stress, chronic illness, and hypothalamic–pituitary–ovarian dysfunction

In amenorrhea from pregnancy, common early symptoms are tenderness, tingling, or increased size of breasts;

Amenorrhea followed by heavy bleeding in threatened abortion or dysfunctional uterine bleeding urinary frequency; nausea and vomiting; easy fatigability; and feelings that the baby is moving (usually noted at about 20 weeks).

See Algorithm 21-1, Approach to the patient with abnormal uterine bleeding, p. 345.

Dysmenorrhea, or painful menses, is common.

Primary dysmenorrhea from increased prostaglandin production; secondary dysmenorrhea from endometriosis, adenomyosis, pelvic inflammatory disease (PID), and endometrial polyps

Premenstrual syndrome criteria for diagnosis include emotional and behavioral symptoms in the 5 days prior to menses for at least three consecutive cycles, cessation of symptoms and signs within 4 days after onset of menses, and interference with daily activities.

Menopause, Postmenopausal Bleeding

Menopause, the absence of menses for 12 consecutive months, usually occurs between age 48 and 55 years. Associated symptoms include hot flashes, flushing, sweating, and sleep disturbances.

Postmenopausal bleeding, or bleeding occurring 6 months or more after cessation of menses, from endometrial cancer, uterine or cervical polyps.

Vulvovaginal Symptoms

For *vaginal discharge* and local *itching,* inquire about amount, color, consistency, and odor of discharge.

See Table 21-1, Lesions of the Vulva, pp. 348–349; and Table 21-2, Vaginal Discharge, p. 350.

See Algorithm 21-2, Approach to the patient with vulvovaginal symptoms, p. 346.

Pelvic Pain

Assess acute and chronic (>6 months) pelvic pain.

Acute pelvic pain in PID, ruptured ovarian cyst, appendicitis; ectopic pregnancy; also mittelschmerz, ruptured ovarian cyst, tubo-ovarian abscess. *Chronic* pelvic pain in endometriosis, PID, adenosis and fibroids, history of sexual abuse; pelvic floor spasm.

See Algorithm 21-3, Approach to the patient with pelvic pain.

TECHNIQUES OF EXAMINATION

Key Components of the Female Genitalia Examination

- Perform an external examination:
  - Assess sexual maturity (if adolescent)
  - Inspect mons pubis, labia, perineum
- Perform an internal examination:
  - Inspect cervix
  - Inspect vagina
- Perform a bimanual examination:
  - Palpate cervix
  - Palpate uterus
  - Palpate ovaries
  - Assess pelvic floor muscles
- Perform a rectovaginal examination (if indicated)

External Genitalia

Observe pubic hair to assess sexual maturity.

Normal or delayed puberty. See Table 25-7, Sex Maturity Ratings in Boys (Tanner Stages), Chapter 25, Children: Infancy through Adolescence, p. 497.

Examine the external genitalia (Fig. 21-1).

See Table 21-1, Lesions of the Vulva, pp. 348–349.

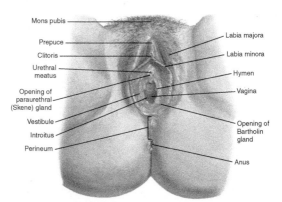

Mons pubis
Prepuce
Clitoris
Urethral meatus
Opening of paraurethral (Skene) gland
Vestibule
Introitus
Perineum

Labia majora
Labia minora
Hymen
Vagina
Opening of Bartholin gland
Anus

FIGURE 21-1. External female genitalia.

TECHNIQUES OF EXAMINATION	POSSIBLE FINDINGS
▪ Labia minora	Ulceration in herpes simplex, syphilitic chancre; inflammation in Bartholin cyst
▪ Clitoris	Enlarged in masculinization
▪ Urethral orifice	Urethral caruncle or prolapse; tenderness in interstitial cystitis
▪ Vaginal opening or introitus	Imperforate hymen
▪ Milk the urethra for discharge if indicated.	Discharge of urethritis

Internal Examination and Pap Smear

A chaperone should accompany the examiner to observe and sometimes assist with this sensitive examination. Whenever possible, the chaperone should be whatever gender the patient feels most comfortable with (Box 21-1).

BOX 21-1. Tips for a Successful Pelvic Examination

Patient	Examiner
▪ Avoids intercourse, douching, or use of vaginal suppositories for 24–48 hours before examination ▪ Empties bladder before examination ▪ Lies supine, with head and shoulders elevated, arms at sides or folded across chest to enhance eye contact and reduce tightening of abdominal muscles	▪ Obtains permission; selects chaperone ▪ Explains each step of the examination in advance ▪ Drapes patient from midabdomen to knees; depresses drape between knees to provide eye contact with patient ▪ Avoids unexpected or sudden movements ▪ Chooses a speculum that is the correct size ▪ Warms speculum with tap water ▪ Monitors comfort of the examination by watching the patient's face ▪ Uses excellent but gentle technique, especially when inserting the speculum

Locate the cervix with a gloved and water-lubricated index finger.

Assess support of vaginal outlet by asking patient to strain down.　　Cystocele, cystourethrocele, rectocele

Enlarge the introitus by pressing its posterior margin downward. Insert a water-lubricated speculum of suitable size. Start with speculum held obliquely (Fig. 21-2), then rotate to horizontal position for full insertion (Fig. 21-3).

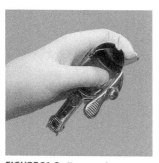

FIGURE 21-2. Entry angle.

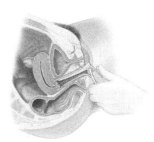

FIGURE 21-3. Carefully inserting the speculum to full length.

Open the speculum gently and inspect cervix:

- Position

  Cervix faces forward if uterus is retroverted.

- Color

  Purplish in pregnancy

- Shape of the cervical os (Fig. 21-4); epithelial surface (squamous–columnar epithelial junction)

  Oval (normal) or slit-like or transverse os from delivery; raised, friable, or lobed wart-like lesions in condylomata or cervical cancer (see Table 21-3, Abnormalities of the Cervix, p. 351)

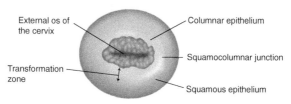

External os of the cervix — Columnar epithelium

Squamocolumnar junction

Transformation zone

Squamous epithelium

FIGURE 21-4. Cervical epithelial surface.

- Any discharge or bleeding

  Discharge from os in mucopurulent cervicitis from Chlamydia or gonorrhea (see Table 21-2, Vaginal Discharge, p. 350)

- Any ulcers, nodules, or masses

  Herpes, polyp, cancer

Obtain specimens for cytology (Pap smears) with:

- An endocervical broom (Fig. 21-5) or brush with scraper (except in pregnant women), to collect both squamous and columnar cells

- Or, if the woman is pregnant, use a cotton-tipped applicator moistened with water

Early cancer before it is clinically evident

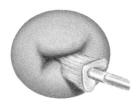

FIGURE 21-5. Endocervical broom.

Inspect the vaginal mucosa as you withdraw the speculum.

Bluish color and deep rugae in pregnancy; vaginal cancer (rare); vaginal discharge from infection from *Candida, Trichomonas vaginalis,* bacterial vaginosis (see Table 21-2, Vaginal Discharge, p. 350)

Palpate, by means of a bimanual examination (Fig. 21-6)

- Cervix and fornices

Pain on moving cervix in PID

- Uterus

Pregnancy, myomas; soft isthmus in early pregnancy (see Table 21-4, Positions of the Uterus and Uterine Myomas, p. 352)

- Right and left adnexa (ovaries)

Ovarian cysts or masses, salpingitis, PID, tubal pregnancy

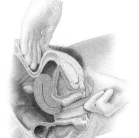

FIGURE 21-6. Palpating the cervix, uterus, and adnexa.

Assess strength of pelvic muscles. With your vaginal fingers clear of the cervix, ask patient to tighten her muscles around your fingers as hard and long as she can.

A firm squeeze that compresses your fingers, moves them up and inward, and lasts more than 3 seconds is full strength (see Table 21-5, Relaxations of the Pelvic Floor, p. 353).

∧∧ When indicated, perform a rectovaginal examination as shown in Figure 21-7 to palpate a retroverted uterus, uterosacral ligaments, cul-de-sac, and adnexa or screen for colorectal cancer in women 50 years or older (see p. 313).

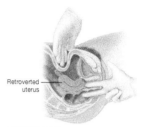

Retroverted uterus

FIGURE 21-7. Examining the rectovaginal area.

Special Techniques

Assessing Hernias. Ask the woman to strain down, as you palpate for a bulge in the:

- Femoral canal

Femoral hernia

- Labia majora up to just lateral to the pubic tubercle

Indirect inguinal hernia

Assessing Urethritis. Insert your index finger into the vagina and milk the urethra gently outward from the inside (Fig. 21-8). Note any discharge.

Discharge in *C. trachomatis* and *Neisseria gonorrhoeae* infection

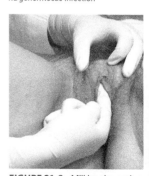

FIGURE 21-8. Milking the urethra, if indicated.

RECORDING YOUR FINDINGS

Recording the Female Genitalia Examination

"No inguinal adenopathy. External genitalia without erythema, lesions, or masses. Vaginal mucosa pink. Cervix parous, pink, and without discharge. Uterus anterior, midline, smooth, and not enlarged. No adnexal tenderness. Pap smear obtained. Rectovaginal wall intact. Rectal vault without masses. Stool brown and occult blood negative."

OR

"Bilateral shotty inguinal adenopathy. External genitalia without erythema or lesions. Vaginal mucosa and cervix coated with thin, white homogeneous discharge with mild fishy odor. After swabbing cervix, no discharge visible in cervical os. Uterus midline; no adnexal masses. Rectal vault without masses. Stool brown and occult blood negative."

These findings suggest bacterial vaginosis.

HEALTH PROMOTION AND COUNSELING: EVIDENCE AND RECOMMENDATIONS

Important Topics for Health Promotion and Counseling

- Cervical cancer prevention
- Cervical cancer screening
- Menopause and hormone replacement therapy

Cervical Cancer Prevention

The most important risk factor for cervical cancer is human papillomavirus (HPV) infection from HPV strains 16, 18, 6, or 11. The three-dose HPV vaccination series prevents HPV infection from these strains when given *before* sexual exposure at age 11 years. The vaccine is also recommended for unvaccinated and immunocompromised females up to age 26 years.

The Advisory Committee on Immunization Practices (ACIP) recommends routine vaccination for females beginning at age 11 or 12 years, though vaccinations can be first given at age 9. Vaccination also recommended for females through age 26 who were not previously adequately vaccinated.

Cervical Cancer Screening

In 2018, the U.S. Preventive Services Task Force (USPSTF) gave a grade A recommendation for screening average-risk women age 21 to 65 years (Box 21-2). They recommended against screening women younger than age 21, average-risk women older than 65 with adequate previous screening, and women who had undergone hysterectomy with removal of the cervix (D recommendations).

BOX 21-2. Current Cervical Cancer Screening Guidelines for Average-Risk Women

Variables	Recommendation
Age to begin screening	21 years
Screening method and interval	Ages 21–65 years: cytology every 3 years OR
	Ages 21–29 years: cytology every 3 years
	Ages 30–65 years: cytology plus HPV testing (for high-risk or oncogenic HPV types) every 5 years; HPV testing alone (age 25 or 30)
Age to end screening	Age >65 years, assuming three consecutive negative results on cytology or two consecutive negative results on cytology plus HPV testing within 10 years before cessation of screening, with the most recent test performed within 5 years
Screening after hysterectomy with removal of the cervix	Not recommended

Average-risk: no history of high-grade, precancerous cervical lesion or cervical cancer; not immunocompromised; and having no in utero exposure to DES.

Source: Curry SJ, Krist AH, Ownes DK, et al. Screening for cervical cancer: U.S. Preventive Services Task Force recommendation statement. *JAMA*. 2018;320:674–686.

Menopause and Hormone Replacement Therapy

Be familiar with the psychologic and physiologic changes of menopause. Help the patient weigh the risks of hormone replacement therapy (HRT) to treat menopausal symptoms, including increased risk of stroke, pulmonary embolism, and breast cancer.

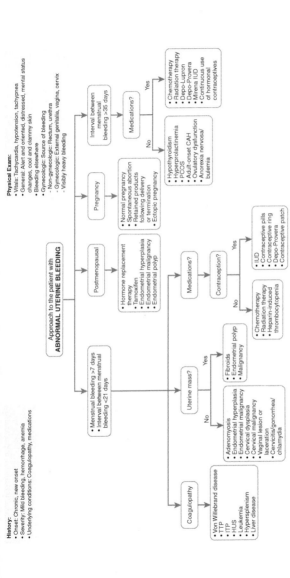

Algorithm 21-1. Approach to the patient with abnormal uterine bleeding. (Note: Although it is not comprehensive, this algorithm may be a helpful starting approach for synthesizing information gathered from the history and physical.) CAH, congenital adrenal hyperplasia; HUS, hemolytic uremic syndrome; ITP, immune/ideopathic thrombocytopenic purpura; IUD, intrauterine device; PCOS, polycystic ovary syndrome; TTP, thrombotic thrombocytopenic purpura.

History:
• Onset: Chronic, new onset
• Severity: Mild bleeding, hemorrhage, anemia
• Underlying conditions: Coagulopathy, medications

Physical Exam:
• Vitals: Tachycardia, hypotension, tachypnea
• General: Alert and oriented, distressed, mental status changes, cool and clammy skin
• Bleeding elsewhere
• Gynecologic: Source of bleeding
  - Non-gynecologic: Rectum, urethra
  - Gynecologic: External genitalia, vagina, cervix
  - Visibly heavy bleeding

Approach to the patient with **ABNORMAL UTERINE BLEEDING**

Coagulopathy
• Von Willebrand disease
• TTP
• HUS
• Leukemia
• Hypersplenism
• Liver disease

• Menstrual bleeding >7 days
• Interval between menstrual bleeding <21 days

Uterine mass?

No:
• Adenomyosis
• Endometrial hyperplasia
• Endometrial malignancy
• Cervical dysplasia
• Cervical malignancy
• Vaginal lesion or laceration
• Cervicitis/gonorrhea/ chlamydia

Yes:
• Fibroids
• Endometrial polyp
• Malignancy

Postmenopausal
• Hormone replacement therapy
• Tamoxifen
• Endometrial hyperplasia
• Endometrial polyp

Medications?

No:
• Chemotherapy
• Radiation therapy
• Heparin-induced thrombocytopenia

Yes — Contraception?

No:
• IUD

Yes:
• Contraceptive pills
• Contraceptive ring
• Depo-Provera
• Contraceptive patch

Pregnancy
• Normal pregnancy
• Spontaneous abortion
• Retained products following delivery or termination
• Ectopic pregnancy

Interval between menstrual bleeding >35 days

Medications?

No:
• Hypothyroidism
• Hyperprolactinemia
• PCOS
• Adult-onset CAH
• Ovulatory dysfunction
• Anorexia nervosa/ bulimia

Yes:
• Chemotherapy
• Radiation therapy
• Depo-Lupron
• Depo-Provera
• Mirena IUD
• Continuous use of hormonal contraceptives

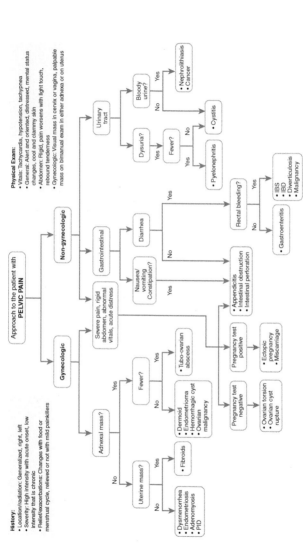

Algorithm 21-2. Approach to the patient with vulvovaginal symptoms. (Note: Although it is not comprehensive, this algorithm may be a helpful starting approach for synthesizing information gathered from the history and physical.) IBD, inflammatory bowel disease; IBS, irritable bowel syndrome; PID, pelvic inflammatory disease.

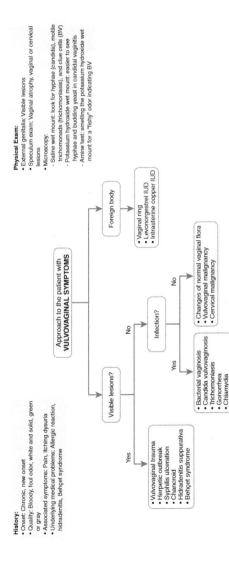

History:
- Onset: Chronic, new onset
- Quality: Bloody, foul odor, white and solid, green or gray
- Associated symptoms: Pain, itching dysuria
- Underlying medical problems: Allergic reaction, hidradenitis, Behçet syndrome

Physical Exam:
- External genitalia: Visible lesions
- Speculum exam: Vaginal atrophy, vaginal or cervical lesions
- Microscopy:
  - Saline wet mount: look for hyphae (candida), motile trichomonads (trichomoniasis), and clue cells (BV)
  - Potassium hydroxide wet mount: easier to see hyphae and budding yeast in candidal vaginitis
  - Amine test: smelling the potassium hydroxide wet mount for a "fishy" odor indicating BV

Approach to the patient with VULVOVAGINAL SYMPTOMS

Visible lesions?

Yes
- Vulvovaginal trauma
- Herpetic outbreak
- Syphilis ulceration
- Chancroid
- Hidradenitis suppurativa
- Behçet syndrome

No

Infection?

Yes
- Bacterial vaginosis
- Candida vulvovaginosis
- Trichomoniasis
- Gonorrhea
- Chlamydia

No
- Changes of normal vaginal flora
- Vulvovaginal malignancy
- Cervical malignancy

Foreign body
- Vaginal ring
- Levonorgestrel IUD
- Intrauterine copper IUD

Algorithm 21-3. Approach to the patient with pelvic pain. (Note: Although it is not comprehensive, this algorithm may be a helpful starting approach for synthesizing information gathered from the history and physical.) BV, bacterial vaginosis; IUD, intrauterine device.

INTERPRETATION AIDS

TABLE 21-1. Lesions of the Vulva

Epidermoid Cyst

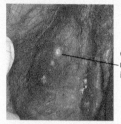

Cystic
nodule
in skin

A small, firm, round cystic nodule in the labia suggests an epidermoid cyst. They are yellowish in color. Look for the dark punctum marking the blocked opening of the gland.

Venereal Wart (*Condyloma Acuminatum*)

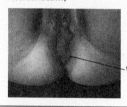

Warts

Warty lesions on the labia and within the vestibule suggest condyloma acuminata from infection with human papillomavirus.

Genital Herpes

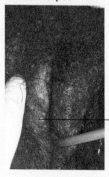

Shallow
ulcers
on red
bases

Shallow, small, painful ulcers on red bases suggest a herpes infection. Initial infection may be extensive, as illustrated here. Recurrent infections are usually confined to a small local patch.

TABLE 21-1. Lesions of the Vulva *(continued)*

Syphilitic Chancre

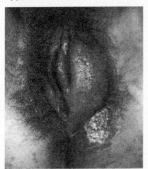

A firm, painless ulcer suggests the chancre of primary syphilis. Because most chancres in women develop internally, they often go undetected.

Secondary Syphilis (*Condyloma Latum*)

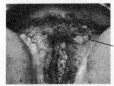

Flat, gray papules

Slightly raised, round or oval flat-topped papules covered by a gray exudate suggest condylomata lata, a manifestation of secondary syphilis. They are contagious.

Carcinoma of the Vulva

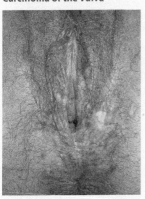

An ulcerated or raised red vulvar lesion in an elderly woman may indicate vulvar carcinoma.

TABLE 21-2. Vaginal Discharge

Accurate diagnosis depends on laboratory assessment and cultures.

Trichomonas **vaginitis**

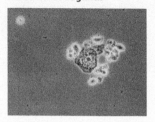

Discharge: Yellowish green, often profuse, may be malodorous

Other Symptoms: Itching, vaginal soreness, dyspareunia

Vulva: May be red

Vagina: May be normal or red, with red spots, petechiae

Laboratory Assessment: Saline wet mount for trichomonads

Candida **vaginitis**

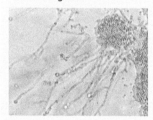

Discharge: White, curdy, often thick, not malodorous

Other Symptoms: Itching, vaginal soreness, external dysuria, dyspareunia

Vulva: Often red and swollen

Vagina: Often red with white patches of discharge

Laboratory Assessment: KOH preparation for branching hyphae

Bacterial vaginosis

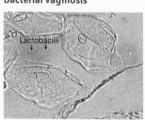

Lactobacilli

Discharge: Gray or white, thin, homogeneous, scant, malodorous

Other Symptoms: Fishy genital odor

Vulva: Usually normal

Vagina: Usually normal

Laboratory Assessment: Saline wet mount for "clue cells," "whiff test" with KOH for fishy odor

TABLE 21-3. Abnormalities of the Cervix

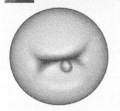

Endocervical polyp. A bright red, smooth mass that protrudes from the os suggests a polyp. It bleeds easily.

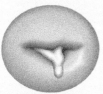

Mucopurulent cervicitis. A yellowish exudate emerging from the cervical os suggests infection from *Chlamydia*, *gonorrhea* (often asymptomatic), or herpes.

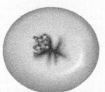

Carcinoma of the cervix. An irregular hard mass suggests carcinoma from HPV infection. Early lesions are best detected by Pap smear and HPV screening, followed by colposcopy.

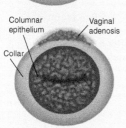

Columnar epithelium

Vaginal adenosis

Collar

Fetal exposure to diethylstilbestrol (DES). Several changes may occur: a collar of tissue around the cervix, columnar epithelium that covers the cervix or extends to the vaginal wall and, rarely, carcinoma of the vagina.

TABLE 21-4. Positions of the Uterus and Uterine Myomas

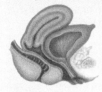

Anteverted uterus lies in a forward position at roughly a right angle to the vagina. This is the most common position. *Anteflexion*—a forward flexion of the uterine body in relation to the cervix—often coexists.

Retroverted uterus is tilted posteriorly with its cervix facing anteriorly.

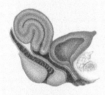

Retroflexed uterus has a posterior tilt that involves the uterine body but not the cervix. A uterus that is retroflexed or retroverted may be felt only through the rectal wall; some cannot be felt at all.

Myoma of the uterus is a very common benign tumor that feels firm and often irregular. There may be more than one. A myoma on the posterior surface of the uterus may be mistaken for a retrodisplaced uterus; one on the anterior surface may be mistaken for an anteverted uterus.

TABLE 21-5. Relaxations of the Pelvic Floor

When the pelvic floor is weakened, various structures may become displaced. These displacements are seen best when the patient strains down.

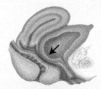

Cystocele is a bulge of the anterior wall of the upper part of the vagina, together with the urinary bladder above it.

Cystourethrocele involves both the bladder and the urethra as they bulge into the anterior vaginal wall throughout most of its extent.

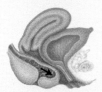

Rectocele is a bulge of the posterior vaginal wall, together with a portion of the rectum.

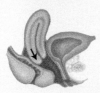

Prolapsed uterus has descended down the vaginal canal. There are three degrees of severity: first, still within the vagina (as illustrated); second, with the cervix at the introitus; and third, with the cervix outside the introitus.

22

Anus, Rectum, and Prostate

HEALTH HISTORY

Common Concerns

- Change in bowel habits
- Blood in stool
- Pain with defecation; rectal tenderness
- Anal warts or fissures
- Weak urinary stream

Familiarize yourself with the anorectal area and its surrounding structures (Fig. 22-1).

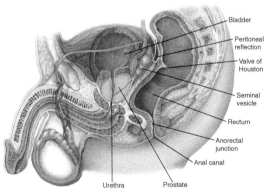

FIGURE 22-1. Anus and rectum—sagittal view.

Change in Bowel Habits

Ask about any change in bowel habits or stool size or caliber, and any diarrhea or constipation.

Change in stool caliber, especially pencil-thin stools, may warn of colon cancer

Blood in Stool

Is there any blood in the stool ranging from black tarry stools (*melena*), to bloody stools (*hematochezia*), to bright-red blood per rectum? Any mucus in the stool?

Dark tarry stools if polyps, carcinoma, gastrointestinal bleeding; mucus in villous adenoma, inflammatory bowel disease (IBD), or irritable bowel syndrome (IBS)

Pain with Defecation, Rectal Tenderness

Any pain with defecation, or rectal bleeding or tenderness?

Hemorrhoids; proctitis from sexually transmitted infections (STIs)

Anal Warts or Fissures

Any anal warts, fissures, or ulcerations?

Human papillomavirus (HPV), condylomata lata in secondary syphilis; fissures in Crohn disease, proctitis from receptive anal intercourse, ulcerations of herpes simplex, or chancres of primary syphilis

Weak Urinary Stream

In men, is there difficulty starting the urine stream or holding back urine? Is the flow weak? What about frequent urination, especially at night? Is there any blood in the urine?

These symptoms suggest urethral obstruction from benign prostatic hyperplasia (BPH) or prostate cancer, especially in men age ≥70 years. The American Urological Association (AUA) Symptom Index helps quantify BPH severity (see Table 22-1, BPH Symptom Score Index: American Urological Association (AUA), p. 360).

See Algorithm 22-1, Approach to the patient with urinary symptoms, p. 359.

TECHNIQUES OF EXAMINATION

Key Components of the Anorectal and Prostate Examination

- Inspect sacrococcygeal and perianal areas
- Inspect anus
- Perform a digital rectal examination:
  - Assess anal sphincter tone
  - Palpate anal canal and rectal surface
  - In men, palpate prostate gland

⚥–♂ Patient with a Prostate

Position the patient on one side or standing leaning forward over the examining table and hips flexed (Fig. 22-2).

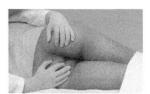

FIGURE 22-2. Position the patient on the left side.

Inspect the:

- Sacrococcygeal area

    Pilonidal cyst or sinus

- Perianal area

    Hemorrhoids, warts, herpes, chancre, cancer, fissures from proctitis, STIs, or Crohn disease, fistula from anorectal abscess

Palpate anal canal and rectum with a lubricated and gloved finger. Palpate the:

Lax sphincter tone in some neurologic disorders; tightness in proctitis

- Walls of the rectum

    Cancer of the rectum, polyps

- Prostate gland, as shown in Figure 22-3, including median sulcus

    Prostate nodule or cancer (Fig. 22-4); BPH; tenderness in prostatitis

- Try to palpate above the prostate for irregularities or tenderness, if indicated.

    See Table 22-2, Abnormalities on Rectal Examination, pp. 361–362.

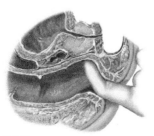

FIGURE 22-3. Palpating the prostate gland.

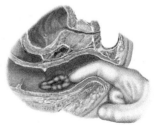

FIGURE 22-4. Rectal cancer.

∿/ↄ̶ Female Patient

The patient is usually in the lithotomy position or lying on one side.	Rectal shelf of peritoneal metastases; tenderness of inflammation
Inspect the anus.	Hemorrhoids
Palpate the anal canal and rectum.	Rectal cancer, normal uterine cervix or tampon (felt through the rectal wall)

RECORDING YOUR FINDINGS

Recording the Anus, Rectum, and Prostate Examination

"No perirectal lesions or fissures. External sphincter tone intact. Rectal vault without masses. Prostate smooth and nontender with palpable median sulcus. (Or in a female, uterine cervix nontender.) Stool brown and occult blood negative."

OR

"No perirectal lesions or fissures. External sphincter tone intact. Rectal vault without masses. Left lateral prostate lobe with 1 × 1 cm firm hard nodule; right lateral lobe smooth; medial sulcus is obscured. Stool brown and occult blood negative."

These findings are suspicious for prostate cancer.

HEALTH PROMOTION AND COUNSELING: EVIDENCE AND RECOMMENDATIONS

Important Topics for Health Promotion and Counseling

- Prostate cancer screening

Prostate Cancer Screening

Prostate cancer is the most frequently diagnosed nonskin cancer in the United States and the second leading cause of death in men. Risk factors are age, family history of prostate cancer, and African American ethnicity. Major professional organizations, including the U.S. Preventive Services Task Force, the

American Cancer Society (ACS), and the American Urological Association (AUA) have all issued guidelines in recent years (Box 22-1).

BOX 22-1. Prostate Cancer Screening Guidelines

	United States Preventive Services Task Force (2018)	American Cancer Society (2012)	American Urological Association (2013)
Shared decision making	Yes	Yes (consider using decision aid)	Yes
Age to begin offering screening			
Average-risk	55	50 years	55 years
High-risk	No recommendation	40–45 years	40 years
Age to stop offering screening	69	Life expectancy <10 years	Life expectancy <10 years
Screening tests	PSA	PSA DRE (optional)	PSA DRE (optional)
Frequency of screening	No recommendation	Annual (biennial when PSA <2.5 ng/mL)	Every two years may be preferable
Biopsy referral criteria	No recommendation	PSA ≥4 ng/mL Abnormal DRE Individualized risk assessment for PSA levels 2.5–4 ng/mL	No specific PSA level, consider using biomarkers, imaging, and risk calculators to inform biopsy decisions

Abbreviations: PSA, prostate-specific antigen; DRE, digital rectal examination.

Encourage men with symptomatic disorders such as incomplete emptying of the bladder, urinary frequency or urgency, weak or intermittent stream or straining to initiate flow, hematuria, nocturia, or even bony pains in the pelvis to seek evaluation and treatment early.

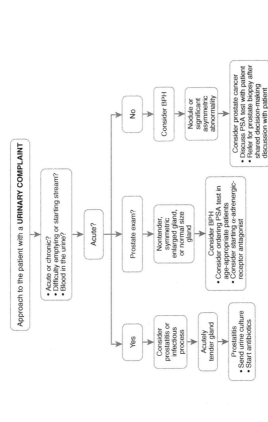

Algorithm 22-1. Approach to the patient with urinary symptoms. (Note: Although it is not comprehensive, this algorithm may be a helpful starting approach for synthesizing information gathered from the history and physical.) BPH, benign prostatic hyperplasia; PSA, prostate-specific antigen.

The following is the content within the algorithm image:

Approach to the patient with a **URINARY COMPLAINT**

- Acute or chronic?
- Difficulty emptying or starting stream?
- Blood in the urine?

Acute?

Yes

Consider prostatitis or infectious process

Acutely tender gland

Prostatitis
- Send urine culture
- Start antibiotics

Prostate exam?

Nontender, symmetric enlarged gland, or normal size gland

Consider BPH
- Consider ordering PSA test in age-appropriate patients
- Consider starting α-adrenergic-receptor antagonist

No

Consider BPH

Nodule or significant asymmetric abnormality

Consider prostate cancer
- Discuss PSA test with patient
- Refer for prostate biopsy after shared decision-making discussion with patient

INTERPRETATION AIDS

TABLE 22-1. BPH Symptom Score Index: American Urological Association (AUA)

PART A	Score

Score or ask the patient to score each of the questions below on a scale of 1 to 5, with 0 = not at all, 1 = less than 1 time in 5, 2 = less than half the time, 3 = about half the time, 4 = more than half the time, and 5 = almost always.

1. **Incomplete emptying:** Over the past month, how often have you had a sensation of not emptying your bladder completely after you finished urinating? _____

2. **Frequency:** Over the past month, how often have you had to urinate again <2 hrs after you finished urinating? _____

3. **Intermittency:** Over the past month, how often have you stopped and started again several times when you urinated? _____

4. **Urgency:** Over the past month, how often have you found it difficult to postpone urination? _____

5. **Weak stream:** Over the past month, how often have you had a weak urinary stream? _____

6. **Straining:** Over the past month, how often have you had to push or strain to begin urination? _____

PART A TOTAL SCORE _____

PART B	Score

0 = none, 1 = 1 time, 2 = 2 times, 3 = 3 times, 4 = 4 times, 5 = 5 times.

7. **Nocturia:** Over the past month, how many times did you most typically get up to urinate from the time you went to bed at night until the time you got up in the morning? (Score 0 to 5 times on night) _____

TOTAL PARTS A and B (maximum 35) _____

Higher scores (maximum 35) indicate more severe symptoms; scores ≤7 are considered mild and generally do not warrant treatment.

Adapted from Madsen FA, Burskewitz RC. Clinical manifestations of benign prostatic hyperplasia. *Urol Clin North Am.* 1995:22(2):291–298. Copyright © 1995 Elsevier. With permission.

TABLE 22-2. Abnormalities on Rectal Examination

External Hemorrhoids (Thrombosed). Dilated hemorrhoidal veins that originate below the pectinate line, covered with skin; a tender, swollen, bluish ovoid mass is visible at the anal margin.

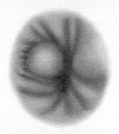

Anal Fissure. Painful longitudinal oval ulceration usually in posterior midline with swollen sentinel tag just below it.

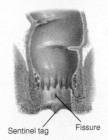

Sentinel tag   Fissure

Anorectal Fistula. An inflammatory tract or tube opening inside the anus or rectum and also onto the perianal area or into another viscus.

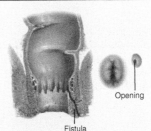

Opening

Fistula

Polyps of the Rectum. A soft mass that may or may not be on a stalk; may not be palpable.

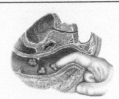

continued

TABLE 22-2. Abnormalities on Rectal Examination *(continued)*

Benign Prostatic Hyperplasia. An enlarged, nontender, smooth, firm but slightly elastic prostate gland; can cause symptoms without palpable enlargement.

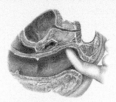

Acute Prostatitis. A prostate that is very tender, swollen, and firm because of acute infection.

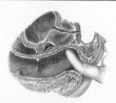

Cancer of the Prostate. A hard area in the prostate that may or may not feel nodular.

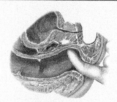

Cancer of the Rectum. Firm, nodular, rolled edge of an ulcerated cancer.

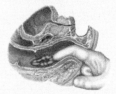

Musculoskeletal System

FUNDAMENTALS FOR ASSESSING JOINTS

Assessing joints requires knowledge of each joint's structure and function. Learn the surface landmarks and underlying anatomy of each of the major joints. Use the descriptive terms below.

Joint Anatomy—Important Terms

- *Articular structures* include the *joint capsule* and *articular cartilage*, the *synovium* and *synovial fluid, intra-articular ligaments,* and *juxta-articular bone.* Articular cartilage is composed of a collagen matrix containing charged ions and water, allowing the cartilage to change shape in response to pressure or load, acting as a cushion for underlying bone. Synovial fluid provides nutrition to the adjacent relatively avascular articular cartilage.
- *Extra-articular structures* include periarticular ligaments, tendons, bursae, muscle, fascia, bone, nerve, and overlying skin.
- *Ligaments* are rope-like bundles of collagen fibrils that connect bone to bone.
- *Tendons* are collagen fibers connecting muscle to bone.
- *Bursae* are pouches of synovial fluid that cushion the movement of tendons and muscles over bone or other joint structures.

Review the three primary types of joint articulation—*synovial, cartilaginous, and fibrous*—and the varying degrees of movement each type allows (Box 23-1). Note that joint anatomy determines its function and degrees of movement.

BOX 23-1. Types of Joints

Type of Joint	Characteristics	Examples
Synovial Bone Ligament Synovial membrane Joint space Joint capsule Synovial cavity Articular cartilage	■ Freely movable within limits of surrounding ligaments ■ Separated by articular cartilage and a synovial cavity ■ Lubricated by synovial fluid ■ Surrounded by a joint capsule	Knee, shoulder
Cartilaginous Vertebral body Nucleus pulposus of the disc Disc Ligament	■ Slightly movable ■ Contain fibrocartilaginous discs that separate the bony surfaces ■ Have a central nucleus pulposus of discs that cushions bony contact	Vertebral bodies of the spine, symphysis pubis, sternomanubrial joint
Fibrous	■ Immovable ■ No appreciable movement ■ Consist of fibrous tissue or cartilage ■ Lack a joint cavity	Skull sutures

Also review the types of synovial joints and their associated features (Box 23-2).

BOX 23-2. Types of Synovial Joints

Type of Synovial Joint	Articular Shape	Movement	Examples
Spheroidal (ball and socket)	Convex surface in concave cavity	Wide-ranging–flexion, extension, abduction, adduction, rotation, circumduction	Shoulder, hip
Hinge	Flat, planar	Motion in one plane; flexion, extension	Interphalangeal joints of hand and foot; elbow
Condylar	Convex or concave	Movement of two articulating surfaces not dissociable	Knee; temporomandibular joint

HEALTH HISTORY

Common Concerns

- Joint pain
- Neck pain
- Low back pain

Joint Pain

Location. Ask "Do you have any pains in your joints?" (Box 23-3) Ask the patient to *point to the pain*. If *localized* and involving only one joint, it is *monoarticular*. Is it *oligo-/pauci-articular* (two to four joints) or *polyarticular*?

See Table 23-1, Patterns of Pain in and Around the Joints, p. 403, and Algorithm 23-1, Approach to the patient with musculoskeletal complaints, p. 399.

Monoarticular arthritis in traumatic, crystalline, or septic arthritis; oligoarticular arthritis gonorrhea or rheumatic fever, connective tissue disease, and OA; polyarthritis if may be viral or inflammatory from RA, SLE, or psoriasis

---

BOX 23-3. Tips for Assessing Joint Pain

- Ask the patient to "point to the pain." This may save considerable time because many patients have trouble pinpointing pain location in words.
- Characterize the pain using the seven attributes of a symptom: *location, quality, quantity or severity, timing, onset, remitting or exacerbating factors, and associated manifestations.*
- Clarify and record the mechanism of injury, particularly if there is a history of trauma.
- Determine whether the pain is articular or extra-articular, acute or chronic, inflammatory or noninflammatory, and localized (monoarticular) or diffuse (polyarticular).

If polyarticular, does it migrate from joint to joint or steadily spread from one joint to multiple joint involvement? Is the involvement *symmetric* (affecting similar joints on both sides of the body) or *asymmetric* (affecting different joints on different sides)?

Migratory pattern in rheumatic fever or gonococcal arthritis; progressive and symmetric pattern in rheumatoid arthritis; asymmetric in psoriatic, reactive, and inflammatory bowel disease (IBD)-associated arthritis

Are there generalized "aches and pains" (*myalgia* if in muscles, *arthralgia* if in joints with no evidence of arthritis)?

Bursitis if inflammation of bursae; *tendinitis* if in tendons, and *tenosynovitis* if in tendon sheaths; also *sprains* from stretching or tearing of ligaments

Ask if there is decreased joint movement or stiffness.

In articular pain, decreased active and passive range of motion and morning stiffness ("gelling"); in nonarticular joint pain, periarticular tenderness and only passive range of motion intact

Quality. What is the pain like? Ask, "Can you describe the pain (what it feels like)?" Patients may describe the pain in many different ways including dull, gnawing, or stiff.

Severity. How bad is the pain? Ask for the severity rating on a scale of 1 to 10.

In general, inflammatory causes of joint pain are considerably more painful than noninflammatory types.

Inflammatory disorders may be infectious (e.g., *Neisseria gonorrhoeae* or *Mycobacterium tuberculosis*), crystal-induced (gout, pseudogout), immune-related (RA, SLE), reactive (rheumatic fever, reactive arthritis), or idiopathic

In noninflammatory disorders, consider trauma (e.g., rotator cuff tear in the shoulder), overuse (bursitis, tendinitis), degenerative changes (OA), or fibro-myalgia.

Onset and Timing. *Acute* joint pain typically lasts up to 6 weeks; *chronic* pain lasts >12 weeks. Assess the timing of joint symptoms.

Severe pain of rapid onset in acute septic arthritis or crystalline arthritis (gout; CPPD).

If from trauma, what was the *mechanism of injury* or series of events that caused the joint pain?

See Table 23-1, Patterns of Pain in and Around the Joints, p. 403.

Remitting or Exacerbating Factors. Ask what aggravates or relieves the pain. What are the effects of exercise, rest, and treatment?

In inflammatory joint disorders (e.g., RA), rest tends to worsen the pain, activity improves it. In mechanical joint disorders (e.g., OA), activity tends to increase the pain and stiffness, and rest improves it.

Associated Manifestations
Inflammation. Is there fever, chills, tenderness, warmth, or redness?

If inflammatory, consider infectious causes (*N. gonorrhoeae* or *M. tuberculosis*), crystal-induced (gout, pseudogout), immune-related (RA, SLE), reactive (rheumatic fever, reactive arthritis), or idiopathic arthritis. If noninflammatory, consider trauma (rotator cuff tear), repetitive use (bursitis, tendinitis), OA, fibromyalgia.

Limitation in Movement and Stiffness.
Assess any stiffness or limitations of
motion.

Morning stiffness that gradually
improves with activity in inflammatory
disorders like RA and PMR; intermittent
stiffness and gelling in OA

Age also provides clues to causes of
joint pain (Box 23-4).

BOX 23-4. Common Causes of Joint Pain by Age

Age <60 Years	Age >60 Years
■ Repetitive strain or overuse syndromes (tendinitis, bursitis) ■ Crystalline arthritis (gout; crystalline pyrophosphate deposition disease [CPPD]) ■ Rheumatoid arthritis (RA), psoriatic arthritis and reactive (Reiter) arthritis (in inflammatory bowel disease [IBD]) ■ Infectious arthritis from gonorrhea, Lyme disease, or viral or bacterial infections	■ Osteoarthritis (OA) ■ Osteoporotic fracture ■ Gout and pseudogout ■ Polymyalgia rheumatica (PMR) ■ Septic bacterial arthritis

---

**Associated Constitutional Symptoms
and Systemic Manifestations from
Other Organ Systems.** Assess *constitutional symptoms* such as fever, chills,
rash, fatigue, anorexia, weight loss, and
weakness.

Common in RA, SLE, PMR, and other
inflammatory arthritides. High fever
and chills suggest an infectious cause.

Neck Pain

Ask about location, radiation into the
shoulders or arms, arm or leg weakness, bladder or bowel dysfunction.

C7 or C6 spinal nerve compression
from foraminal impingement is more
common than disc herniation. See
Table 23-2, Pains in the Neck, p. 404.

If the patient reports neck trauma,
common in motor vehicle accidents,
ask about neck tenderness and consider
clinical decision rules that identify risk
of cervical cord injury (e.g., NEXUS
criteria and Canadian C-Spine Rule).

Low Back Pain

Ask, "Do you have any pains in your back?" and "Is the pain in the midline over the vertebrae, or off midline?"

See Table 23-3, Low Back Pain, p. 405. Midline back pain in vertebral collapse, disc herniation, epidural abscess, spinal cord compression, or spinal cord metastases. Pain off the midline in muscle strain, sacroiliitis, trochanteric bursitis, sciatica, hip arthritis, renal conditions such as pyelonephritis or renal stones

If the pain radiates into the legs, ask about any associated numbness, tingling, or weakness. Ask about history of trauma.

Sciatica if radicular gluteal and posterior leg pain in the S1 distribution that increases with cough or Valsalva

Check for bladder or bowel dysfunction.

Present in cauda equina syndrome from S2–S4 tumor or disc herniation, especially if "saddle anesthesia" from perianal numbness

Elicit any red flags for serious underlying systemic disease (Box 23-5).

BOX 23-5. Red Flags for Low Back Pain from Underlying Systemic Disease

- Age <20 years or >50 years
- History of cancer
- Unexplained weight loss, fever, or decline in general health
- Pain lasting more than 1 month or not responding to treatment
- Pain at night or present at rest
- History of intravenous drug use, addiction, or immuno-suppression
- Presence of active infection or human immunodeficiency virus (HIV) infection
- Long-term steroid therapy
- Saddle anesthesia
- Bladder or bowel incontinence
- Neurologic symptoms or progressive neurologic deficit
- Lower extremity weakness

TECHNIQUES OF EXAMINATION

Steps for Examining Joints

The approach can be divided into three broad sections: visual inspection, palpation, and the evaluation of joint motion (Look, Feel and Move). This systematic approach can best be remembered by the mnemonic *IPROMS* (*"I promise…"*), which includes *Inspection, Palpation, Range of Motion, and Special maneuvers.*

1. **I**nspect: *Look*—evaluate visually for signs of deformity, asymmetry, swelling, scars, inflammation or muscle atrophy.
2. **P**alpate: *Feel*—surface anatomy landmarks used for localization of points of tenderness, *crepitus* (palpable crunching on movement of tendons or ligaments over bone, cartilage loss or fluid collection).
3. **R**ange **o**f **M**otion: *Move*—involved joints are moved *actively* by the patient, then *passively* by the examiner.
4. **S**pecial Maneuvers: *Move*—if indicated, stress maneuvers are performed to evaluate stability and integrity of ligaments, tendons, and bursae.

In addition, inspect and palpate any joints with signs of inflammation (Box 23-6).

BOX 23-6. Four Signs of Inflammation

- *Swelling.* Palpable swelling may involve: (1) the synovial membrane, which can feel boggy or doughy; (2) effusion from excess synovial fluid within the joint space; or (3) soft tissue structures, such as bursae, tendons, and tendon sheaths.

  Palpable bogginess or doughiness indicates synovitis, tenderness over the tendon sheath in tendinitis

- *Warmth.* Use the backs of your fingers to compare the involved joint with its unaffected contralateral joint, or with nearby tissues if both joints are involved.

  Increased warmth can be seen in arthritis, tendinitis, bursitis, osteomyelitis.

- *Redness.* Redness of the overlying skin is the least common sign of inflammation near the joints and is usually seen in more superficial joints like fingers, toes, and knees.

  Diffuse tenderness and warmth suggest arthritis or infection; focal tenderness suggests injury or trauma

- *Pain or tenderness.* Try to identify the specific anatomic structure that is tender.

  Redness over a tender joint suggests acute inflammation seen in septic, crystalline, or RA.

Temporomandibular Joint

Key Components of the Temporomandibular Joint Examination

- Inspect the face and TMJ
- Palpate the TMJ and muscles of mastication (masseters, temporal muscles, pterygoid muscles)
- Assess range of motion: opening, closing; protrusion, retraction; lateral, or side-to-side, motions

Inspect the temporomandibular joint (TMJ) for swelling or redness.

Palpate:

- TMJ as the patient opens and closes the mouth (Fig. 23-1).
- Muscles of mastication: the *masseters*, *temporal muscles*, and *pterygoid muscles.*

Assess range of motion (Box 23-7).

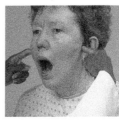

FIGURE 23-1. Palpating the TMJ while asking the patient to open and close the mouth.

BOX 23-7. Temporomandibular Joint Range of Motion

Jaw Movement	Primary Muscles Affecting Movement	Patient Instructions
Opening	Inferior head of lateral pterygoid, anterior digastric, mylohyoid	"Open your mouth wide."
Closing	Masseter, anterior and middle temporalis, medial pterygoid, superior head lateral pterygoid	"Close your mouth."
Protrusion	Lateral pterygoid	"Move your lower jaw by sticking it out (jutting it out)."
Retraction (Retrusion)	Middle and posterior temporalis	"Move your lower jaw by moving it in towards you."
Side-to-side (Laterotrusion)	Ipsilateral middle and posterior temporalis, contralateral inferior head lateral pterygoid	"Move your lower jaw from side to side."

Shoulders

Key Components of the Shoulder Joint Examination

- Inspect shoulder and shoulder girdle anteriorly and scapulae and related muscles posteriorly
- Palpate sternoclavicular joint, clavicle, acromioclavicular joint, coracoid process, greater tubercle, biceps tendon, subacromial and subdeltoid bursae, and underlying palpable SITS muscles
- Assess range of motion: flexion, extension, abduction, adduction, and internal and external rotations
- Perform special maneuvers (if indicated): painful arc test, Neer test, Hawkins test, drop arm test, empty can test

Inspect the contour of shoulders and shoulder girdles from front and back. When the shoulder muscles appear atrophic, inspect for scapular winging.

Muscle atrophy; anterior or posterior dislocation of humeral head; scoliosis if shoulder heights asymmetric

See Table 23-4, Painful Shoulders, p. 406 and Algorithm 23-2, Approach to the patient with shoulder pain, p. 400.

Palpate:

- Clavicle from the sternoclavicular joint to the acromioclavicular joint

"Step-offs" if fracture from trauma

- Bicipital tendon (Fig. 23-2)

- Subacromial and subdeltoid bursae after lifting arm posteriorly (Fig. 23-3)

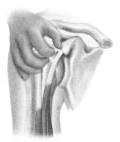

FIGURE 23-2. Palpating the bicipital tendon along the bicipital groove in the right shoulder.

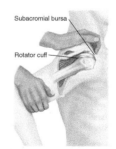

Subacromial bursa

Rotator cuff

FIGURE 23-3. Extending the right humerus posteriorly to palpate the SITS muscle insertions and bursae.

Assess range of motion (Box 23-8).   Shoulder arthritis

BOX 23-8. Shoulder Joint Range of Motion

Shoulder Movement	Primary Muscles Affecting Movement	Patient Instructions
Flexion 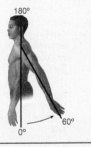	Anterior deltoid, pectoralis major (clavicular head), coracobrachialis, biceps brachii	"Raise your arms in front of you and overhead."
Extension 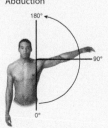	Latissimus dorsi, teres major, posterior deltoid, triceps brachii (long head)	"Raise your arms behind you."
Abduction	Supraspinatus, middle deltoid, serratus anterior (via upward rotation of the scapula)	"Raise your arms out to the side and overhead."

continued

Adduction 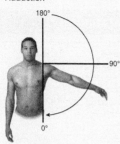	Pectoralis major, coracobrachialis, latissimus dorsi, teres major, subscapularis	"Bring your raised arm from overhead down to your side."
Internal Rotation 	Subscapularis, anterior deltoid, pectoralis major, teres major, latissimus dorsi	"Place one hand behind your back and try to touch your shoulder blade."
External Rotation 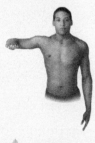 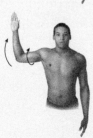	Infraspinatus, teres minor, posterior deltoid, supraspinatus (especially with arm overhead)	"Raise your arm to shoulder level; bend your elbow and rotate your forearm toward the ceiling." OR "Place one hand behind your neck or head as if you are brushing your hair."

TECHNIQUES OF EXAMINATION	POSSIBLE FINDINGS

Perform special maneuvers (Box 23-9) to assess the "SITS" muscles of the *rotator cuff* and the bicipital tendon (if indicated).

Subacromial or subdeltoid bursitis; tenderness over the SITS (**S**upraspinatus, **I**nfraspinatus, **T**eres minor, and **S**ubscapularis) muscle insertions and difficulty abducting the arm above shoulder level occurs in sprains, tears, tendon rupture of rotator cuff.

Pain or inability to perform these maneuvers in rotator cuff sprains, tendinitis, rupture

BOX 23-9. Special Maneuvers for SITS Muscle Assessment

Pain Provocation Tests

■ *Painful arc test.* Fully adduct the patient's arm from 0 to 180 degrees.

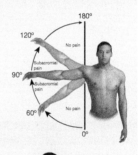

■ *Hawkins impingement sign.* Flex the patient's shoulder and elbow to 90 degrees with the palm facing down. Then, with one hand on the forearm and one on the arm, rotate the arm internally. This compresses the greater tuberosity against the supraspinatus tendon and coracoacromial ligament.

■ *Neer impingement sign.* Press on the scapula to prevent scapular motion with one hand and raise the patient's arm with the other. This compresses the greater tuberosity of the humerus against the acromion.

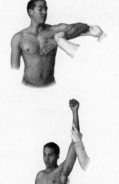

continued

Strength Test

Drop-arm test. Ask the patient to fully abduct the arm to shoulder level, up to 90 degrees, and lower it slowly. Note that abduction above shoulder level, from 90 to 120 degrees, reflects action of the deltoid muscle.

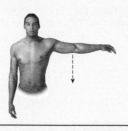

Composite Test

Empty can test. Elevate the arms to 90 degrees and internally rotate the arms with the thumbs pointing down, as if emptying a can. Ask the patient to resist as you place downward pressure on the arms.

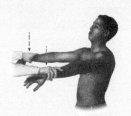

Elbows

Key Components of the Elbow Joint Examination

- Inspect contours of elbow, extensor surfaces of ulna, olecranon process
- Palpate olecranon process, medial and lateral epicondyles
- Assess range of motion: flexion, extension, pronation and supination
- Perform special maneuvers (if indicated): Cozen test (lateral epicondylitis)

Inspect and palpate:

- Olecranon process

  Olecranon bursitis; posterior dislocation from direct trauma or supracondylar fracture

- Medial and lateral epicondyles

  Tenderness distal to epicondyle in epicondylitis (*medial* → "tennis elbow"; *lateral* → "pitcher's elbow")

- Extensor surface of the ulna

  Rheumatoid nodules

- Grooves between the epicondyles and the olecranon

Assess range of motion (Box 23-10).   Tender in arthritis

BOX 23-10. Elbow Joint Range of Motion

Elbow Movement	Primary Muscles Affecting Movement	Patient Instructions
Flexion	Biceps brachii, brachialis, brachioradialis	"Bend your elbow."
Extension	Triceps brachii, anconeus	"Straighten your elbow."
Supination	Biceps brachii, supinator	"Turn your palms up."
Pronation	Pronator teres, pronator quadratus	"Turn your palms down."

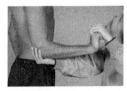

Perform special maneuver (if indicated)

■ *Cozen test:* Stabilize the patient's elbow and palpate the lateral epicondyle. Then ask the patient to pronate and extend the wrist against resistance. Pain should be reproduced along the lateral aspect of the elbow (Fig. 23-4).

FIGURE 23-4. Testing for lateral epicondylitis or "tennis elbow" (Cozen test). (From Anderson MK. *Foundations of Athletic Training: Prevention, Assessment, and Management.* 6th ed. Wolters Kluwer; 2017. Figure 18-11a.)

Wrists and Hands

Key Components of Wrist Joint and Hand Examination

■ Inspect wrist, hand, and finger bones; thenar and hypothenar eminences; and flexor tendons

continued

- Palpate radius, ulna, radial styloid bone, and anatomic snuffbox; carpal bones; metacarpals and proximal, middle, and distal phalanges, wrist joint, MCPs, and PIPs
- Assess range of motion. *Wrist:* flexion, extension, abduction (radial deviation) and adduction (ulnar deviation). *Fingers (MCP, PIP, DIP):* flexion, extension, abduction and adduction. *Thumb:* flexion, extension, abduction, adduction, and opposition
- Perform special maneuvers (if indicated): hand grip strength, tests for thumb tenosynovitis (Finkelstein test), and nerve entrapment neuropathy (sensation, thumb abduction and opposition, Tinel sign, Phalen sign)

Inspect:

- Movement of wrist, hands, and fingers

  Guarded movement in injury

- Contours of wrists, hands, and fingers

  Asymmetric DIP, PIP deformities in OA; symmetric deformities in PIP, MCP, wrist joints in RA; swelling in arthritis, ganglia; impaired alignment of fingers in flexor tendon damage; flexion contractures in Dupuytren contractures

- Contours of palms

  Thenar atrophy in median nerve compression (carpal tunnel syndrome); hypothenar atrophy in ulnar nerve compression

Palpate:

- Wrist joints (Fig. 23-5)

  Swelling and tenderness in rheumatoid arthritis, gonococcal infection of joint or extensor tendon sheaths

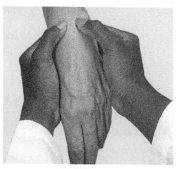

FIGURE 23-5. Palpating the left wrist joint.

- Distal radius and ulna

  Tenderness over ulnar styloid in Colles fracture

- "Anatomic snuffbox," the hollow space distal to the radial styloid bone; thumb extensor and abductor tendons (Fig. 23-6).

  Tenderness suggests scaphoid fracture. Tenderness over extensor and abductor tendons in de Quervain tenosynovitis.

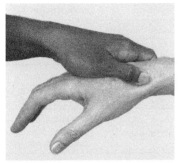

FIGURE 23-6. Palpating the anatomic snuffbox.

- Metacarpophalangeal joints (Fig. 23-7)

  Swelling in rheumatoid arthritis

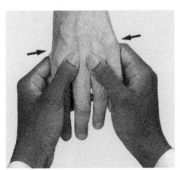

FIGURE 23-7. Palpating the MCP joints of the left hand.

- Proximal and distal interphalangeal joint

  Proximal nodules in RA; Bouchard (PIP) and Heberden (DIP) nodes in OA

Assess range of motion (Box 23-11).

- Wrists: Arthritis, tenosynovitis

BOX 23-11. Wrist Joint Range of Motion

Wrist Movement	Primary Muscles Affecting Movement	Patient Instructions
Flexion	Flexor carpi radialis, flexor carpi ulnaris	"With palms down, point your fingers toward the floor."
Extension	Extensor carpi ulnaris, extensor carpi radialis longus, extensor carpi radialis brevis	"With palms down, point your fingers toward the ceiling."
Adduction (ulnar deviation)	Flexor carpi ulnaris Extensor carpi ulnaris	"With palms down, move your fingers toward the midline."
Abduction (radial deviation)	Flexor carpi radialis Extensor carpi radialis longus and brevis Occasional contribution from abductor pollicis longus	"With palms down, move your fingers away from the midline."

- Fingers: Flexions, extension, abduc-   Trigger finger, Dupuytren contracture
  tion/adduction (spread fingers apart
  and back)

- Thumbs (Figs. 23-8 to 23-11)

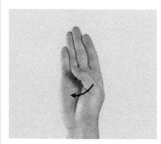

FIGURE 23-8. Testing thumb flexion.

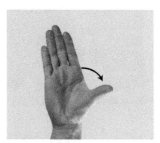

FIGURE 23-9. Testing thumb extension.

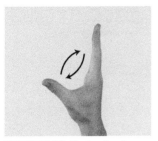

FIGURE 23-10. Testing thumb abduction and adduction.

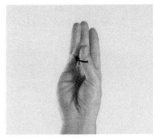

FIGURE 23-11. Testing thumb opposition.

Perform special maneuvers (if indicated).

- Hand grip strength (Fig. 23-12)

- Thumb movement (Fig. 23-13)

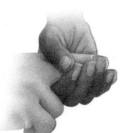

FIGURE 23-12. Testing hand grip strength.

Decreased grip strength if weakness of finger flexors or intrinsic hand muscles

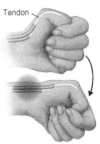

FIGURE 23-13. Testing for thumb tenosynovitis (Finkelstein test).

Pain if de Quervain tenosynovitis

- Carpal tunnel testing

  - *Tinel sign:* Tap lightly over median nerve at volar wrist (Fig. 23-14)

Aching, tingling, and numbness in second, third, and fourth fingers is a positive Tinel sign.

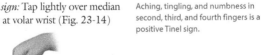

FIGURE 23-14. Testing for carpal tunnel syndrome (Tinel sign).

Chapter 23 ▪ Musculoskeletal System   **381**

■ *Phalen sign:* Patient flexes wrists for 60 seconds (Fig. 23-15)

Aching, tingling, and numbness in second, third, and fourth volar fingers is a positive Phalen sign.

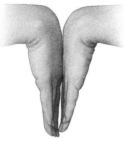

FIGURE 23-15. Testing for carpal tunnel syndrome (Phalen sign).

Spine

Key Components of the Vertebral Spine Examination

- Inspect posture; inspect cervical, thoracic, and lumbar curves laterally; alignment of shoulders, iliac crests, and gluteal folds posteriorly
- Palpate vertebral spinous processes, paravertebral muscles, facet joints, lumbosacral vertebra, sacroiliac joint, iliac crests, and posterior superior iliac spines
- Assess range of motion. *Cervical spine*: flexion, extension, rotation, and lateral bending. *Thoracolumbosacral spine*: flexion, extension, rotation, and lateral bending
- Perform special maneuver (if indicated): cervical radiculopathy (Spurling test)

Inspect the spine from the side and back, noting any abnormal curvatures.

Kyphosis, scoliosis, lordosis, gibbus, list curvatures

Look for asymmetric heights of shoulders, iliac crests, or buttocks.

Scoliosis, pelvic tilt, unequal leg length

Palpate (Fig. 23-16):

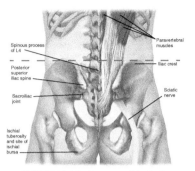

Spinous process
of L4

Posterior
superior
iliac spine

Sacroiliac
joint

Ischial
tuberosity
and site of
ischial
bursa

Paravertebral
muscles

Iliac crest

Sciatic
nerve

FIGURE 23-16. Anatomy of the back.

■ Spinous processes of each vertebra	Tender if trauma, infection; "step-offs" in spondylolisthesis, fracture
■ Sacroiliac joints	Sacroiliitis, ankylosing spondylitis
■ Paravertebral muscles, if painful	Paravertebral muscle spasm in abnormal posture, degenerative and inflammatory muscle disorders, over-use; see Algorithm 23-3, Approach to the patient with back pain, p. 401.
Assess range of motion in the neck and spine (Boxes 23-12 and 23-13).	Decreased mobility in arthritis

BOX 23-12. Cervical Spine Range of Motion

Movement	Primary Muscles Affecting Movement	Patient Instructions
Flexion	Sternocleidomastoid, scalene, and prevertebral muscles	*"Bring your chin to your chest."*
Extension	Splenius capitis and cervicis and small intrinsic neck muscles	*"Look up toward the ceiling."*
Rotation	Sternocleidomastoid and small intrinsic neck muscles	*"Look over one shoulder and then the other."*
Lateral Bending	Scalenes and small intrinsic neck muscles	*"Bring your ear to your shoulder."*

BOX 23-13. Thoracolumbosacral Spine Range of Motion

Movement	Primary Muscles Affecting Movement	Patient Instructions
Flexion ↓	Psoas major, psoas minor, and quadratus lumborum; abdominal muscles attaching to the anterior vertebrae, such as the internal and external obliques and rectus abdominis	"Bend forward and try to touch your toes."
Extension	Deep intrinsic muscles of the back, such as the erector spinae, transversospinalis group, iliocostalis, longissimus, and spinalis	"Bend back as far as possible."
Rotation	Abdominal muscles and intrinsic muscles of the back	"Rotate from side to side."
Lateral Bending	Abdominal muscles and intrinsic muscles of the back	"Bend to the side from the waist."

Hips

Key Components of the Hip Joint Examination

- Inspect gait and inspect the lumbar spine, legs, and anterior and posterior hip
- Palpate *anterior landmarks:* iliac crest, iliac tubercle, anterior–superior iliac spine, greater trochanter of femur, and the pubic tubercle. *posterior landmarks:* posterior–superior iliac spine, greater trochanter laterally, ischial tuberosity, and the sacroiliac joint. Palpate inguinal ligament, psoas bursa, trochanteric bursa, and ischiogluteal bursa
- Assess range of motion: flexion, extension, abduction, adduction, internal and external rotations
- Perform special maneuvers (if indicated): groin strain (FABER or Patrick test)

Inspect gait (Fig. 23-17) for:

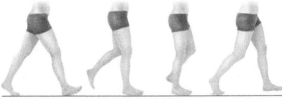

Heelstrike	Foot flat	Midstance	Push-off

FIGURE 23-17. Stance phase of gait.

- *Stance* (see Fig. 23-17) and *swing* (foot moves forward, does not bear weight)

  Most problems arise during the weight-bearing stance phase.

- *Width of base* (usually 2 to 4 inches from heel to heel), shift of pelvis, flexion of knee

  Cerebellar disease or foot problems if wide base; impaired shift of pelvis in arthritis, hip dislocation, abductor weakness; disrupted gait if poor knee flexion

Palpate:

- Bony landmarks: anterior—iliac crest and tubercle, anterior-superior iliac spine, greater trochanter, pubic tubercle; posterior—posterior-superior iliac spine, greater trochanter, ischial tuberosity, sacroiliac joint

- Along the inguinal ligament. Identify the **N**erve–**A**rtery–**V**ein–**E**mpty space–**L**ymph node (NAVEL).

Bulges in inguinal hernia, aneurysm

- *Trochanteric bursa*, on the greater trochanter of the femur (Fig. 23-18)

Focal tenderness in trochanteric bursitis, often described by patients as "low back pain"

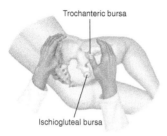

Trochanteric bursa

Ischiogluteal bursa

FIGURE 23-18. Palpating the trochanteric bursa.

- *Ischiogluteal bursa*, superficial to the ischial tuberosity

Tender in bursitis ("weaver's bottom") from prolonged sitting

Assess range of motion (Box 23-14).

BOX 23-14. Hip Joint Range of Motion

Hip Movement	Primary Muscles Affecting Movement	Patient Instructions	
Flexion	Iliopsoas and rectus femoris (especially when knee is in extension)	"Bring your knee to your chest and pull it against your abdomen."	Flexion of opposite leg suggests deformity of that hip.
Extension	Gluteus maximus, gluteus medius, adductor magnus, and hamstrings (especially when knee is in extension)	"Lying flat, move your lower leg away from the midline and down over the side of the table."	Painful in iliopsoas abscess

Abduction	Gluteus medius and minimus, tensor fascia latae (TFL)	"Lying flat, move your lower leg away from the midline."	
Adduction	Adductor brevis, adductor longus, adductor magnus, pectineus, and gracilis	"Lying flat, bend your knee and move your lower leg toward the midline."	Restricted in hip arthritis
External Rotation	Internal and external obturators, quadratus femoris, and superior and inferior gemelli	"Lying flat, bend your knee and turn your lower leg and foot across the midline."	
Internal Rotation	Gluteus medius and minimus, TFL, and some assistance from the adductors	"Lying flat, bend your knee and turn your lower leg and foot away from the midline."	Restricted in hip arthritis

Perform special maneuvers (if indicated)

- FABER (**F**lexion, **A**bduction, **E**xternal **R**otation) or Patrick test for groin strain. With the patient supine, position the leg into 90 degrees of flexion and externally rotate and abduct it so that the ipsilateral ankle rests distal to the knee of the contralateral leg (Fig. 23-19).

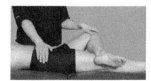

FIGURE 23-19. Testing for groin strain (FABER or Patrick test). (From Anderson MK. *Foundations of Athletic Training: Prevention, Assessment, and Management.* 6th ed. Wolters Kluwer; 2017. Figure 16-19.)

Knees

Key Components of the Knee Joint Examination

- Inspect gait, knee, hollows around patella and quadriceps muscles
- Palpate tibiofemoral joint. *Medial compartment*: medial femoral condyle, adductor tubercle, medial tibial plateau, and MCL. *Lateral compartment:* lateral femoral condyle, lateral tibial plateau, and LCL. *Patellofemoral compartment*: patella, patellar tendon, tibial tuberosity, prepatellar bursa, anserine bursa, and popliteal fossa
- Assess range of motion: flexion and extension
- Perform special maneuvers (if indicated): McMurray test (meniscus), abduction or valgus test (MCL), adduction or varus test (LCL), anterior drawer sign or Lachman test (ACL), and posterior drawer sign (PCL). Effusions: bulge sign, balloon sign, and balloting the patella

Identify the medial (Fig. 23-20) and lateral structures of the knee.

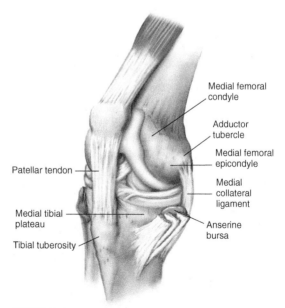

FIGURE 23-20. Structures in the medial compartment of the right knee.

Inspect:

- Gait for knee extension at heel strike, flexion during all other phases of swing and stance

  Stumbling or "giving way" during heel strike in quadriceps weakness or abnormal patellar tracking

- Alignment of knees

  Bowlegs, knock-knees; flexion contractures in limb paralysis or hamstring tightness.

- Contours of knees, including any atrophy of the quadriceps muscles

  Quadriceps atrophy with patellofemoral disorder; swelling over the patella in prepatellar bursitis (housemaid's knee), over the tibial tubercle in infrapatellar or if more medial anserine bursitis

Inspect and palpate:

See Table 23-5, Painful Knees, pp. 407–408 and Algorithm 23-4, Approach to the patient with knee pain, p. 402.

Tibiofemoral joint—with knees flexed, including:

- Joint line—place thumbs on either side of patellar tendon.

  Irregular, bony ridges in osteoarthritis.

- Medial and lateral meniscus

  Tenderness if meniscus tear

- Medial and lateral collateral ligaments

  Tenderness if MCL tear (LCL injuries less common)

- Patellofemoral compartment:

  - Patella

    Swelling over the patella in prepatellar bursitis ("housemaid's knee")

    - Palpate patellar tendon and ask patient to extend the leg.

      Tenderness or inability to extend the leg in partial or complete tear of the patellar tendon

    - Press patella against the underlying femur.

      Pain, crepitus, and a history of knee pain in *patellofemoral disorder*

    - Push patella distally and ask patient to tighten knee against table.

      Pain during contraction of quadriceps in *chondromalacia*

  - Suprapatellar pouch

    Swelling in synovitis and arthritis

  - Infrapatellar spaces (hollow areas adjacent to patella)

    Swelling in arthritis

  - Medial tibial condyle

    Swelling in pes anserine bursitis

  - Popliteal surface

Assess range of motion (Box 23-15).

BOX 23-15. Knee Joint Range of Motion

Knee Movement	Primary Muscles Affecting Movement	Patient Instructions
Flexion	Hamstring group: biceps femoris, semitendinosus, and semimembranosus	"Bend your knee."
Extension	Quadriceps: rectus femoris, vastus medialis, lateralis, and intermedius	"Straighten your leg."

Perform special maneuvers to assess menisci, ligaments and effusions

- *Medial meniscus and lateral meniscus—McMurray test* (Fig. 23-21): With the patient supine, grasp the heel and flex the knee. Cup your other hand over the knee joint with fingers and thumb along the medial joint line. From the heel, externally rotate the lower leg, then push on the lateral side to apply a valgus stress on the medial side of the joint. Slowly extend the lower leg in external rotation.

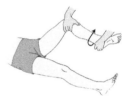

FIGURE 23-21. McMurray test.

The same maneuver with internal rotation stresses the lateral meniscus.

Click or pop along the medial joint with valgus stress, external rotation, and leg extension in tear of posterior medial meniscus.

- *Medial collateral ligament* (Fig. 23-22): With knee slightly flexed, push medially against lateral surface of knee with one hand and pull laterally at the ankle with the other hand (*abduction* or *valgus stress*).

Pain or a gap in the medial joint line points to a partial or complete MCL tear.

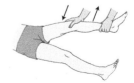

FIGURE 23-22. Medial collateral ligament test.

■ *Lateral collateral ligament (LCL)* (Fig. 23-23): With knee slightly flexed, push laterally along medial surface of knee with one hand and pull medially at the ankle with the other hand (an *adduction* or *varus stress*).

Pain or a gap in the lateral joint line points to a partial or complete LCL tear.

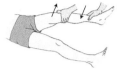

FIGURE 23-23. Lateral collateral ligament test.

■ *Anterior cruciate ligament (ACL):* (1) *Anterior drawer sign* (Fig. 23-24): With knee flexed, place thumbs on medial and lateral joint line and place fingers on hamstring insertions. Pull tibia forward, observe if tibia slides forward "like a drawer." Compare to opposite knee.

Forward slide of proximal tibia is a positive *anterior drawer sign* in ACL laxity or tear.

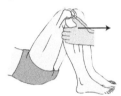

FIGURE 23-24. Anterior cruciate ligament test (anterior drawer sign).

(2) *Lachman test* (Fig. 23-25): Grasp the distal femur with one hand and the proximal tibia with the other (place the thumb on the joint line). Move the femur forward and the tibia back.

Significant forward excursion of tibia in ACL tear

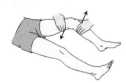

FIGURE 23-25. Lachman test.

■ *Posterior cruciate ligament (PCL): Posterior drawer sign* (Fig. 23-26): Position patient and hands as in the ACL test. Push the tibia posteriorly and observe for posterior movement, like a drawer sliding posteriorly.

Isolated PCL tears are rare.

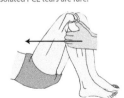

FIGURE 23-26. Posterior cruciate ligament test (posterior drawer sign).

Assess any effusions.

Popliteal or Baker cyst

- *Bulge sign* (minor effusions): Compress the suprapatellar pouch, stroke downward on medial surface (Fig. 23-27), apply pressure to force fluid to lateral surface (Fig. 23-28), and then tap knee behind lateral margin of patella (Fig. 23-29).

A fluid wave returning to the medial surface after a lateral tap confirms an effusion—a positive "bulge sign."

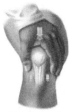

Milk downward

FIGURE 23-27. Bulge sign—Step 1: Displace ("milk") fluid downward from suprapatellar recess.

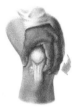

Apply medial pressure

FIGURE 23-28. Bulge sign—Step 2: Then force fluid to lateral area by applying pressure on medial aspect of knee.

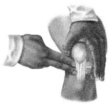

Tap and watch for fluid wave

FIGURE 23-29. Bulge sign—Step 3: Tap bulge formed by accumulated fluid on the lateral margin of the patella.

- *Balloon sign* (major effusions): Compress suprapatellar pouch with one hand; with thumb and finger of other hand, feel for fluid entering the spaces next to the patella (Fig. 23-30).

A palpable fluid wave is a positive sign.

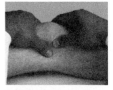

FIGURE 23-30. Test for the balloon sign.

- *Ballotte the patella* (major effusion): Push the patella sharply against the femur; watch for fluid returning to the suprapatellar space.

Ankles and Feet

Key Components of Ankle Joint and Foot Examination

- Inspect ankle and foot
- Palpate ankle joint, Achilles tendon, calcaneus, plantar fascia, medial and lateral ankle ligaments, medial and lateral malleolus, metatarsophalangeal (MTP) joints, metatarsals, gastrocnemius, and soleus
- Assess range of motion: flexion (plantar flexion), extension (dorsiflexion), inversion and eversion
- Perform special maneuvers (if indicated). *Tests for joint integrity:* tibiotalar, subtalar or talocalcaneal, talocrural, transverse tarsal, and metatarsophalangeal. Test for Achilles tendon integrity

Inspect ankles and feet.

Hallux valgus, corns, calluses

Palpate:

- Ankle joint

Tender in arthritis

- Ankle ligaments: medial-deltoid; lateral-anterior and posterior talofibular, calcaneofibular

Tenderness in sprain: lateral ligaments weaker, making inversion injuries (ankle bows outward, heel bows inward) more common

- Achilles tendon

Rheumatoid nodules, tenderness in tendinitis

- Compress the metatarsophalangeal joints; then palpate each joint between the thumb and forefinger (Figs. 23-31 and 23-32).

Tenderness in arthritis, Morton neuroma third and fourth MTP joints; inflammation of first MTP joint in gout

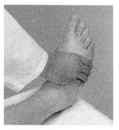

FIGURE 23-31. Palpating metatarsophalangeal joints.

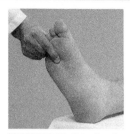

FIGURE 23-32. Palpating the metatarsal heads and grooves.

Assess range of motion (Box 23-16).

BOX 23-16. Ankle Joint and Foot Range of Motion

Ankle and Foot Movement	Primary Muscles Affecting Movement	Patient Instructions	
Ankle Flexion (Plantar Flexion)	Gastrocnemius, soleus, plantaris, and tibialis posterior	"Point your foot toward the floor."	Arthritic joint often painful when moved in any direction; sprain, when injured ligament is stretched.
Ankle Extension (Dorsiflexion)	Tibialis anterior, extensor digitorum longus, and extensor hallucis longus	"Point your foot toward the ceiling."	
Inversion	Tibialis posterior and anterior	"Bend your heel inward."	Ankle sprain
Eversion	Fibularis longus and brevis	"Bend your heel outward."	Trauma, arthritis

Special Techniques

Measuring Leg Length. The patient's legs should be aligned symmetrically. With a tape, measure distance from anterior-superior iliac spine to medial malleolus. Tape should cross the knee medially (Fig. 23-33).

Unequal leg length may be the cause of *scoliosis*.

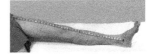

FIGURE 23-33. Measuring leg length from anterior superior iliac spine to medial malleolus.

Measuring Range of Motion. To measure range of motion precisely, a simple pocket goniometer is needed. Estimates may be made visually. Movement in the elbow at the right is limited to range indicated by red lines (Fig. 23-34).

Flexion deformity of 45 degrees and further flexion to 90 degrees (45 degrees → 90 degrees)

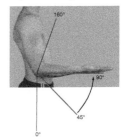

FIGURE 23-34. Normal (black) and patient's measured (red) range of motion of elbow flexion.

RECORDING YOUR FINDINGS

Recording the Musculoskeletal System Examination

"Full range of motion in all joints. No evidence of swelling or deformity."

OR

"Full range of motion in all joints. Hand with degenerative changes of Heberden nodes at the distal interphalangeal joints, Bouchard nodes at proximal interphalangeal joints. Mild pain with flexion, extension, and rotation of both hips. Full range of motion in the knees, with moderate crepitus; no effusion but boggy synovium and osteophytes along the tibiofemoral joint line bilaterally. Both feet with hallux valgus at the first metatarsophalangeal joints."

These findings suggest OA.

HEALTH PROMOTION AND COUNSELING: EVIDENCE AND RECOMMENDATIONS

> **Important Topics for Health Promotion and Counseling**
>
> - Low back pain
> - Osteoporosis: risk factors, screening, and assessing fracture risk
> - Treating osteoporosis and preventing falls

Low Back Pain

The estimated lifetime prevalence of low back pain in the US population is over 80%. Most patients with acute low back pain get better within 6 weeks; for patients with nonspecific symptoms, clinical guidelines emphasize reassurance, staying active, analgesics, muscle relaxants, and spinal manipulation therapy. About 10% to 15% of these patients develop chronic symptoms, often associated with long-term disability. Poor outcomes are linked to inappropriate beliefs about low back pain as a serious clinical condition, maladaptive pain-coping behaviors (avoiding work, movement, or other activities for fear of causing back damage), multiple nonorganic physical examination findings, psychiatric disorders, poor general health, high levels of baseline functional impairment, and low work satisfaction. (See Box 23-5 in Low Back Pain, p. 369.)

Osteoporosis: Risk Factors, Screening, and Assessing Fracture Risk

Osteoporosis is a major public health threat and a common US health problem—10% of adults over age 50 years have osteoporosis at the femoral neck or lumbar spine, including 16% of women and 4% of men. Half of all postmenopausal women sustain an osteoporosis-related fracture during their lifetime; 25% develop vertebral deformities, and 15% suffer hip fractures that increase risk of chronic pain, disability, loss of independence, and increased mortality (Box 23-17).

The U.S. Preventive Services Task Force (USPSTF) gives a grade B recommendation supporting osteoporosis screening for women age ≥65 years and for younger women whose 10-year fracture risk equals or exceeds that of an average-risk 65-year-old white woman.

> ### BOX 23-17. Risk Factors for Osteoporosis
>
> - Postmenopausal status in women
> - Age ≥50 years
> - Prior fragility fracture
> - Low body mass index
> - Low dietary calcium
> - Vitamin D deficiency
> - Tobacco and excessive alcohol use
> - Immobilization
> - Inadequate physical activity
> - Family history of fracture in a first-degree relative, particularly with history of fragility fracture
> - Clinical conditions such as thyrotoxicosis, celiac sprue, IBD, cirrhosis, chronic renal disease, organ transplantation, diabetes, HIV, hypogonadism, multiple myeloma, anorexia nervosa, and rheumatologic and autoimmune disorders
> - Medications such as oral and high-dose inhaled corticosteroids, anticoagulants (long-term use), aromatase inhibitors for breast cancer, methotrexate, selected antiseizure medications, immunosuppressive agents, proton-pump inhibitors (long-term use), and androgen deprivation therapy for prostate cancer

- Use the country specific FRAX calculator to assess fracture risk: https://www.sheffield.ac.uk/FRAX/
- Use the World Health Organization scoring criteria to determine bone density (Box 23-18).

> ### BOX 23-18. World Health Organization Bone Density Criteria
>
> - **Osteoporosis:** T score < −2.5 (>2.5 SDs below the young adult mean)
> - **Osteopenia:** T score between −1.0 and −2.5 (1.0 to 2.5 SDs below the young adult mean)

Treating Osteoporosis and Preventing Falls

More than one in three adults over age 65 years fall each year. Risk factors for falls include increasing age, impaired gait and balance, postural hypotension, loss of strength, medication use, comorbid illness, depression, cognitive impairment, and visual deficits.

Learn the therapeutic uses of agents that inhibit bone resorption: calcium and vitamin D (Box 23-19); antiresorptive agents such as bisphosphonates, selective estrogen-receptor modulators (SERMs), and postmenopausal estrogen; anabolic agents such as PTH; and the anti-RANK ligand agent denosumab.

BOX 23-19. Recommended Dietary Intakes of Calcium and Vitamin D for Adults (Institute of Medicine 2010)

Age Group	Calcium (Elemental) mg/day	Vitamin D IU/day
19–50 years	1,000	600
51–70 years		
Women	1,200	600
Men	1,000	600
71 and older	1,200	800

The USPSTF gives a grade B recommendation for exercise or providing physical therapy and/or vitamin D supplementation to prevent falls among at-risk community-dwelling adults age ≥65 years. It recommends personalized decision making (grade C) regarding *multifactorial fall-prevention interventions* for at-risk community-dwelling adults ages 65 and older. Urge patients to correct poor lighting, dark or steep stairs, chairs at awkward heights, slippery or irregular surfaces, and ill-fitting shoes. Scrutinize any medications affecting balance, especially benzodiazepines, vasodilators, and diuretics.

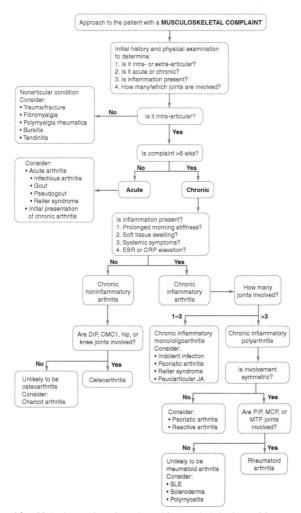

Algorithm 23-1. Approach to the patient with musculoskeletal complaints. (Note: Although it is not comprehensive, this algorithm may be a helpful starting approach for synthesizing information gathered from the history and physical.) CMC, carpometacarpal; CRP, C-reactive protein; DIP, distal interphalangeal; ESR, erythrocyte sedimentation rate; JA, juvenile arthritis; MCP, metacarpophalangeal; MTP, metatarsophalangeal; PIP, proximal interphalangeal; PMR, polymyalgia rheumatica; SLE, systemic lupus erythematosus. (Adapted from Cooper G, Herrera J. *Manual of Musculoskeletal Medicine.* Wolters Kluwer; 2015.)

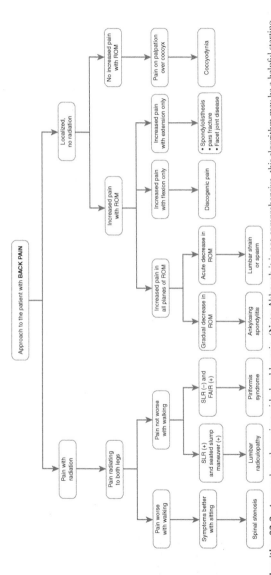

Algorithm 23-2. Approach to the patient with shoulder pain. (Note: Although it is not comprehensive, this algorithm may be a helpful starting approach for synthesizing information gathered from the history and physical.) AC, acromioclavicular; MI, myocardial infarction; ROM, range of motion. (Adapted from Cush JJ, Lipsky PE. Chapter 331, Approach to articular and musculoskeletal disorders. In: Longo DL, et al., eds. *Harrison's Principles of Internal Medicine.* 18th ed. McGraw-Hill; 2012.)

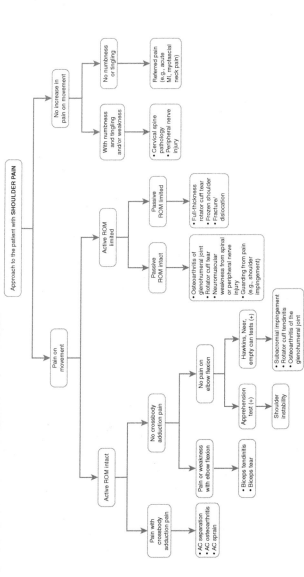

Algorithm 23-3. Approach to the patient with back pain. (Note: Although it is not comprehensive, this algorithm may be a helpful starting approach for synthesizing information gathered from the history and physical.) FAIR, flexion, adduction, internal rotation; ROM, range of motion; SLR, straight leg raise. (Adapted from Cooper G, Herrera J. *Manual of Musculoskeletal Medicine*. Wolters Kluwer; 2015.)

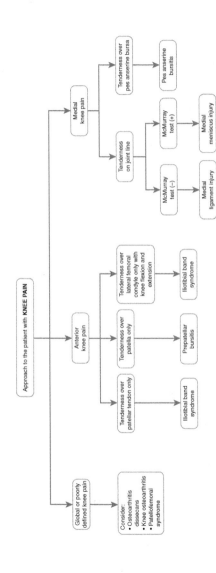

Algorithm 23-4. Approach to the patient with knee pain. (Note: Although it is not comprehensive, this algorithm may be a helpful starting approach for synthesizing information gathered from the history and physical.) FAIR, flexion, adduction, internal rotation; ROM, range of motion; SLR, straight leg raise. (Adapted from Cooper G, Herrera J. *Manual of Musculoskeletal Medicine*. Wolters Kluwer; 2015.)

INTERPRETATION AIDS

TABLE 23-1. Patterns of Pain in and Around the Joints

	Rheumatoid Arthritis	Osteoarthritis (Degenerative Joint Disease [DJD])
Process	Chronic inflammation of synovial membranes with secondary erosion of adjacent cartilage and bone, damage to ligaments and tendons	Degeneration and progressive loss of cartilage within joints, damage to underlying bone, formation of new bone at margins of cartilage
Common Locations	Hands (proximal interphalangeal and metacarpophalangeal joints), feet (metatarsophalangeal joints), wrists, knees, elbows, ankles	Knees, hips, hands (distal, sometimes proximal interphalangeal joints), cervical and lumbar spine, and wrists (first carpometacarpal joint); also joints previously injured or diseased
Pattern of Spread	Symmetrically additive: progresses to other joints; persists in initial ones	Additive; however, sometimes only one joint affected
Onset	Usually insidious	Usually insidious
Progression and Duration	Often chronic, with remissions and exacerbations	Slowly progressive, with exacerbations after overuse
Associated Symptoms	Frequent swelling of synovial tissue in joints or tendon sheaths; also subcutaneous nodules Tender, often warm but seldom red Prominent stiffness, often for >1 hr in mornings	Small joint effusions may be present, especially in knees; also bony enlargement Tender, seldom warm or red Frequent but brief stiffness in the morning

TABLE 23-2. Pains in the Neck

Patterns	Physical Signs
Mechanical Neck Pain Aching pain in the cervical paraspinal muscles and ligaments with associated muscle spasm, stiffness, and tightness in the upper back and shoulder, lasting up to 6 wks. No associated radiation, paresthesia, or weakness. Headache may be present.	Local muscle tenderness; pain on movement. No neurologic deficits. Possible trigger points in fibromyalgia. Torticollis if prolonged abnormal neck posture and muscle spasm.
Mechanical Neck Pain—Whiplash Also mechanical neck pain with aching paracervical pain and stiffness, often beginning the day after injury. Occipital headache, dizziness, malaise, and fatigue may be present. Chronic whiplash syndrome if symptoms last more than 6 mo, present in 20–40% of injuries.	Localized paracervical tenderness, decreased neck range of motion, perceived weakness of the upper extremities. Causes of cervical cord compression such as fracture, herniation, head injury, or altered consciousness are excluded.
Cervical Radiculopathy—from nerve root compression Sharp burning or tingling pain in the neck and one arm, with associated paresthesia and weakness. Sensory symptoms often in myotomal pattern, deep in muscle, rather than dermatomal pattern.	C7 nerve root affected most often (45–60%), with weakness in triceps and finger flexors and extensors. C6 nerve root involvement also common, with weakness in biceps, brachioradialis, wrist extensors.
Cervical Myelopathy—from cervical cord compression Neck pain with bilateral weakness and paresthesia in both upper and lower extremities, often with urinary frequency. Hand clumsiness, palmar paresthesia, and gait changes may be subtle. Neck flexion often exacerbates symptoms.	Hyperreflexia; clonus at the wrist, knee, or ankle; extensor plantar reflexes (positive Babinski signs); and gait disturbances. May also see *Lhermitte sign*: neck flexion with resulting sensation of electrical shock radiating down the spine. Confirmation of cervical myelopathy warrants neck immobilization and neurosurgical evaluation.

TABLE 23-3. Low Back Pain

Patterns	Physical Signs
Mechanical Low Back Pain Aching pain in lumbosacral area; may radiate into lower leg, along L5 or S1 dermatomes. Usually acute, work related, in age group 30 to 50 yrs; no underlying pathology	Paraspinal muscle or facet tenderness, muscle spasm or pain with back movement, loss of normal lumbar lordosis but no motor or sensory loss or reflex abnormalities. In osteoporosis, check for thoracic kyphosis, percussion tenderness over a spinous process, or fractures in the thoracic spine or hip.
Sciatica (Radicular Low Back Pain) Usually from disc herniation; more rarely from nerve root compression, primary or metastatic tumor	Disc herniation most likely if calf wasting, weak ankle dorsiflexion, absent ankle jerk, positive *crossed straight-leg raise* (pain in affected leg when healthy leg tested); negative straight-leg raise makes diagnosis highly unlikely.
Lumbar Spinal Stenosis Pseudoclaudication pain in the back or legs that improves with rest, forward lumbar flexion. Pain vague but usually bilateral, with paresthesia in one or both legs; usually from arthritic narrowing of spinal canal	Posture may be flexed forward with lower extremity weakness and hyporeflexia; straight-leg raise usually negative
Chronic Back Stiffness Consider ankylosing spondylitis in inflammatory polyarthritis, most common in men younger than 40 yrs. Diffuse idiopathic skeletal hyperostosis (DISH) affects men more than women, usually age older than 50 yrs.	Loss of the normal lumbar lordosis, muscle spasm, limited anterior and lateral flexion; improves with exercise. Lateral immobility of the spine, especially thoracic segment
Nocturnal Back Pain, Unrelieved by Rest Consider metastasis to spine from cancer of the prostate, breast, lung, thyroid, and kidney, and multiple myeloma.	Findings vary with the source. Local vertebral tenderness may be present.
Pain Referred from the Abdomen or Pelvis Usually a deep, aching pain, the level of which varies with the source (~2% of low back pain)	Spinal movements are not painful and range of motion is not affected. Look for signs of the primary disorder, such as peptic ulcer, pancreatitis, dissecting aortic aneurysm.

TABLE 23-4. Painful Shoulders

Acromioclavicular Arthritis

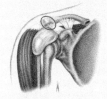

Tenderness over the acromioclavicular joint, especially with adduction of the arm across the chest. Pain often increases with shrugging the shoulders, due to movement of scapula.

Subacromial and Subdeltoid Bursitis

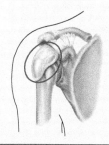

Pain over anterior-superior aspect of shoulder, particularly when raising the arm overhead. Tenderness common anterolateral to the acromion, in hollow recess formed by the acromiohumeral sulcus. Often seen in overuse syndromes.

Rotator Cuff Tendinitis

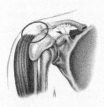

Tenderness over the rotator cuff, when elbow passively lifted posteriorly or with maneuvers (pp. 376–377).

Bicipital Tendinitis

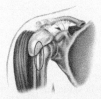

Tenderness over the long head of the biceps when rolled in the bicipital groove or when flexed arm is supinated against resistance suggests bicipital tendinitis.

TABLE 23-5. Painful Knees

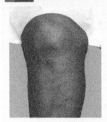

Arthritis. Degenerative arthritis usually occurs after age 50; associated with obesity. Often with medial joint line tenderness, palpable osteophytes, bowleg appearance, suprapatellar bursae and joint effusion. Systemic involvement, swelling, and subcutaneous nodules in rheumatoid arthritis.

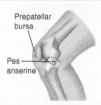
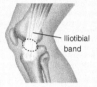

Prepatellar bursa

Pes anserine

Iliotibial band

Bursitis. Inflammation and thickening of bursa seen in repetitive motion and overuse syndromes. Can involve prepatellar bursa ("housemaid's knee"), pes anserine bursa medially (runners, osteoarthritis), iliotibial band laterally (over lateral femoral condyle), especially in runners.

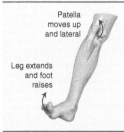

Patella moves up and lateral

Leg extends and foot raises

Patellofemoral instability. During flexion and extension of knee, due to subluxation and/or malalignment, patella tracks laterally instead of centrally in trochlear groove of femoral condyle. Inspect or palpate for lateral motion with leg extension. May lead to chondromalacia, osteoarthritis.

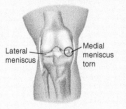

Lateral meniscus

Medial meniscus torn

Meniscal tear. Commonly arises from twisting injury of knee; in older patients may be degenerative, often with clicking, popping, or locking sensation. Check for tenderness along joint line over medial or lateral meniscus and for effusion. May have associated tears of medial collateral of anterior cruciate ligaments.

continued

TABLE 23-5. Painful Knees *(continued)*

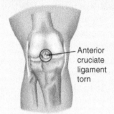

Anterior cruciate tear or sprain. In twisting injuries of the knee, often with popping sensation, immediate swelling, pain with flexion/extension, difficulty walking, and sensation of knee "giving way." Check for anterior drawer sign, swelling of hemarthrosis, injuries to medial meniscus or medial collateral ligament. Consider evaluation by an orthopedic surgeon.

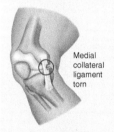

Collateral ligament sprain or tear. From force applied to medial or lateral surface of knee (valgus or varus stress), producing localized swelling, pain, stiffness. Patients able to walk but may develop an effusion. Check for tenderness over affected ligament and ligamentous laxity during valgus or varus stress.

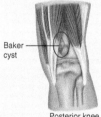

Posterior knee

Baker cyst. Cystic swelling palpable on the medial surface of the popliteal fossa, prompting complaints of aching or fullness behind the knee. Inspect, palpate for swelling adjacent to medial hamstring tendons. If present, suggests involvement of posterior horn of medial meniscus. In rheumatoid arthritis, cyst may expand into calf or ankle.

Nervous System

FUNDAMENTALS FOR ASSESSING THE NERVOUS SYSTEM

When neurologic disease is suspected, two complementary questions should be addressed throughout your assessment. These questions are not answered separately, but iteratively as you learn about the patient during the interview and establish your neurologic findings.

- What is the localization of the responsible lesion(s) in the nervous system?
- What is the underlying pathophysiology causing the disease?

The nervous system can be divided into the central nervous system (CNS) and the peripheral nervous system (PNS), as shown in Figure 24-1.

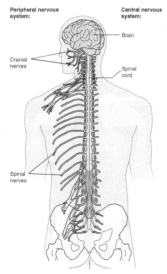

Peripheral nervous system:

Cranial nerves

Spinal nerves

Central nervous system:

Brain

Spinal cord

FIGURE 24-1. Central nervous system (CNS) and peripheral nervous system (PNS), coronal section. (Modified from Cohen BJ, Hull K. *Memmler's The Human Body in Health and Disease.* 14th ed. Jones & Bartlett Learning; 2019. Figure 9-1.)

Central Nervous System

The *central nervous system* (CNS) consists of the brain and spinal cord.

Brain. The brain has four regions: the *cerebrum*, the *diencephalon*, the *brainstem*, and the *cerebellum* (Fig. 24-2). Each cerebral hemisphere is subdivided into *frontal, parietal, temporal,* and *occipital lobes.* The brain consists of gray matter and myelinated neuronal axons, or white matter. Important structures include the *basal ganglia*, the *thalamus*, the *hypothalamus*, the *brainstem (midbrain, pons,* and *medulla)*, which connects the cortex with the spinal cord, the *reticular activating (arousal) system* linked to consciousness, and the *cerebellum.*

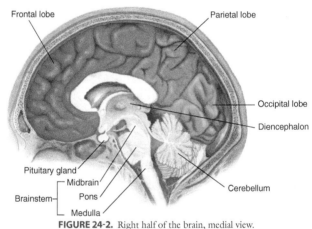

Frontal lobe

Parietal lobe

Occipital lobe

Diencephalon

Pituitary gland

Midbrain

Cerebellum

Brainstem — Pons

Medulla

FIGURE 24-2. Right half of the brain, medial view.

Spinal Cord. The spinal cord extends from the medulla to the first or second lumbar vertebrae. The spinal cord:

- is divided into five segments: *cervical* (C1–C8), *thoracic* (T1–T12), *lumbar* (L1–L5), *sacral* (S1–S5), and *coccygeal.* Its roots fan out like a horse's tail at L1–L2, the *cauda equina.*
- contains important motor and sensory nerve pathways that exit and enter the cord via anterior and posterior nerve roots and spinal and peripheral nerves.
- mediates the monosynaptic muscle stretch reflexes.

Peripheral Nervous System

The peripheral nervous system consists of the 12 pairs of cranial nerves and the spinal and peripheral nerves. Most peripheral nerves contain both motor and sensory fibers.

Cranial Nerves. The twelve pairs of cranial nerves (CNs) emerge from the cranial vault through skull foramina and canals to structures in the head and neck (Box 24-1).

BOX 24-1. Cranial Nerves and Function

No.	Cranial Nerve	Function
I	Olfactory	Sense of smell
II	Optic	Vision
III	Oculomotor	Pupillary constriction, opening the eye (lid elevation), most extraocular movements
IV	Trochlear	Downward, internal rotation of the eye
V	Trigeminal	*Motor*—temporal and masseter muscles (jaw clenching), lateral pterygoids (lateral jaw movement) *Sensory*—facial; the nerve has three divisions: (1) ophthalmic, (2) maxillary, and (3) mandibular
VI	Abducens	Lateral deviation of the eye
VII	Facial	*Motor*—facial movements, including those of facial expression, closing the eye, closing the mouth *Sensory*—taste for salty, sweet, sour, and bitter substances on anterior two-thirds of tongue; sensation from the ear
VIII	Acoustic	Hearing (*cochlear* division) and balance (*vestibular* division)
IX	Glossopharyngeal	*Motor*—pharynx *Sensory*—posterior portions of the eardrum and ear canal, the pharynx, and the posterior tongue, including taste (salty, sweet, sour, bitter)
X	Vagus	*Motor*—palate, pharynx, and larynx *Sensory*—pharynx and larynx
XI	Spinal accessory	*Motor*—sternocleidomastoid; upper portion of the trapezius
XII	Hypoglossal	*Motor*—tongue

Peripheral Nerves. Thirty-one pairs of nerves carry impulses to and from the cord: 8 cervical, 12 thoracic, 5 lumbar, 5 sacral, and 1 coccygeal. Each nerve has an anterior (ventral) root containing motor fibers, and a posterior (dorsal) root containing sensory fibers. These merge to form a short (<5 mm) *spinal nerve*. Spinal nerve fibers commingle with similar fibers in plexuses outside the cord—from these emerge *peripheral nerves*. Most peripheral nerves contain both sensory (*afferent*) and motor (*efferent*) fibers.

HEALTH HISTORY

Common Concerns

- Headache
- Dizziness or vertigo
- Numbness, abnormal or lost sensations
- Weakness (generalized, proximal, or distal)
- Fainting or blacking out (near-syncope and syncope)
- Seizures
- Tremors or involuntary movements

Headache

Ask about location, severity, duration, and any associated symptoms, such as visual changes, weakness, or loss of sensation. Always elicit unusual headache warning signs, such as sudden onset "like a thunderclap," onset after age 50 years, and associated symptoms such as fever and stiff neck, which warrant examination for papilledema and focal neurologic signs.

See Table 24-1, Primary Headaches, p. 438, Table 24-2, Secondary Headaches, pp. 439–441, and Algorithm 24-1, Approach to the patient with new headache, p. 435.

Subarachnoid hemorrhage may evoke "the worst headache of my life." Dull headache especially on awakening and in the same location, especially when affected by examination maneuvers, may arise from mass lesions like a brain tumor or abscess.

Dizziness or Vertigo

Dizziness or vertigo can have many meanings. Is the patient lightheaded or feeling faint (*presyncope*)? Is there unsteady gait from disequilibrium or ataxia, or true *vertigo*, a perception that the room is spinning or rotating?

See Peripheral and Central Vertigo, p. 200, for distinguishing symptoms and time course.

Lightheadedness in palpitations; near-syncope from vasovagal stimulation, low blood pressure, febrile illness, and others; vertigo in benign positional vertigo, Ménière disease, brainstem tumor

Are any medications contributing to dizziness?

Are associated symptoms present, such as double vision (*diplopia*), difficulty forming words (*dysarthria*), or difficulty with gait or balance (*ataxia*)? Is there any weakness?

Diplopia, dysarthria, ataxia in vertebrobasilar transient ischemic attack (TIA) or stroke

See Table 24-3, Types of Stroke, pp. 442–443, and Table 24-4, Disorders of Speech, pp. 444–445.

Weakness or paralysis in TIA or stroke

Numbness, Abnormal or Lost Sensations

Is there any loss of sensation or altered sensation such as tingling or pins and needles without an obvious stimulus (*paresthesia*)? *Dysesthesias*, or disordered sensations in response to a stimulus, may last longer than the stimulus itself.

Consider paresthesia in hands and around the mouth in hyperventilation; local nerve compression or "entrapment," seen in hand numbness from median, ulnar, or radial nerve disorders; nerve root compression with dermatomal sensory loss from vertebral bone spurs or herniated discs; or central lesions from stroke or multiple sclerosis. See Algorithm 24-2, Approach to the patient with numbness, p. 436.

Weakness

Distinguish proximal from distal weakness. For *proximal* weakness, ask about combing hair, reaching for things on a high shelf, difficulty getting out of a chair.

Bilateral proximal limb weakness with intact sensation in myopathies from alcohol, drugs like glucocorticoids, and inflammatory muscle disorders like polymyositis and dermatomyositis; see Algorithm 24-3, Approach to the patient with weakness, p. 437.

In myasthenia gravis, weakness is asymmetric and gets worse with effort (fatigability), and often has bulbar symptoms such as diplopia, ptosis, dysarthria, and dysphagia.

For *distal* weakness, ask about hand movements such as opening a jar or can or using hand tools (e.g., scissors, pliers, screwdriver). Ask about frequent tripping.

Bilateral predominantly distal weakness, often with sensory loss, in polyneuropathy, as in diabetes

Near Syncope or Syncope

"Have you ever fainted or passed out?" leads to discussion of any *loss of consciousness* (*syncope*).

Syncope is complete but temporary loss of consciousness from decreased cerebral blood flow, commonly called *fainting*.

Get a complete description of the event including setting and triggers, any warning signs, position (standing, sitting, lying down), and duration. What brought on the episode? Could voices be heard while passing out and coming to? How rapid was recovery? Were onset and offset slow or fast?

Young people with emotional stress and warning symptoms of flushing, warmth, or nausea may have vasodepressor (or vasovagal) syncope of slow onset, slow offset.

Consider seizures; "neurocardiogenic" conditions such as vasovagal syncope, postural tachycardia syndrome, carotid sinus syncope, and orthostatic hypotension; arrhythmias, especially ventricular tachycardia and bradyarrhythmias, often with syncope of sudden onset and offset

Also ask if anyone observed the episode. What did the patient look like before, during, and after the episode? Was there any seizure-like movement of the arms or legs? Any incontinence of the bladder or bowel?

Tonic–clonic motor activity, incontinence, and *postictal state* in generalized *seizures*. Unlike in syncope, tongue biting or bruising of limbs may occur.

Depending on the type of seizure, there may be loss of consciousness or abnormal feelings, thought processes, and sensations, including smells, as well as abnormal movements.

Seizure

A *seizure* is a sudden excessive electrical discharge from cortical neurons, and may be symptomatic, with an identifiable cause, or idiopathic. Elicit a careful history.

If acute symptomatic seizures, consider head trauma; alcohol, cocaine, and other drugs; withdrawal from alcohol, benzodiazepines, and barbiturates; metabolic insults from low or high glucose or low calcium or sodium; acute stroke; and meningitis or encephalitis.

Tremors or Involuntary Movements

Ask about any tremor, shaking, or body movements that the patient is unable to control. Does the tremor occur at rest? Get worse with voluntary intentional movement or with sustained postures?

Low-frequency unilateral resting tremor, rigidity, and bradykinesia in Parkinson disease.

Essential tremors if high-frequency, bilateral, upper extremity tremors that occur with both limb movement and sustained posture and subside when the limb is relaxed.

TECHNIQUES OF EXAMINATION

Key Components of the Examination of the Nervous System

- Assess mental status
- Test cranial nerves:
  - Test sense of smell (I)
  - Test visual acuity in each eye (II)
  - Inspect optic fundi with an ophthalmoscope (II)
  - Test visual fields by confrontation (II)
  - Inspect size and shape of pupils (II, III)
  - Test pupillary reactions to light (II, III)
  - Check pupillary constriction, convergence, and lens accommodation (II, III)
  - Test extraocular movements (III, IV, VI)
  - Palpate temporal and masseter muscles (V)
  - Test sensation in face (V)
  - Inspect face (VII)
  - Test muscles of facial expression (VII)
  - Assess gross hearing (VIII)
  - Assess swallowing and palate/uvula movement (IX, X)
  - Assess speech (V, VII, IX, X, XII)
  - Test trapezii or sternocleidomastoid strength against resistance (XI)
  - Inspect and test tongue movement (XII)
- Assess motor system
  - Test muscle strength:
    - Shoulder abduction (C5, C6)
    - Elbow flexion (C5, C6)/extension (C6, C7, C8)
    - Wrist flexion/extension (C6, C7, C8, radial nerve)
    - Finger extension (C7, C8, radial nerve)/abduction (C8, T1, ulnar nerve)
    - Thumb abduction (C8, T1, median nerve)
    - Hip flexion (L2, L3, L4)/extension (S1)
    - Knee flexion (L5, S1, S2)/extension (L2, L3, L4)
    - Ankle dorsiflexion (L4, L5)/plantar flexion (S1)
  - Assess coordination:
  - Assess position sense (Romberg test)
- Assess sensory system
- Elicit muscle stretch reflexes:
  - Biceps reflex (C5, C6)
  - Triceps reflex (C6, C7)
  - Brachioradialis reflex (C5, C6)
  - Quadriceps (patellar) reflex (L2, L3, L4)
  - Achilles (ankle) reflex (primarily S1)
- Elicit cutaneous or superficial stimulation reflexes

Mental Status

Check level of alertness, language function (fluency, comprehension, repetition, and naming), memory (short-term and long-term), calculation, visuospatial processing and abstract reasoning.

See Box 24-4, Levels of Consciousness, p. 430 and Chapter 9, Cognition, Behavior, and Mental Status, pp. 136–139.

Cranial Nerves

CN I (Olfactory). Test sense of smell on each side.

Loss of smell in sinus conditions, head trauma, smoking, aging, cocaine use, Parkinson disease

CN II (Optic). Assess visual acuity.

Blindness

Check visual fields.

Hemianopsia

Inspect optic discs.

Papilledema, optic atrophy, glaucoma

CN II, III (Optic and Oculomotor). Inspect size and shape of pupils.

Test pupillary reactions to light. If abnormal, test reactions to near effort.

Blindness, CN III paralysis, tonic pupils; Horner syndrome may affect light reactions

CN III, IV, VI (Oculomotor, Trochlear, and Abducens). Assess extraocular movements.

Strabismus and binocular diplopia in CN III, IV, and VI neuropathy; diplopia in eye muscle disorders from myasthenia gravis, trauma, thyroid ophthalmopathy, and internuclear ophthalmoplegia; nystagmus

CN V (Trigeminal). Palpate the contractions of temporal and masseter muscles (*motor component*). Test pain and light touch on face (*sensory component*) in (1) ophthalmic, (2) maxillary, and (3) mandibular zones (Fig. 24-3).

Motor or sensory loss from lesions of CN V or its higher motor pathways.

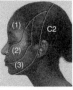

FIGURE 24-3. Areas for testing sensation of the three divisions of CN V.

TECHNIQUES OF EXAMINATION	POSSIBLE FINDINGS

CN VII (Facial). Ask the patient to raise both eyebrows, frown, close eyes tightly, show teeth, smile, and puff out cheeks.

Weakness from lesion of peripheral nerve, as in Bell palsy, or of CNS, as in a stroke. See Table 24-5, Types of Facial Paralysis, p. 446.

CN VIII (Vestibulocochlear). Test hearing of whispered voice. If decreased:

■ Test for lateralization if unilateral hearing loss (*Weber test*).

In unilateral sensorineural loss, sound is heard in the good ear where AC > BC. In conductive loss lateralization is to the affected ear where BC > AC. See Patterns of Hearing Loss, p. 204 in Chapter 13, Ears and Nose.

■ Compare air and bone conduction (*Rinne test*).

In sensorineural hearing loss, sound is heard longer through air than bone (AC > BC). In conductive loss sound is heard through bone longer than air (BC = AC or BC > AC). See Patterns of Hearing Loss, p. 204 in Chapter 13, Ears and Nose.

CNs IX, X (Glossopharyngeal and Vagus). Observe any difficulty swallowing.

A weakened palate or pharynx impairs swallowing.

Listen to the voice.

Hoarseness in vocal cord paralysis; nasal voice in paralysis of palate

Watch soft palate rise with "ah."

In unilateral paralysis, one side of the palate fails to rise and, together with the uvula, is pulled toward the normal side. Deviated uvula, palatal paralysis in CVA

Test gag reflex on each side.

Absent reflex is often normal.

CN XI (Spinal Accessory). *Trapezius muscles.* Assess muscles for bulk, involuntary movements, and strength of shoulder shrug (Fig. 24-4).

Atrophy, fasciculations, weakness

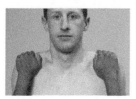

FIGURE 24-4. Testing trapezius strength.

Sternocleidomastoid muscles. Assess strength as head turns against your hand.	Weakness of sternocleidomastoid muscle when head turns to *opposite* side
CN XII (Hypoglossal). Listen to patient's articulation.	Dysarthria from damage to CN X or CN XII
Inspect the resting tongue.	Atrophy, fasciculations in ALS, polio
Inspect the protruded tongue.	In a unilateral cortical lesion, the protruded tongue deviates away from the side of cortical lesion; in CN XII lesion, tongue deviates to the weak side.

Motor System

	See Table 24-6, Motor Disorders, p. 447.
Body Position. Observe the patient's body position during movement and at rest.	Hemiplegia in stroke
Involuntary Movements. If present, observe location, quality, rate, rhythm, amplitude, and setting.	Tremors, fasciculations, tics, chorea, athetosis, oral–facial dyskinesias. See Table 24-7, Involuntary Movements, p. 448.
Muscle Bulk and Tone. Inspect muscle contours.	Atrophy of bulk. See Table 24-8, Disorders of Muscle Tone, p. 449.
Assess resistance to passive stretch of arms and legs.	Marked floppiness indicates muscle hypotonia or flaccidity. *Spasticity* is increased tone that is velocity-dependent and worsens at the extremes of range of motion. *Rigidity* is increased tone that remains the same throughout the range of motion; it is not velocity dependent.
Muscle Strength. Test and grade the major muscle groups (Box 24-2), with the examiner trying to overcome the strength of the *patient's resistance.*	
Is the pattern focal, from a lower motor neuron lesion in peripheral nerve or nerve root? Is there unilateral paralysis from an upper motor neuron cortical or subcortical lesion? Is there a symmetric distal weakness from polyneuropathy, or proximal weakness from myopathy?	

BOX 24-2. Scale for Grading Muscle Strength

Grade	Description
0	No muscular contraction detected
1	A barely detectable trace of contraction
2	Active movement with gravity eliminated (planar movement)
3	Active movement against gravity
4	Active movement against gravity and some resistance
5	Active movement against full resistance (normal)

- *Flexion* (C5, C6—biceps and brachioradialis) and *extension* (C6, C7, C8—triceps) *at the elbow*

  Peripheral radial nerve damage; central *stroke* or *multiple sclerosis* if hemiplegia.

- Wrist *extension* (C6, C7, C8, radial nerve—extensor carpi radialis longus and brevis, extensor carpi ulnaris), as shown in Figure 24-5

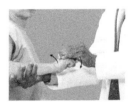

FIGURE 24-5. Testing wrist extension (C6, C7, C8, radial nerve)

- Finger *extension* (C7, C8, radial nerve—extensor digitorum), as shown in Figure 24-6.

  Weak in cervical radiculopathy, de Quervain tenosynovitis, carpal tunnel syndrome

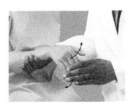

FIGURE 24-6. Testing finger extension (C7, C8, radial nerve—extensor digitorum)

- Finger *abduction* (C8, T1, ulnar nerve—first dorsal interosseous and abductor digiti minimi), as shown in Figure 24-7.

Weak in ulnar nerve disorders

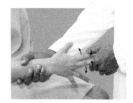

FIGURE 24-7. Testing finger abduction (C8, T1, ulnar nerve).

- Thumb *abduction* (C8, T1, median nerve—abductor pollicis brevis), as shown in Figure 24-8.

Weak in carpal tunnel syndrome

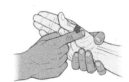

FIGURE 24-8. Testing abduction of the thumb (C8, T1, median nerve). (MediClip image copyright (c) 2003 Lippincott Williams & Wilkins. All rights reserved.)

- Hip flexion (L2, L3, L4—iliopsoas), as shown in Figure 24-9.

- Hip extension (S1)—gluteus maximus

- Hip adduction (L2, L3, L4—adductors)

- Hip abduction (L4, L5, S1—gluteus medius and minimus)

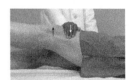

FIGURE 24-9. Testing hip flexion (L2, L3, L4—iliopsoas).

- Knee extension (L2, L3, L4—quadriceps)

- Knee flexion (L5, S1, S2—hamstrings)

- Ankle dorsiflexion (L4, L5—tibialis anterior)

- Ankle plantar flexion (S1—gastrocnemius, soleus)

Coordination. Test *rapid alternating movements* in hands (tap fingers), arms, and legs (tap foot), as shown in Figure 24-10.

Clumsy, slow movements in cerebellar disease

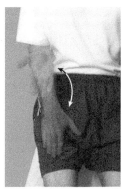

FIGURE 24-10. Testing coordination with rapid alternating arm movement.

Point-to-point movements in arms and legs—finger-to-nose, heel-to-shin

Clumsy, unsteady movements in cerebellar disease

Gait. Ask patient to:

- Walk away, turn, and come back

CVA, cerebellar ataxia, parkinsonism, or loss of position sense may affect performance.

- Walk heel-to-toe or tandem walking (Fig. 24-11)

Ataxia

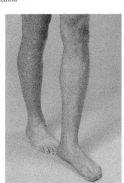

FIGURE 24-11. Testing tandem gait (heel-to-toe).

- Walk on toes, then on heels

Corticospinal tract injury

- Hop in place on each foot; do one-leg shallow knee bends. Substitute rising from a chair and climbing on a stool for hops and bends as indicated.

Proximal hip girdle weakness increases risk of falls.

Position Sense or Station

- Do a *Romberg test* (a sensory test of stance). Ask patient to stand with feet together and eyes open, then closed for 20 to 30 seconds. Mild swaying may occur. Stand close by to prevent falls.

Loss of balance when eyes are closed is a *positive* Romberg test, suggesting poor position sense.

- Inspect for a *pronator drift* as patient holds arms forward, with eyes closed, for 20 to 30 seconds (Fig. 24-12).

Flexion and pronation at elbow and downward drift of arm from *contralateral* corticospinal tract lesion (Fig. 24-13)

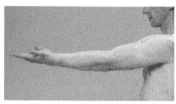

FIGURE 24-12. Testing for pronator drift.

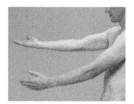

FIGURE 24-13. Positive test for pronator drift.

- Ask patient to keep arms up and tap them downward. A smooth return to position is normal.

Weakness, incoordination, poor position sense

♎/☞ Sensory System

Use an object like a sharp stick portion of a broken cotton swab to test sharp and dull sensation; Do not reuse the object on another patient. *Compare symmetric areas on the two sides of the body. Vary the pace of your testing* so that the patient does not merely respond to your repetitive rhythm.

A hemisensory loss pattern suggests a contralateral cortical lesion.

Compare proximal and distal areas of arms and legs for *pain, temperature,* and *touch sensation.* Scatter stimuli to sample most dermatomes and major peripheral nerves (Figs. 24-14 and 24-15).

"Glove-and-stocking" loss of peripheral neuropathy, often seen in alcoholism and diabetes

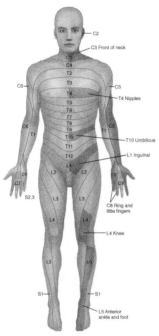

FIGURE 24-14. Dermatomes innervated by posterior roots (anterior view).

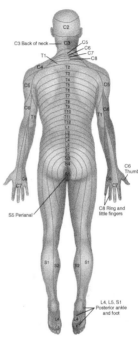

FIGURE 24-15. Dermatomes innervated by posterior roots (anterior view).

Map any area of abnormal response, including dermatomes, if present.

Dermatomal sensory loss in herpes zoster, nerve root compression.

Assess response to the following stimuli, with the patient's eyes closed.

■ *Pain.* Use the sharp end of a pin or other suitable tool. The dull end serves as a control.

Analgesia, hypalgesia, hyperalgesia

- *Temperature* (if indicated). Use test tubes with hot and cold water, or other objects of suitable temperature.

Temperature and pain sensation usually correlate.

- *Light touch.* Use a fine wisp of cotton.

Anesthesia, hyperesthesia

- Test for *vibration* and *proprioception* (*joint position sense*). If responses are abnormal, test more proximally. Vibration and position senses, both carried in the posterior columns, often correlate.

Loss of vibration and position senses in peripheral neuropathy from diabetes or alcoholism and in posterior column disease from tertiary syphilis or vitamin B$_{12}$ deficiency

- *Vibration.* Use a 128-Hz tuning fork, held on a *bony* prominence at the ankle and wrist (Fig. 24-16).

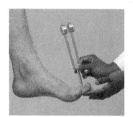

FIGURE 24-16. Testing vibration sense.

- *Proprioception (joint position sense).* Holding patient's finger or big toe by its sides, move it up or down (Fig. 24-17).

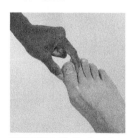

FIGURE 24-17. Testing joint position sense (proprioception).

Assess *discriminative* sensations:

- *Stereognosis.* Ask for identification of a common object placed in patient's hand.

Lesions in the posterior columns or sensory cortex impair stereognosis, number identification, and two-point discrimination.

- *Number identification (graphesthesia).* Draw a number on patient's palm with blunt end of a pen and ask the patient to identify the number.

- *Two-point discrimination* (Fig. 24-18). Use two pins of the sides of a paper clip to find minimal distance on pad of patient's finger at which two points can be distinguished (normally <5 mm).

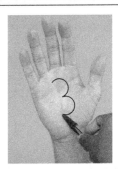

FIGURE 24-18. Testing discriminative sensation using number identification (*graphesthesia*).

- *Point localization.* Touch skin briefly and ask patient to open both eyes and identify the place touched.

A lesion in the sensory cortex may impair point localization on the contralateral side and cause contralateral extinction of the touch sensation.

- *Extinction.* Simultaneously touch opposite, corresponding areas of the body; ask whether the patient feels one touch or two.

⚕/⚕ Muscle Stretch Reflexes

Hold the reflex hammer loosely between your thumb and index finger so that it swings freely in an arc within the limits set by your palm and other fingers. Reflexes are usually graded on a 0 to 4 scale (Box 24-3).

Hyperactive deep tendon reflexes, absent abdominal reflexes, and a positive Babinski response in *upper* motor neuron lesions.

BOX 24-3. Grading Reflexes

Grade	Description
4+	Very brisk, with *clonus* (rhythmic oscillations between flexion and extension)
3+	Brisker than average, not necessarily indicative of disease
2+	Average, normal
1+	Diminished, or requires reinforcement
0	No response

ᕲ Biceps reflex (C5, C6); Figure 24-19

ᕲ Triceps reflex (C6, C7); Figure 24-20

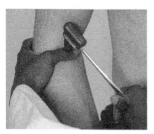

FIGURE 24-19. Biceps reflex (C5, C6).

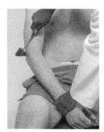

FIGURE 24-20. Triceps reflex (C6, C7).

ᕲ Brachioradialis reflex (C5, C6); Figure 24-21

ᵒᕋ/ᕋ Quadriceps or patellar reflex (L2, L3, L4); Figure 24-22

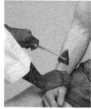

FIGURE 24-21. Brachioradialis reflex (C5, C6).

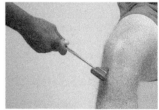

FIGURE 24-22. Quadriceps/patellar reflex (L2, L3, L4).

Achilles or ankle reflex (primarily S1); Figure 24-23

Check for clonus if reflexes seem hyperactive (Fig. 24-24).

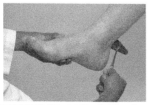

FIGURE 24-23. Achilles/ankle reflex (S1).

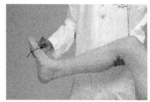

FIGURE 24-24. Testing for ankle clonus.

Ankle jerks symmetrically, decreased or absent in peripheral polyneuropathy; slowed ankle jerk in hypothyroidism.

⌀ Cutaneous or Superficial Stimulation Reflexes

Abdominal reflexes (upper T8, T9, T10; lower T10, T11, T12); Figure 24-25

May be absent in both central and peripheral nerve disorders

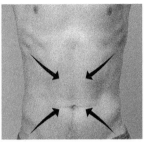

FIGURE 24-25. Direction of light touch while testing for abdominal reflexes.

Plantar response (L5, S1), normally flexor (Fig. 24-26)

Babinski extensor response (big toe fans up) from corticospinal tract lesion (Fig. 24-27)

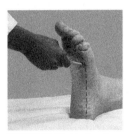

FIGURE 24-26. Testing the plantar response.

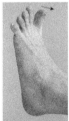

FIGURE 24-27. Abnormal plantar response (Babinski response). Note dorsiflexion of big toe.

⌀ *Anal (anocutaneous) reflex.* With a dull object, stroke outward from anus in four quadrants. Watch for anal contraction.

Loss of reflex suggests cauda equina lesion at the S2, S3, S4 level.

Special Techniques

⌀ **Meningeal Signs.** Make sure there is no injury or fracture to the cervical vertebrae or cervical cord. This often requires radiologic evaluation.

Brudzinski sign. With patient supine, flex head and neck toward chest. Note resistance or pain and watch for flexion of hips and knees.

Inflammation in the subarachnoid space causes resistance to movement that stretches the spinal nerves (neck flexion), the femoral nerve (Brudzinski sign), and the sciatic nerve (Kernig sign).

Kernig sign. Flex one of patient's legs at hip and knee, then straighten knee (Fig. 24-28). Note resistance or pain.

A compressed lumbosacral nerve root also causes pain on straightening the knee of the raised leg.

The frequency of Brudzinski and Kernig signs in meningitis ranges from 5% to 60%.

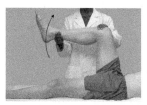

FIGURE 24-28. Testing for Kernig sign.

Jolt accentuation of headache (JAH). Have the patient rotate their head side to side (as if nodding no) at a speed of 2 to 3 times per second. Note any worsening of headache.

Although a positive JAH strongly increases the possibility of meningitis, a negative result is not able to rule out the presence of acute meningitis.

o— Lumbosacral Radiculopathy: Straight Leg Raise. With patient supine, raise relaxed and straightened leg, flexing the leg at the hip. Then dorsiflex the foot (Fig. 24-29).

Pain radiating into the ipsilateral leg is a positive straight-leg test for lumbosacral radiculopathy. Foot dorsiflexion can further increase leg pain in lumbosacral radiculopathy, sciatic neuropathy, or both. Increased pain when the contralateral healthy leg is raised is a positive *crossed straight leg raise sign.*

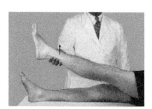

FIGURE 24-29. Testing for lumbosacral radiculopathy with the straight leg raise.

ᛃ Asterixis (Flapping Tremor). Ask patient to hold both arms forward, with hands cocked up and fingers spread, like "stopping traffic." Watch for 1 to 2 minutes.

Sudden brief flexions in liver disease, uremia, and hypercapnia

ᛁ Scapular Winging. Ask the patient to push against the wall of your hand with a partially straightened arm (Fig. 24-30). Inspect scapula. It should stay close to the chest wall.

Winging of scapula away from chest wall suggests weakness of the serratus anterior muscle, seen in muscular dystrophy or injury to long thoracic nerve (Fig. 24-31).

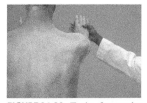

FIGURE 24-30. Testing for scapular winging.

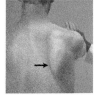

FIGURE 24-31. Presence of scapular winging.

Assessing the Patient Who Is Comatose

∘— Assess ABCs (airway, breathing, and circulation)

See Table 24-9, Metabolic and Structural Coma, p. 450, Table 24-10, Glasgow Coma Scale, p. 451, and Table 24-11, Pupils in Comatose Patients, p. 452.

- Take pulse, blood pressure, and rectal temperature.

Level of Consciousness (Arousal). Establish level of consciousness with escalating stimuli (Box 24-4). However, do not dilate pupils, and do not flex the patient's neck if any suspicion of cervical cord injury.

Lethargy, obtundation, stupor, coma

BOX 24-4. Levels of Consciousness

Alertness	Patient is awake and aware of self and environment. When spoken to in a *normal* voice, patient looks at you and responds fully and appropriately to stimuli.
Lethargy	When spoken to in a *loud* voice, patient appears drowsy but opens eyes and looks at you, responds to questions, and then falls asleep.
Obtundation	When *tactile* stimuli is applied like being shaken gently, patient opens eyes and looks at you but responds slowly and is somewhat confused. Alertness and interest in environment are decreased.
Stupor	Patient arouses from sleep only after *painful* stimuli. Verbal responses are slow or absent. Patient lapses into unresponsiveness when stimulus stops. Patient has minimal awareness of self or environment.
Coma	Despite repeated painful stimuli, patient remains unarousable with eyes closed. No evident response to inner need or external stimuli is shown.

Neurologic Examination. Conduct neurologic examination, looking for asymmetric findings.

Observe:

- Breathing pattern

  Cheyne–Stokes, ataxic breathing

- Pupils

  Asymmetrical pupils and loss of the light reaction in structural lesions from stroke, abscess, or tumor

- Ocular movements

  Deviation to affected side in hemispheric stroke

Check for the *oculocephalic reflex* (*doll's eye movements*). Holding upper eyelids open, turn head quickly to each side, and then flex and extend patient's neck. As seen in Figure 24-32, the eyes move toward left on head turn toward right (doll's eye movement) which indicates an intact brainstem.

In a comatose patient with an intact brainstem, the eyes move in the opposite direction, in this case to her left (doll's eye movements) as in Figure 24-33.

Very deep coma or a lesion in the midbrain or pons abolishes this reflex, so eyes do not move.

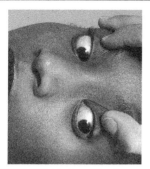

FIGURE 24-32. Oculocepahlic reflex present; thus patient's head will be turned to her right. Note movement of eyes toward left on head turn toward right (doll's eye movement).

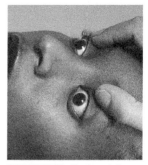

FIGURE 24-33. Oculocephalic reflex absent. Note loss of movement of eyes toward left on head turn toward right.

Note posture of body.

Decorticate rigidity, decerebrate rigidity, flaccid hemiplegia

- Test for flaccid paralysis.

- Hold forearms vertically; note wrist positions.

A flaccid hand droops to the horizontal.

- From 12 to 18 in above bed, drop each arm.

A flaccid arm drops more rapidly.

- Support both knees in a somewhat flexed position, and then extend each knee and let leg drop to the bed.

The flaccid leg drops more rapidly.

- From a similar starting position, release both legs.

A flaccid leg falls into extension and external rotation.

- Complete the neurologic and general physical examination.

RECORDING YOUR FINDINGS

Recording the Nervous System Examination

"Mental Status: Alert, relaxed, and cooperative. Thought process coherent. Oriented to person, place, and time. Detailed cognitive testing deferred. *Cranial Nerves:* I—not tested; II through XII intact.

continued

Motor: Good muscle bulk and tone. Strength 5/5 throughout.
Cerebellar: Rapid alternating movements (RAMs), finger-to-nose
(F→N), heel-to-shin (H→S) intact. Gait with normal base. Romberg—
maintains balance with eyes closed. No pronator drift. *Sensory:*
Pinprick, light touch, position, and vibration intact. *Reflexes:* 2+ and
symmetric with plantar reflexes downgoing."

OR

"*Mental Status:* The patient is alert and tries to answer questions
but has difficulty finding words. *Cranial Nerves:* I—not tested;
II—visual acuity intact; visual fields full; III, IV, VI—extraocular
movements intact; V motor—temporal and masseter strength
intact, sensory corneal reflexes present; VII motor—prominent
right facial droop and flattening of right nasolabial fold, left facial
movements intact, sensory—taste not tested; VIII—hearing intact
bilaterally to whispered voice; IX, X—gag intact; XI—strength
of sternocleidomastoid and trapezius muscles 5/5; XII—tongue
midline. *Motor:* strength in right biceps, triceps, iliopsoas, gluteals,
quadriceps, hamstring, and ankle flexor and extensor muscles
3/5 with good bulk but increased tone and spasticity; strength
in comparable muscle groups on the left 5/5 with good bulk and
tone. Gait—unable to test. Cerebellar—unable to test on right due
to right arm and leg weakness; RAMs, F→N, H→S intact on left.
Romberg—unable to test due to right leg weakness. Right pronator
drift present. *Sensory:* decreased sensation to pinprick over right
face, arm, and leg; intact on the left. Stereognosis and two-point
discrimination not tested. *Reflexes* (can record in two ways):

	Biceps	Triceps	Brach	Knee	Ankle	PI
RT	4+	4+	4+	4+	4+	↑
LT	2+	2+	2+	2+	1+	↓

OR

These findings suggest left hemispheric CVA in distribution of the left middle cerebral
artery, with right-sided hemiparesis.

HEALTH PROMOTION AND COUNSELING: EVIDENCE AND RECOMMENDATIONS

Important Topics for Health Promotion and Counseling

- Preventing cerebrovascular disease
- Screening for asymptomatic carotid artery stenosis
- Screening for diabetic peripheral neuropathy

Preventing Cerebrovascular Disease

Cerebrovascular disease is the fourth leading cause of death in the United States. *Stroke* is a sudden neurologic deficit caused by cerebrovascular ischemia (87%) or hemorrhage (13%). Hemorrhagic strokes may be *intra-cerebral* (10% of all strokes) or *subarachnoid* (3% of all strokes). Decreased vascular perfusion results in sudden focal but transient brain dysfunction in *TIA*, or in permanent neurologic deficits in stroke, as determined by neurodiagnostic imaging. Detecting a *transient ischemic attack (TIA)*, an episode of neurologic dysfunction that resolves within 24 hours, is important—in the first 3 months after a TIA, subsequent stroke occurs in approximately 15% of patients (Box 24-5).

BOX 24-5. AHA/ASA Stroke Warning Signs and Symptoms

F – Face Drooping—Does one side of the face droop or is it numb? Ask the person to smile. Is the person's smile uneven or lopsided?

A – Arm Weakness—Is one arm weak or numb? Ask the person to raise both arms. Does one arm drift downward?

S – Speech Difficulty—Is speech slurred? Is the person unable to speak or hard to understand? Ask the person to repeat a simple sentence, like *"The sky is blue."* Is the sentence repeated correctly?

T – Time to call 9-1-1—If someone shows any of these symptoms, even if the symptoms go away, call 9-1-1 and get the person to the hospital immediately. Check the time so you'll know when the first symptoms appeared.

continued

Beyond FAST: Other important symptoms
- Sudden numbness or weakness of the leg, arm, or face, especially on one side of the body
- Sudden confusion or trouble speaking or understanding speech
- Sudden trouble seeing in one or both eyes
- Sudden trouble walking, dizziness, loss of balance or coordination
- Sudden severe headache with no known cause

AHA, American Heart Association; ASA, American Stroke Association.

Source: https://www.heart.org/en/about-stroke/stroke-symptoms

Primary prevention of stroke requires aggressive management of risk factors and patient education.

- Target modifiable risk factors: hypertension, smoking, dyslipidemia, excess weight, diabetes, poor diet and nutrition, physical inactivity, and alcohol use.
- Address disease-specific risk factors: atrial fibrillation, carotid artery disease, sickle cell disease and sleep apnea.

Screening for Asymptomatic Carotid Artery Stenosis

The U.S. Preventive Services Task Force recommends against screening asymptomatic patients in the general population (grade D). Furthermore, it found no evidence that ultrasound screening reduced the risk for ipsilateral stroke.

Screening for Diabetic Peripheral Neuropathy

In diabetics, promote optimal glucose control to reduce risk of sensorimotor polyneuropathy, autonomic dysfunction, mononeuritis multiplex, or diabetic neuropathy. Examine diabetics regularly for neuropathy, including testing pinprick sensation, ankle reflexes, vibration perception (with a 128-Hz tuning fork) and plantar light touch sensation (with a 10-g *monofilament*), as well as checking for skin breakdown, poor circulation, and musculoskeletal abnormalities.

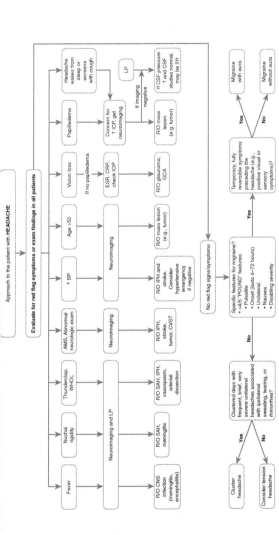

Algorithm 24-1. Approach to the patient with new headache. (Note: Although it is not comprehensive, this algorithm may be a helpful starting approach for synthesizing information gathered from the history and physical.) AMS, altered mental status; BP, blood pressure; CNS, central nervous system; CRP, C-reactive protein; CSF, cerebrospinal fluid; CVST, cerebral venous sinus thrombosis; ESR, erythrocyte sedimentation rate; GCA, giant cell arteritis (also called temporal arteritis); ICP, intracranial pressure; IIH, idiopathic intracranial hypotension; IOP, intraocular pressure; IPH, intraparenchymal hemorrhage; LP, lumbar puncture; SAH, subarachnoid hemorrhage. (Adapted from Detsky ME et al. *JAMA.* 2006; 296(10):1274–1283; Michel P et al. *Cephalalgia.* 1993;13:(suppl 12):54–59.)

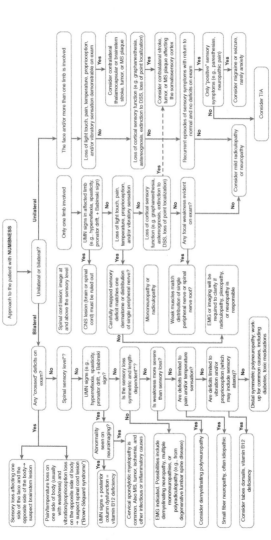

Algorithm 24-2. Approach to the patient with numbness. (Note: Although it is not comprehensive, this algorithm may be a helpful starting approach for synthesizing information gathered from the history and physical. CNS, central nervous system; EMG, electromyography; MS, multiple sclerosis; TIA, transient ischemic attack; UMN, upper motor neuron. *Spinal sensory level = sensory loss involves all dermatomes below a particular level on one or both sides of the body, best detected on the trunk. **Length dependent = longest nerves are affected most, in a "stocking glove" distribution.

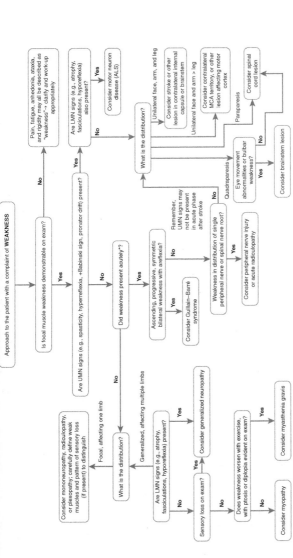

Algorithm 24-3. Approach to the patient with weakness. (Note: Although it is not comprehensive, this algorithm may be a helpful starting approach for synthesizing information gathered from the history and physical.) ALS, amyotrophic lateral sclerosis; LMN, lower motor neuron; MCA, middle cerebral artery; UMN, upper motor neuron. *Stroke is a medical emergency. Patients presenting with acute onset focal weakness <24 hours should be emergently evaluated for possibility of stroke, as they may be candidates for thrombolytic or endovascular therapies.

INTERPRETATION AIDS

TABLE 24-1. Primary Headaches

Problem	Common Characteristics	Associated Symptoms, Provoking and Relieving Factors
Tension	**Location:** variable **Quality:** pressing or tightening **pain;** mild-to-moderate intensity **Onset:** gradual **Duration:** minutes to days	Sometimes photophobia, phonophobia; nausea absent ↑ by sustained muscle tension, as in driving or typing ↓ possibly by massage, relaxation
Migraine ■ With aura ■ Without aura ■ Variants	**Location:** unilateral in ~70%; bifrontal or global in ~30% **Quality:** throbbing or aching, variable in severity **Onset:** fairly rapid, peaks in 1–2 hrs **Duration:** 4–72 hrs	Nausea, vomiting, photophobia, phonophobia, visual auras (flickering zig-zagging lines), motor auras affecting hand or arm, sensory auras (numbness, tingling usually precede headache) ↑ by alcohol, certain foods, tension, noise, bright light. More common premenstrually ↓ by quiet dark room, sleep
Cluster	**Location:** unilateral, usually behind or around the eye **Quality:** deep, continuous, severe **Onset:** abrupt, peaks within minutes **Duration:** up to 3 hrs	Lacrimation, rhinorrhea, miosis, ptosis, eyelid edema, conjunctival infection ↑ sensitivity to alcohol during some episodes

Sources: Headache Classification Committee of the International Headache Society (IHS). The International Classification of Headache Disorders, 3rd edition (beta version). *Cephalalgia.* 2013;33:629. Lipton RB, Bigal ME, Steiner TJ, et al. Classification of primary headaches. *Neurology.* 2004;63:427; Sun-Edelstein C, Bigal ME, Rappoport AM. Chronic migraine and medication overuse headache: clarifying the current International Headache Society classification criteria. *Cephalalgia.* 2009;29:445. Lipton RB, Stewart WF, Seymour D, et al. Prevalence and burden of migraine in the United States: data from the American Migraine Study II. *Headache.* 2001;41:646; Fumal A, Schoenen J. Tension-type headache: current research and clinical management. *Lancet Neurol.* 2008;7:70; Nesbitt AD, Goadsby PJ. Cluster headache. *BMJ.* 2012;344:e2407.

TABLE 24-2. Secondary Headaches

Problem	Common Characteristics	Associated Symptoms, Provoking and Relieving Factors
Analgesic Rebound	**Location:** previous headache pattern **Quality:** variable **Onset:** variable **Duration:** depends on prior headache pattern	Depends on prior headache pattern ↑ by fever, carbon monoxide, hypoxia, withdrawal of caffeine, other headache triggers ↓—depends on cause
Headaches from Eye Disorders *Errors of Refraction (farsightedness and astigmatism, but not nearsightedness)*	**Location:** around and over the eyes; may radiate to the occipital area **Quality:** steady, aching, dull **Onset:** gradual **Duration:** variable	Eye fatigue, "sandy" sensation in eyes, redness of the conjunctiva ↑ by prolonged use of the eyes, particularly for close work ↓ by resting the eyes
Acute Glaucoma	**Location:** in and around one eye **Quality:** steady, aching, often severe **Onset:** often rapid **Duration:** variable, may depend on treatment	Diminished vision, sometimes nausea and vomiting ↑—sometimes by drops that dilate the pupils
Headache from Sinusitis	**Location:** usually above eye (frontal sinus) or over maxillary sinus **Quality:** aching or throbbing, variable in severity; consider possible migraine **Onset:** variable **Duration:** often several hours at a time, recurring over days or longer	Local tenderness, nasal congestion, tooth pain, discharge, and fever ↑ by coughing, sneezing, or jarring the head, ↓ by nasal decongestants, antibiotics

continued

TABLE 24-2. Secondary Headaches *(continued)*

Problem	Common Characteristics	Associated Symptoms, Provoking and Relieving Factors
Meningitis	**Location:** generalized **Quality:** steady or throbbing, very severe **Onset:** fairly rapid **Duration:** variable, usually days	Fever, stiff neck, photophobia, change in mental status Can ↓ from immediate antibiotics until viral versus bacterial cause identified
Subarachnoid Hemorrhage— "Thunderclap Headache"	**Location:** generalized **Quality:** severe, "the worst of my life" **Onset:** usually abrupt; prodromal symptoms may occur **Duration:** variable, usually days	Nausea, vomiting, possibly loss of consciousness, neck pain ↑ rebleeding, ↑ intracranial pressure, cerebral edema ↓ by subspecialty treatments
Brain Tumor	**Location:** varies with the location of the tumor **Quality:** aching, steady, variable in intensity **Onset:** variable **Duration:** often brief	↑ by coughing, rebleeding, ↑ intracranial pressure, cerebral edema ↓ by subspecialty treatments
Giant Cell (Temporal) Arteritis	**Location:** near the involved artery, often the temporal, also the occipital; age related **Quality:** throbbing, generalized, persistent, often severe **Onset:** gradual or rapid **Duration:** variable	Tenderness of the adjacent scalp; fever (in ~50%), fatigue, weight loss; new headache (~60%), jaw claudication (~50%), visual loss or blindness (~15–20%), polymyalgia rheumatica (~50%) ↑ by movement of neck and shoulders Often ↓ by steroids

TABLE 24-2. Secondary Headaches *(continued)*

Problem	Common Characteristics	Associated Symptoms, Provoking and Relieving Factors
Postconcussion Headache	**Location:** often but not always localized to the injured area **Quality:** generalized, dull, aching, constant **Onset:** within hours to 1–2 days of the injury **Duration:** weeks, months, or even years	Drowsiness, poor concentration, confusion, memory loss, blurred vision, dizziness, irritability, restlessness, fatigue ↑ by mental and physical exertion, straining, stooping, emotional excitement, alcohol ↓ by rest
Cranial Neuralgias: Trigeminal Neuralgia (CN V)	**Location:** cheek, jaws, lips, or gums; trigeminal nerve divisions 2 and 3 >1 **Quality:** shocklike, stabbing, burning, severe **Onset:** abrupt, paroxysmal **Duration:** each jab lasts seconds but recurs at intervals of seconds or minutes	Exhaustion from recurrent pain ↑ by touching certain areas of the lower face or mouth; chewing, talking, brushing teeth ↓ by medication; neurovascular decompression

Sources: Headache Classification Committee of the International Headache Society (IHS). The International Classification of Headache Disorders, 3rd edition (beta version). *Cephalalgia*. 2013; 33:629. Schwedt TJ, Matharu MS, Dodick DW. Thunderclap headache. *Lancet Neurol*. 2006;5:621; Van de Beek D, de Gans J, Spanjaard L, et al. Clinical features and prognostic factors in adults with bacterial meningitis. *N Engl J Med*. 2004;351:1849; Salvarini C, Cantini F, Hunder GG. Polymyalgia rheumatica and giant cell arteritis. *Lancet*. 2008;372:234; Smetana GW, Shmerling RH. Does this patient have temporal arteritis? *JAMA*. 2002;287:92; Ropper AH, Gorson KC. Clinical practice. Concussion. *N Engl J Med*. 2007;356:166. American College of Physicians. *Neurology—MKSAP 16*. Philadelphia.

TABLE 24-3. Types of Stroke

Clinical Features and Vascular Territories of Stroke

Assessment of stroke requires careful history taking and a detailed physical examination. Focus on three fundamental questions: *What brain area and related vascular territory explain the patient's findings? Is the stroke ischemic or hemorrhagic? If ischemic, is the mechanism thrombosis or embolus?* This brief overview is intended to prompt further study and practice.

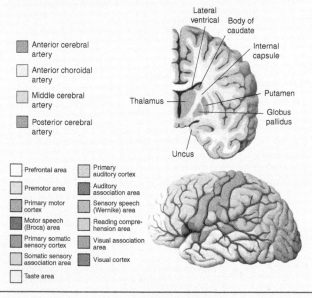

Major Clinical Features	Vascular Territory
Contralateral leg weakness	*Anterior circulation*—anterior cerebral artery (ACA)
	Includes stem of circle of Willis connecting internal carotid artery to ACA, and the segment distal to ACA and its anterior choroidal branch

TABLE 24-3. Types of Stroke *(continued)*

Major Clinical Features	Vascular Territory
Contralateral face, arm > leg weakness, sensory loss, field cut, aphasia (left MCA) or neglect, apraxia (right MCA)	*Anterior circulation*—middle cerebral artery (MCA) Largest vascular bed for stroke
Contralateral motor or sensory deficit without cortical signs	*Subcortical circulation*—lenticulostriate deep penetrating branches of MCA Small vessel subcortical *lacunar infarcts* in internal capsule, thalamus, or brainstem. Four common syndromes: pure motor hemiparesis; pure sensory hemianesthesia; ataxic hemiparesis; clumsy hand—dysarthria syndrome
Contralateral field cut	*Posterior circulation*—posterior cerebral artery (PCA) Includes paired vertebral arteries, the basilar artery, paired posterior cerebral arteries. Bilateral PCA infarction causes cortical blindness but preserved pupillary light reaction.
Dysphagia, dysarthria, tongue/palate deviation and/or ataxia with crossed sensory/motor deficits (= ipsilateral face with contralateral body)	*Posterior circulation*—brainstem, vertebral, or basilar artery branches
Oculomotor deficits and/ or ataxia with crossed sensory/motor deficits	*Posterior circulation*—basilar artery Complete basilar artery occlusion—"locked-in syndrome" with intact consciousness but inability to speak and quadriplegia

TABLE 24-4. Disorders of Speech

Disorders of speech fall into three groups affecting: (1) phonation of the voice, (2) the articulation of words, and (3) the production and comprehension of language.

- *Aphonia* refers to a loss of voice that accompanies disease affecting the larynx or its nerve supply. *Dysphonia* refers to less severe impairment in the volume, quality, or pitch of the voice. For example, a person may be hoarse or only able to speak in a whisper. Causes include laryngitis, laryngeal tumors, and unilateral vocal cord paralysis (CN X).

- *Dysarthria* refers to a defect in the muscular control of the speech apparatus (lips, tongue, palate, or pharynx). Words may be nasal, slurred, or indistinct, but the central symbolic aspect of language remains intact. Causes include motor lesions of the central or peripheral nervous system, parkinsonism, and cerebellar disease.

- *Aphasia* refers to a disorder in producing or understanding language. It is often caused by lesions in the dominant cerebral hemisphere, usually the left.

Compared below are two common types of aphasia: (1) Wernicke, a fluent (receptive) aphasia, and (2) Broca, a nonfluent (or expressive) aphasia. There are other less common kinds of aphasia, which are distinguished by differing responses on the specific tests listed. Neurologic consultation is usually indicated.

	Wernicke Aphasia	Broca Aphasia
Qualities of Spontaneous Speech	Fluent; often rapid, voluble, and effortless. Inflection and articulation are good, but sentences lack meaning, and words are malformed (*paraphasias*) or invented (*neologisms*). Speech may be totally incomprehensible.	Nonfluent; slow, with few words and laborious effort. Inflection and articulation are impaired, but words are meaningful, with nouns, transitive verbs, and important adjectives. Small grammatical words are often dropped.
Word Comprehension	Impaired	Fair to good

TABLE 24-4. Disorders of Speech *(continued)*

	Wernicke Aphasia	Broca Aphasia
Repetition	Impaired	Impaired
Naming	Impaired	Impaired, though the patient recognizes objects
Reading Comprehension	Impaired	Fair to good
Writing	Impaired	Impaired
Location of Lesion	Posterior superior temporal lobe	Posterior inferior frontal lobe

Although it is important to recognize aphasia early in your encounter with a patient, integrate this information with your neurologic examination as you generate your differential diagnosis.

TABLE 24-5. Types of Facial Paralysis

Distinguish peripheral from central lesions of CN VII by closely observing movements of the *upper face*. Because of innervation from both hemispheres, the upper facial movements are *preserved* in central lesions.

CN VII—Peripheral Lesion	CN VII—Central Lesion

Peripheral nerve damage to CN VII paralyzes the entire right side of the face, including the forehead.

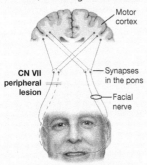

Motor cortex

CN VII peripheral lesion

Synapses in the pons

Facial nerve

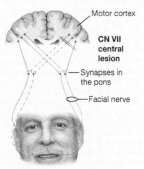

Motor cortex

CN VII central lesion

Synapses in the pons

Facial nerve

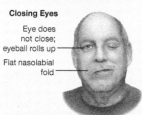

Closing Eyes
Eye does not close; eyeball rolls up
Flat nasolabial fold

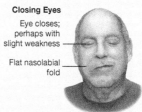

Closing Eyes
Eye closes; perhaps with slight weakness
Flat nasolabial fold

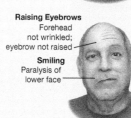

Raising Eyebrows
Forehead not wrinkled; eyebrow not raised
Smiling
Paralysis of lower face

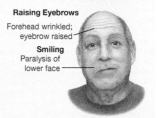

Raising Eyebrows
Forehead wrinkled; eyebrow raised
Smiling
Paralysis of lower face

	Peripheral Nervous System Disorder	Central Nervous System Disorder[a]	Parkinsonism (Basal Ganglia Disorder)	Cerebellar Disorder
Involuntary movements	Often fasciculations	No fasciculations	Resting tremors	Intention tremors
Muscle bulk	Atrophy	Normal or mild atrophy (disuse)	Normal	Normal
Muscle tone	Decreased or absent	Increased, spastic	Increased, rigid	Decreased
Muscle strength	Decreased or lost	Decreased or lost	Normal or slightly decreased	Normal or slightly decreased
Coordination	Unimpaired, though limited by weakness	Slowed and limited by weakness	Good, though slowed and often tremulous	Impaired, ataxic
Reflexes				
Deep tendon	Decreased or absent	Increased	Normal or decreased	Normal or decreased
Plantar	Flexor or absent	Extensor	Flexor	Flexor
Abdominals	Absent	Absent	Normal	Normal

TABLE 24-6. Motor Disorders

[a]Upper motor neuron.

TABLE 24-7. Involuntary Movements

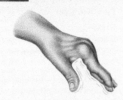

Resting static tremors. Fine, "pill-rolling" tremor seen at rest, usually disappear with movement; seen in basal ganglia disorders like Parkinson disease.

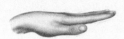

Postural tremor. Seen when maintaining active posture; in anxiety, hyperthyroidism; also familial. From basal ganglia disorder.

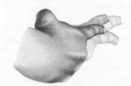

Intention tremor. Seen with intentional movement, absent at rest; in cerebellar disorders, including multiple sclerosis

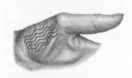

Fasciculations. Fine, rapid flickering of muscle bundles in lower motor neuron disorders.

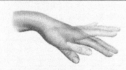

Chorea. Brief, rapid, irregular, jerky; face, head, arms, or hands (e.g., Huntington disease)

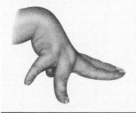

Athetosis. Slow, twisting, writhing; face, distal limbs, often with associated spasticity (e.g., cerebral palsy)

TABLE 24-8. Disorders of Muscle Tone

Spasticity	Rigidity
Location. Upper motor neuron or corticospinal tract systems.	**Location.** Basal ganglia system
Description. Increased muscle tone (*hypertonia*) that is rate dependent. Tone is greater when passive movement is rapid, and less when passive movement is slow. Tone is also greater at the extremes of the movement arc. During rapid passive movement, initial hypertonia may give way suddenly as the limb relaxes. This spastic "catch" and relaxation is known as "clasp-knife" resistance.	**Description.** Increased resistance that persists throughout the movement arc, independent of rate of movement, is called *lead-pipe rigidity*. With flexion and extension of the wrist or forearm, a superimposed ratchet-like jerkiness is called *cogwheel rigidity*.
Common Cause. Stroke, especially late or chronic stage	**Common Cause.** Parkinsonism

Flaccidity	Paratonia
Location. Lower motor neuron at any point from the anterior horn cell to the peripheral nerves	**Location.** Both hemispheres, usually in the frontal lobes
Description. Loss of muscle tone (*hypotonia*), causing the limb to be loose or floppy. The affected limbs may be hyperextensible or even flail-like.	**Description.** Sudden changes in tone with passive range of motion. Sudden loss of tone that increases the ease of motion is called *mitgehen* (moving with). Sudden increase in tone making motion more difficult is called *gegenhalten* (holding against).
Common Cause. Guillain–Barré syndrome; also initial phase of spinal cord injury (spinal shock) or stroke	**Common Cause.** Dementia

TABLE 24-9. Metabolic and Structural Coma

Toxic–Metabolic	Structural
Pathophysiology	
Arousal centers poisoned or critical substrates depleted	Lesion destroys or compresses brainstem arousal areas, either directly or secondary to more distant expanding mass lesions.
Clinical Features	
■ *Respiratory pattern.* If regular, may be normal or hyperventilation. If irregular, usually Cheyne–Stokes	*Respiratory pattern.* Irregular, especially Cheyne–Stokes or ataxic breathing. Also with selected stereotypical patterns like "apneustic" respiration (peak inspiratory arrest) or central hyperventilation.
■ *Pupillary size and reaction.* Equal, reactive to light. If *pinpoint* from opiates or cholinergics, you may need a magnifying glass to see the reaction.	*Pupillary size and reaction.* Unequal or unreactive to light (fixed)
May be unreactive if *fixed and dilated* from anticholinergics or hypothermia	*Midposition, fixed*—suggests midbrain compression
■ *Level of consciousness.* Changes *after* pupils change	*Dilated, fixed*—suggests compression of CN III from herniation
	Level of consciousness. Changes *before* pupils change
Examples of Cause	
Uremia, hyperglycemia	Epidural, subdural, or intracerebral hemorrhage
Alcohol, drugs, liver failure	
Hypothyroidism, hypoglycemia	Cerebral infarct or embolus
Anoxia, ischemia	Tumor, abscess
Meningitis, encephalitis	Brainstem infarct, tumor, or hemorrhage
Hyperthermia, hypothermia	Cerebellar infarct, hemorrhage, tumor, or abscess

TABLE 24-10. Glasgow Coma Scale

Activity		Score
Eye Opening		
None	1 = Even to supraorbital pressure	
To pain	2 = Pain from sternum/limb/ supraorbital pressure	
To speech	3 = Nonspecific response, not necessarily to command	
Spontaneous	4 = Eyes open, not necessarily aware	＿＿＿
Motor Response		
None	1 = To any pain; limbs remain flaccid	
Extension	2 = Shoulder adducted and shoulder and forearm internally rotated	
Flexor response	3 = Withdrawal response or assumption of hemiplegic posture	
Withdrawal	4 = Arm withdraws to pain, shoulder abducts	
Localizes pain	5 = Arm attempts to remove supraorbital/chest pressure	
Obeys commands	6 = Follows simple commands	＿＿＿
Verbal Response		
None	1 = No verbalization of any type	
Incomprehensible	2 = Moans/groans, no speech	
Inappropriate	3 = Intelligible, no sustained sentences	
Confused	4 = Converses but confused, disoriented	
Oriented	5 = Converses and is oriented	＿＿＿
	TOTAL (3–15)[a]	＿＿＿

[a]Interpretation: Patients with scores of 3–8 usually are considered to be in a coma.

Source: Reprinted from Teasdale G, Jennett B. Assessment of coma and impaired consciousness. A practical scale. *Lancet.* 1974;304(7872):81–84. Copyright © 1974 Elsevier. With permission.

TABLE 24-11. Pupils in Comatose Patients

Small or Pinpoint Pupils 	*Bilaterally small pupils* (1–2.5 mm) suggest (1) damage to the sympathetic pathways in the hypothalamus or (2) metabolic encephalopathy (a diffuse failure of cerebral function from drugs and other causes). Light reactions are usually normal. *Pinpoint pupils* (<1 mm) suggest (1) a hemorrhage in the pons or (2) the effects of morphine, heroin, or other narcotics. Use a magnifying glass to see the light reactions.
Midposition Fixed Pupils 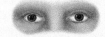	*Midposition* or *slightly dilated pupils* (4–6 mm) and *fixed to light* suggest damage in the midbrain.
Large Pupils 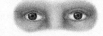	*Bilaterally fixed and dilated pupils* in severe anoxia with sympathomimetic effects, may be seen with cardiac arrest. They also result from atropine-like agents, phenothiazines, or tricyclic antidepressants.
One Large Pupil 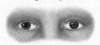	*One fixed and dilated pupil* warns of herniation of the temporal lobe, causing compression of the oculomotor nerve and midbrain. Also seen in diabetes with CN III infarction.

Children: Infancy through Adolescence

GENERAL PRINCIPLES OF CHILD DEVELOPMENT

Children display tremendous variations in physical, cognitive, and social development compared with adults.

Key Principles of Child Development

- Child development proceeds along a predictable pathway.
- The range of normal development is wide.
- Various physical, psychological, social, and environmental factors, as well as diseases, can affect child development and health.
- The child's developmental level affects how you conduct the history and physical examination.

Surveillance of Development

Understanding the normal physical, cognitive, and social development of children facilitates effective interviews and physical examinations and is the basis for distinguishing normal from abnormal findings.

- *Physical development* encompasses both *gross* and *fine motor* abilities.
- *Cognitive development* is a measure of the child's ability to problem solve through intuition, perception, and verbal and nonverbal reasoning
- *Language development* consists of the ability of a child to articulate, receive and express information. It also involves nonverbal modes of communication such as waving and head nodding.
- *Social and emotional development* encompasses the child's ability to form and maintain relationships.

The American Academy of Pediatrics (AAP) recommends the use of standardized screening instruments to assess these developmental domains.

PEDIATRIC CLINICAL ENCOUNTER

General Outline

As with an adult encounter, the relationships between the clinician, the child and the parents are viewed as a partnership. The goal is to recognize the importance of the family's strength in caring for their children. The encounter follows the same outline as an adult's but with certain *unique sections* highlighted here (Box 25-1).

BOX 25-1. Bright Futures Health Supervision Visit Outline, Using a Strength-Based Approach

Context

Priorities for the Visit

Health Supervision
- History
  - General questions
  - Past medical history
  - Family history
  - Social history
- Surveillance of development
- Review of systems
- Observation of parent-child/youth interaction
- Physical examination
  - Assessment of growth
    - <2 years: weight, length, head circumference, and weight-for-length
    - ≥2 years: weight, height, and BMI
  - Listing of particular components of the examination that are important for the child at each age visit
- Screening
  - Universal screening
  - Selective screening
    - Risk assessment
- Immunizations

Anticipatory Guidance
- Information for the health care professional
- Health promotion questions for the priorities for the visit
- Anticipatory guidance for the parent and child

Source: Republished with permission of American Academy of Pediatrics from Bright Futures: *Guidelines for Health Supervision of Infants, Children, and Adolescents.* 4th ed. Elk Grove Village: Bright Futures/American Academy of Pediatrics, 2017:266; permission conveyed through Copyright Clearance Center, Inc.

Pediatric Health History

Context. This is intended to gather information about the child that makes him/her unique compared to other children of his/her age. Include the date and place of birth, nickname, and first and last names of parents. Assess the child's developmental environment including observing the parent-child/youth interaction.

Chief Complaints or Concerns. Expert panels note that "the first priority is to address the concerns of the parents and the child/adolescent and parent." Determine if they are the concerns of the child, the parent(s), a schoolteacher, or some other person.

Initial or Interval Health History. Include information that is relevant and specific to the child's age. Determine how each family member responds to the child's symptoms, why he or she is concerned, and impact on the child's functioning. These may include gathering information related to past medical history, pertinent family history and on occasion relevant social history. If age-appropriate, may include:

Prenatal history, labor, and delivery

- Prenatal—maternal health: medications; tobacco, drug, and alcohol use; weight gain; duration of pregnancy
- Natal—nature of labor and delivery, birth weight, Apgar scores at 1 and 5 minutes (p. 457)
- Neonatal—resuscitation efforts, cyanosis, jaundice, infections, bonding

Feeding history

- Breastfeeding—frequency and duration of feeds, difficulties, timing and method of weaning
- Bottle-feeding—type; amount; frequency; vomiting; colic; diarrhea
- Vitamins, and iron or fluoride supplements; introduction of solid foods
- Eating habits—types and amounts of food eaten, parental attitudes and responses to feeding problems

Allergies

Pay particular attention to history of eczema, urticaria, perennial allergic rhinitis, asthma, food intolerance, insect hypersensitivity, and recurrent wheezing.

Surveillance of Development

- Physical growth—weight and height at all ages; head circumference at birth and younger than 2 years; periods of slow or rapid growth; BMI after age 2 years (see below)
- Developmental milestones, speech development, performance in preschool and school
- Social development—day and night sleeping patterns; toilet training; habitual behaviors; discipline problems; school behavior; relationships

with family and peers; social risks such as poverty, food insecurity and adverse childhood experiences

Physical Examination. This is a critical component of the pediatric evaluation. This also provides the opportunity for discussion of the physical changes associated with the child's development. See pp. 457–459.

The physical examination always should include an assessment of growth:

- Younger than 2 years: weight, length, head circumference, and weight-for-length
- 2 years and older: weight, height, and body mass index (BMI)

The sequence of examination varies according to the child's age and comfort level.

- For infants and young children, *perform nondisturbing maneuvers early and potentially distressing maneuvers toward the end.* For example, palpate the head and neck and auscultate the heart and lungs early; examine the ears and mouth and palpate the abdomen near the end. If the child reports pain in an area, examine that part last.
- For older children and adolescents, use the same sequence as with adults, except examine the most painful areas last.

Please check with your institution about a chaperone policy. In many settings, chaperones are recommended during the examination of school-aged children and adolescents (irrespective of the gender of the examiner) when examining the genitalia of either boys or girls and the breasts of girls.

Screening. Certain screening is *universal*—applied to each child at that visit. Other screening is *selective*. These vary according to the child's medical, developmental, and social conditions. Include newborn screening results, anemia screening, blood lead levels, sickle cell disease, vision, hearing, developmental screening, and others (e.g., tuberculosis).

Immunizations. Include dates given and any untoward reactions. Discussion regarding parental anxiety and misinformation regarding immunization must be addressed.

Anticipatory Guidance. Key areas cover a broad range of topics, from clinical to developmental, social, and emotional health.

NEWBORNS AND INFANTS
HEALTH HISTORY: GENERAL APPROACH

The newborn visit is a critical opportunity for the health care provider to engage with the family, learn about the newborn's family and environment, understand key aspects of the pregnancy, bond with the family, and observe the family's interactions with the newborn. Experienced clinicians learn to combine history-taking with anticipatory guidance as outlined previously (p. 455), so that the history feels like a conversation with new parents.

TECHNIQUES OF EXAMINATION

Assessment at Birth

Physical growth during infancy is faster than at any other age.

Listen to the anterior thorax with your stethoscope. Palpate the abdomen. Inspect the head, face, oral cavity, extremities, genitalia, and perineum.

Apgar Score. Score each newborn according to the following table, at 1 and 5 minutes after birth, according to the 3-point scale (0, 1, or 2) for each component (Box 25-2).

If the 5-minute score is 8 or more, proceed to a more complete examination.

BOX 25-2. Apgar Scoring System

Clinical Sign	Assigned Score		
	0	**1**	**2**
Heart rate	Absent	<100	>100
Respiratory effort	Absent	Slow and irregular	Good; strong
Muscle tone	Flaccid	Some flexion of the arms and legs	Active movement
Reflex irritability[a]	No responses	Grimace	Crying vigorously, sneeze, or cough
Color	Blue, pale	Pink body, blue extremities	Pink all over

1-Minute Apgar Score		5-Minute Apgar Score	
8–10	Normal	8–10	Normal
5–7	Some nervous system depression	0–7	High risk for subsequent central nervous system and other organ system dysfunction
0–4	Severe depression, requiring immediate resuscitation		

[a]Reaction to suction of nares with bulb syringe.

Gestational Age and Birth Weight.
Classify newborns according to their
gestational age and birth weight (Boxes
25-3 and 25-4).

See Table 25-1, Newborn Classification,
p. 488.

BOX 25-3. Classification by Gestational Age and Birth Weight

Gestational Age Classification	Gestational Age
Preterm	<37 weeks
Late preterm	34–36 weeks
Term	37–41 weeks
Post-term	>42 weeks
Birth Weight Classification	**Weight**
Extremely low birth weight	<1,000 g
Very low birth weight	<1,500 g
Low birth weight	<2,500 g
Normal birth weight	≥2,500 g

BOX 25-4. Newborn Classifications

Category	Abbreviation	Percentile
Small for gestational age	SGA	<10th
Appropriate for gestational age	AGA	10–90th
Large for gestational age	LGA	>90th

Assessment Several Hours After Birth

During the first day of life, newborns should have a comprehensive examination following the technique outlined under Infants starting on p. 456. Wait until 1 or 2 hours after a feeding, when a newborn is more responsive. Ask parents to remain.

Observe the baby's color, size, body proportions, nutritional status, posture, respirations, and movements of the head and extremities.	Most newborns are bowlegged, reflecting their curled up intrauterine position.
Inspect the newborn's *umbilical cord* to detect abnormalities. Normally, there are two thick-walled umbilical arteries and one larger but thin-walled umbilical vein, which is usually located at the 12-o'clock position.	A single umbilical artery may be associated with congenital anomalies. Umbilical hernias in infants are from a defect in the abdominal wall.
The neurologic screening examination of all newborns should include assessment of mental status, gross and fine motor function, tone, cry, deep tendon reflexes, and primitive reflexes.	Signs of severe neurologic disease include extreme irritability; persistent asymmetry of posture or extension of extremities; constant turning of head to one side; marked extension of head, neck, and extremities (*opisthotonus*); severe flaccidity; and limited pain response.

Box 25-5 provides helpful techniques for the infant examination.

BOX 25-5. Tips for Examining Infants

- Approach the infant gradually, using a toy or object for distraction.
- Perform as much of the examination as possible with the infant in the parent's lap.
- Speak softly to the infant or mimic the infant's sounds to attract attention.
- If the infant is cranky, make sure he or she is well fed before proceeding.
- Ask a parent about the infant's strengths to elicit useful developmental and parenting information.
- Do not expect to do a head-to-toe examination in a specific order. Work with what the infant gives you and save the mouth and ear examination for last.

Mental and Physical Status

Observe the parents' affect when talking about the baby and their manner of holding, moving, and dressing the baby. Observe a breast- or bottle-feeding. Determine attainment of developmental milestones, optimally using a standardized developmental screening test.	Common causes of developmental delay include abnormalities in embryonic development, hereditary and genetic disorders, environmental and social problems, other pregnancy or perinatal problems, childhood diseases such as infection (e.g., meningitis), trauma, and severe chronic disease.

General Survey

Growth, reflected in increases in height and weight within expected limits, is an excellent indicator of health during infancy and childhood. Deviations from normal may be early indications of an underlying problem. To assess growth, compare a child's parameters with respect to:

Failure to thrive is a condition reflecting significantly low weight gain (e.g., below second percentile) for gestational age–corrected age and sex. Causes can be environmental or psychosocial or various gastrointestinal, neurologic, cardiac, endocrine, renal, or other diseases.

■ Normal values according to age and sex

Measures above the 97th or below the 3rd percentile, or recent rises or falls from prior levels, require investigation.

■ Prior readings to assess trends

Height and Weight

Plot each child's height and weight on standard growth charts to determine progress.

Reduced growth in height may indicate endocrine disease, other causes of short stature, or, if weight is also low, other chronic diseases.

Head Circumference

Determine head circumference at every physical examination during the first 2 years (Fig. 25-1).

Premature closure of the sutures or microcephaly may cause small head size. Hydrocephalus, subdural hematoma, or, rarely, brain tumor or inherited syndromes may cause an abnormally large head size.

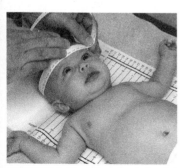

FIGURE 25-1. Head circumference is a vital metric during early childhood.

Vital Signs

Blood Pressure. Measure blood pressure at least once during infancy. Although the hand-held method is shown in Figure 25-2, the most easily used measure of systolic blood pressure in infants and young children is obtained with the *Doppler method*.

See Table 25-2, Causes of Sustained Hypertension in Children, p. 488.

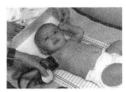

FIGURE 25-2. Practice is required to accurately measure blood pressure in early childhood.

Pulse. The heart rate is quite variable (Box 25-6) and will increase markedly with excitement, crying, or anxiety. Therefore, measure the pulse when the infant or child is quiet.

Tachycardia (>180 to 200 beats per minute) usually indicates paroxysmal supraventricular tachycardia. Bradycardia may result from serious underlying disease.

BOX 25-6. Heart Rates of Healthy Children from Birth to 1 Year

Age	Average Heart Rate (per minute)	Range (1st to 99th percentile) per minute
Birth–1 month	140	90–165
1–6 months	130	80–175
6–12 months	115	90–170

Respiratory Rate. The respiratory rate has a very wide range and is more responsive to illness, exercise, and emotion than in adults.

Respiratory diseases such as bronchiolitis or pneumonia may cause rapid respirations (up to 80 to 90 breaths per minute), and increased work of breathing. Peaceful tachypnea (without increased work of breathing) may be a sign of cardiac failure.

Temperature. Body temperature in infants and children is less constant than in adults. Rectal temperatures are the most accurate for infants. The average rectal temperature is higher in infancy and early childhood, usually above 99°F (37.2°C) until after age 3 years.

Skin

Assess:

- Texture and appearance

  Cutis marmorata

- Vasomotor changes

  Acrocyanosis; cyanotic congenital heart disease

- Pigmentation

  Café-au-lait spots

- Hair (e.g., lanugo)

  Midline hair tuft on back

- Common skin conditions (e.g., milia, erythema toxicum)

  Herpes simplex

- Color

  Jaundice can be from hemolytic disease.

- Turgor

  Dehydration

Head

Examine *sutures* and *fontanelles* carefully. The *anterior fontanelle* at birth measures 4 to 6 cm in diameter and will close by 18 to 22 months of age. The *posterior fontanelle* measures 1 to 2 cm at birth and usually closes by 2 months (Fig. 25-3).

Head small with microcephaly, enlarged with hydrocephaly; fontanelles full and tense with meningitis, closed with microcephaly, separated with increased intracranial pressure (hydrocephaly, subdural hematoma, and brain tumor)

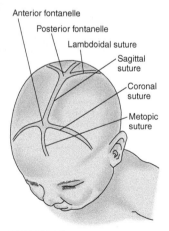

Anterior fontanelle
Posterior fontanelle
Lambdoidal suture
Sagittal suture
Coronal suture
Metopic suture

FIGURE 25-3. Sutures and fontanelles.

Palpate the infant's skull with care. The cranial bones generally appear "soft" or pliable; they will normally become firmer with increasing gestational age.	Swelling from subperiosteal hemorrhage (cephalohematoma) does not cross suture lines; swelling from bleeding associated with a fracture does.
Check the *face* for symmetry. Examine for an overall impression of the *facies* (Box 25-7). Comparing with the faces of the parents is helpful.	Abnormal facies occurs in a child with a constellation of facial features that appear abnormal. A variety of syndromes can cause abnormal facies (see Box 25-7). Examples include Down syndrome and fetal alcohol syndrome.

BOX 25-7. Pearls to Evaluate Potentially Abnormal Facies

- Carefully review the history, especially the *family history, pregnancy,* and *perinatal history.*
- Note abnormalities of growth/development or dysmorphic somatic features.
- Measure and plot percentiles, especially of *head circumference, height,* and *weight.*
- Consider the three mechanisms of facial dysmorphogenesis:
  - Deformations from intrauterine constraint
  - Disruptions from amniotic bands or fetal tissue
  - Malformations from intrinsic abnormality (either face/head or brain)
- Examine parents and siblings (similarity may be reassuring but might also point to a familial disorder).
- Determine whether facial features fit a recognizable syndrome. Compare against references, pictures, tables, and databases.

Eyes

Newborns and young infants may look at your face and follow a bright light if you catch them while alert (Box 25-8).	Nystagmus, strabismus
For the ophthalmoscopic examination, with the newborn awake and eyes open, examine the *red retinal (fundus) reflex* by setting the ophthalmoscope at 0 diopters and viewing the pupil from about 10 in.	*Leukocoria* is a white papillary reflex (instead of the normal red papillary reflex). It can be a sign of a rare tumor called retinoblastoma.
	Papilledema is rare in infants because the fontanelles and open sutures accommodate any increased intracranial pressure, sparing the optic discs.

BOX 25-8. Visual Milestones of Infancy

Birth	Blinks, may regard face
1 month	Fixes on objects
1½–2 months	Coordinated eye movements
3 months	Eyes converge, baby reaches
12 months	Acuity around 20/60–20/80

Ears

Check position, shape, and features.

Small, deformed, or low-set auricles may indicate associated congenital defects, especially renal disease.

Assess hearing (Box 25-9).

BOX 25-9. Signs that an Infant Can Hear

Age	Signs
0–2 months	Startle response and blink to a sudden noise Calming down with soothing voice or music
2–3 months	Change in body movements in response to sound Change in facial expression to familiar sounds Turning eyes and head to sound
3–4 months	Turning to listen to voices and conversation
6–7 months	Appropriate language development

Nose

Test patency of the nasal passages by occluding alternately each nostril while holding the infant's mouth closed.

With choanal atresia, the baby cannot breathe if one nostril is occluded.

Mouth and Pharynx

Inspect (with a tongue blade and flash-light) and palpate.

Supernumerary teeth, Epstein pearls

You may see a whitish covering on the tongue. If this coating is from milk, you can easily remove it by scraping or wiping it away.

Oral candidiasis (thrush)

Vesicles in the mouth can be caused by enteroviral infections and herpes simplex virus infections.

Assess the teeth. *Natal* teeth are teeth that are present at birth.

Neck

Palpate the *lymph nodes,* and assess for any additional masses (e.g., congenital cysts), as shown in Figure 25-4.

Lymphadenopathy is usually from viral or bacterial infections.

Other neck masses include malignancy, branchial cleft or thyroglossal duct cysts, and periauricular cysts and sinuses.

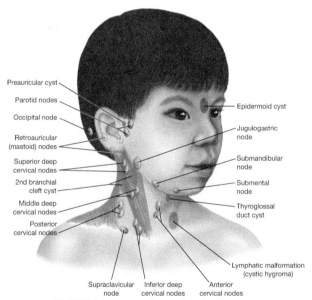

Preauricular cyst
Parotid nodes
Occipital node
Retroauricular (mastoid) nodes
Superior deep cervical nodes
2nd branchial cleft cyst
Middle deep cervical nodes
Posterior cervical nodes
Epidermoid cyst
Jugulogastric node
Submandibular node
Submental node
Thyroglossal duct cyst
Lymphatic malformation (cystic hygroma)
Supraclavicular node
Inferior deep cervical nodes
Anterior cervical nodes

FIGURE 25-4. Nodes and cysts of the head and neck.

Thorax and Lungs

Carefully assess respirations and breathing pattern (Box 25-10).

Apnea

Do not rush to the stethoscope but observe the patient carefully first.

Upper respiratory infections may cause nasal flaring.

BOX 25-10. Observing Respiration

Assessment	Possible Findings	Explanation
General appearance	■ Inability to feed or smile ■ Lack of consolability	■ Lower respiratory infections (e.g., bronchiolitis, pneumonia) are common in infants.
Respiratory rate	■ Tachypnea	■ Cardiac or respiratory disease (e.g., pneumonia)
Color	■ Pallor or cyanosis	■ Cardiac or pulmonary disease
Nasal component of breathing	■ Nasal flaring (enlargement of both nasal openings during inspiration)	■ Upper or lower respiratory infection
Audible breath sounds	■ *Grunting* (repetitive, short expiratory sound) ■ *Wheezing* (musical expiratory sound) ■ *Stridor* (high-pitched, inspiratory noise) ■ *Obstruction* (lack of breath sounds)	■ Lower respiratory disease Asthma or bronchiolitis Croup, epiglottitis, bacterial tracheitis Foreign body

Work of breathing	■ Nasal flaring
	■ Grunting
	■ *Retractions* (chest indrawing):
	  ■ Supraclavicular (motion of soft tissue above clavicles)
	  ■ Intercostal (indrawing of the skin between ribs)
	  ■ Substernal (at xiphoid process)
	  ■ Subcostal (just below the costal margin)
		■ In infants, abnormal work of breathing combined with abnormal findings on auscultation is the best finding for ruling in pneumonia.

Auscultate the chest and try to distinguish upper airway from lower airway sounds (Box 25-11).

Thoracoabdominal paradox, or paradoxical breathing, is inward movement of the chest and outward movement of the abdomen during inspiration (abdominal breathing). This is a normal finding in newborns (but not older infants).

BOX 25-11. Distinguishing Upper Airway from Lower Airway Sounds

Technique	Upper Airway	Lower Airway
Compare sounds from nose/stethoscope	Same sounds	Often different sounds
Listen to harshness of sounds	Harsh and loud	Variable
Note symmetry (left/right)	Symmetric	Often asymmetric
Compare sounds at different locations (higher or lower)	Sounds louder as stethoscope is moved up chest	Sounds louder lower in chest
Inspiratory versus expiratory	Almost always inspiratory	Often has expiratory phase
Hold stethoscope above infant's mouth	Inspiratory sounds remain loud	Often quieter than by auscultation of the chest

Heart and Peripheral Vascular System

Inspection. Observe carefully for any cyanosis. The best body part to assess cyanosis is the tongue or inside of the mouth.

At birth: transposition of the great arteries; pulmonary valve atresia or stenosis

Within a few days of birth: The above; also, total anomalous pulmonary venous return, hypoplastic left heart

Palpation. The point of maximal impulse (PMI) is not always palpable in infants. Palpate the *peripheral pulses*. *Thrills* are palpable when enough turbulence is within the heart or great vessels.

Absent or diminished femoral pulses suggest coarctation of the aorta. Weak or thready, difficult-to-feel pulses may reflect myocardial dysfunction and heart failure.

Auscultation. Heart *rhythm* is evaluated more easily in infants by listening to the heart than by feeling the peripheral pulses.

Infants and children commonly have a normal sinus dysrhythmia, with the heart rate increasing on inspiration and decreasing on expiration, sometimes quite abruptly.

The most common dysrhythmia in children is paroxysmal supraventricular tachycardia.

Evaluate S_1 and S_2 carefully. They are normally crisp with intermittent splitting of S_1 and S_2 (fused in expiration).

A louder-than-normal pulmonic component suggests pulmonary hypertension. Persistent splitting of S_2 may indicate atrial septal defect.

Listen for heart murmurs. Two common benign systolic murmurs are from a closing ductus or peripheral pulmonary flow murmur.

Most infants with cardiac pathology have signs beyond heart murmurs such as poor feeding, failure to thrive, irritability, poor overall appearance, weakness, tachypnea, clubbing, hepatomegaly and fatigue.

Breasts

The breasts of males and females may be enlarged for months after birth as a result of maternal estrogen.

Abdomen

You will find it easy to palpate an infant's abdomen, because infants like being touched. Palpate the liver and spleen and assess for hepatosplenomegaly (Box 25-12).

Abnormal abdominal masses can be associated with kidney, bladder, or bowel tumors. In pyloric stenosis, deep palpation in the right upper quadrant or midline can reveal an "olive," or a 2-cm firm pyloric mass.

BOX 25-12. Liver Size in Healthy Term Newborns

By palpation and percussion	Mean, 5.9 ± 0.7 cm
Projection below right costal margin	Mean, 2.5 ± 1.0 cm

Male Genitalia

Inspect with the infant supine. The foreskin of a newborn is nonretractable at birth or just enough to visualize the urethral meatus.

Common scrotal masses are hydroceles and inguinal hernias.

In 3% of infants, one or both testes cannot be felt in the scrotum or inguinal canal. Try to milk the testes into the scrotum.

Inability to palpate testes, even with maneuvers, indicates undescended testicles.

Female Genitalia

In females, genitalia may be prominent for several months after birth from the effects of maternal estrogen. This decreases during the first year (Fig. 25-5).

Ambiguous genitalia involves masculinization of the female external genitalia.

Rectum and Anus

In general, a digital rectal examination is *not performed* on infants or children unless there is question of patency of the anus or an abdominal mass.

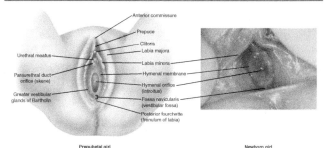

FIGURE 25-5. Highly estrogenized hymen of a newborn with thickening and hypertrophy of hymenal tissue.

Musculoskeletal System

Examine the extremities by inspection and palpation to detect congenital abnormalities, particularly in the hands, spine, hips, legs, and feet.

Skin tags, remnants of digits, *polydactyly* (extra fingers), or *syndactyly* (webbed fingers) are congenital defects. Fracture of the clavicle can occur during a difficult delivery.

Examine the *hips* carefully at each visit for signs of dislocation. There are two major techniques: one to test for a posteriorly dislocated hip (*Ortolani test*), as shown in Figure 25-6, and the other to test for the ability to sublux or dislocate an intact but unstable hip (*Barlow test*), as shown in Figure 25-7.

Congenital hip dysplasia may have a positive Ortolani or Barlow test, particularly during the first 3 months of age. With a hip dysplasia, you feel a "clunk."

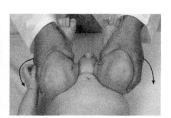

FIGURE 25-6. Ortolani test, overhead view.

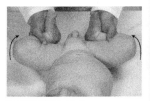

FIGURE 25-7. Barlow test, overhead view.

Some infants exhibit normal twisting or *torsion of the tibia* inwardly or outwardly on its longitudinal axis.

Pathologic tibial torsion occurs only in association with deformities of the feet or hips.

Nervous System

Evaluate the developing central nervous system by assessing *infantile automatisms*, called *primitive reflexes*.

See Table 25-3, Primitive Reflexes, pp. 489–492.

Suspect a neurologic or developmental abnormality if primitive reflexes are absent at appropriate age, present longer than normal, asymmetric, or associated with posturing or twitching.

Neurologic abnormalities in infants often present as developmental abnormalities such as failure to perform age-appropriate tasks.

Hypotonia can be a sign of a variety of neurologic abnormalities.

YOUNG AND SCHOOL-AGED CHILDREN, HEALTH HISTORY: GENERAL APPROACH

- *Establish rapport.* Refer to children by name and meet them on their own level. Maintain eye contact at their level (e.g., sit on the floor if needed). Participate in play and talk about their interests.
- *Work with families.* Ask simple, open-ended questions such as "Are you sick? Tell me about it," followed by more specific questions. Once the parent has started the conversation, direct questions back to the child. Also observe how parents interact with the child.
- *Identify multiple agendas.* Your job is to discover as many perspectives and agendas as possible.
- *Use the family as the key resource.* View parents as experts in the care of their child and you as their consultant.
- *Note hidden agendas.* As with adults, the chief complaint may not relate to the real reason the parent has brought the child to see you.

TECHNIQUES OF EXAMINATION

The following discussion focuses on those areas of the comprehensive physical examination that are different for children than for infants and for adults. Techniques for adolescents are shown below.

Mental and Physical Status

- In *children age 1 to 5 years,* observe the degree of sickness or wellness, mood, nutritional state, speech, cry, facial expression, and developmental

This overall examination can uncover evidence of chronic disease, developmental delay, social or environmental disorders, and family problems.

skills. Note parent–child interaction, including separation tolerance, affection, and response to discipline.

- In *children 6 to 10 years,* determine orientation to time and place, factual knowledge, and language and number skills. Observe motor skills used in writing, tying laces, buttoning, cutting, and drawing.

Observing children performing tasks can reveal signs of inattentiveness or impulsivity, which may indicate attention deficit disorder.

Body Mass Index for Age. Age- and sex-specific charts are now available to assess BMI in children.

Underweight is <5th percentile, *at risk of overweight* is ≥85th percentile, and *overweight* is ≥95th percentile.

Blood Pressure. Hypertension during childhood is more common than previously thought. Recognizing, confirming, and appropriately managing it is important. Blood pressure readings should be part of the physical examination of every child older than 2 years. *Proper cuff size is essential for accurate determination of blood pressure in children.*

Most errors in blood pressure readings in children are due to using an incorrect cuff size.

Causes of sustained hypertension in childhood include renal disease, coarctation of the aorta, and primary hypertension. Hypertension is often related to childhood obesity.

Eyes

Test visual acuity in each eye (Box 25-13) and determine whether the gaze is conjugate or symmetric.

Any difference in visual acuity between eyes is abnormal.

Myopia or hyperopia often present in school-aged children.

Special Techniques

The corneal light reflex test (Fig. 25-8) and the cover–uncover test (Fig. 25-9) are particularly useful in young children.

Strabismus can lead to amblyopia.

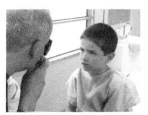

FIGURE 25-8. Corneal light reflex test.

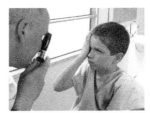

FIGURE 25-9. Cover–uncover test.

BOX 25-13. Visual Acuity in Children

Age	Visual Acuity
3 months	Eyes converge, baby reaches
12 months	20/60–20/80
Younger than 4 years	20/40
4 years and older	20/30

Ears

Examine the ear canal and drum. There are two positions for the child (lying down or sitting), and also two ways to hold the otoscope, as shown in Figures 25-10 and 25-11.

Pain on movement of the pinna occurs with otitis externa.

FIGURE 25-10. Gently holding the child's arms reduces reactions to the otoscope.

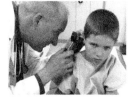

FIGURE 25-11. Gently pulling up on the auricle gives a better otoscope view with many children.

Insert the speculum, obtaining a proper seal.

Acute otitis media involves a red and bulging tympanic membrane.

Pneumatic Otoscope. It may be helpful to learn to use a *pneumatic otoscope* (Fig. 25-12) to improve accuracy of

Diminished movement of tympanic membrane with acute otitis media; no movement with otitis media with effusion.

FIGURE 25-12. Pneumatic otoscope.

diagnosis of otitis media (Box 25-14). When air is introduced into the normal ear canal, the tympanic membrane and its light reflex move inward. When air is removed, the tympanic membrane moves outward toward you.

BOX 25-14. Tips for Conducting the Otoscopic Examination in Children

- Use the best angle of the otoscope.
- Use the largest possible speculum.
  - A larger speculum allows you to better visualize the tympanic membrane and is less painful since it is not inserted as far as a smaller speculum.
  - A small speculum may not provide a seal for pneumatic otoscopy.
- Don't apply too much pressure which will cause the child to cry and may cause false-positive results on pneumatic otoscopy.
- Insert the speculum ¼ to ½ in into the canal.
- First find the landmarks.
  - Careful—sometimes the ear canal resembles the tympanic membrane.
- Note whether the tympanic membrane is abnormal.
- Remove cerumen if it is blocking your view, using one of the following:
  - Special plastic curettes
  - A moistened microtipped cotton swab
  - Flushing of ears for older children
  - Special instruments that can also be purchased.

Mouth and Pharynx

For anxious or young children, leave this examination toward the end. The best technique for a tongue blade is to push down and pull slightly forward toward you while the child says "ah." Do not place the blade too far posteriorly, eliciting a gag reflex.

A common cause of a strawberry tongue, red uvula, and pharyngeal exudate is streptococcal pharyngitis.

Tonsils. Note the size, position, symmetry, and appearance of the *tonsils*. The size of the tonsils varies considerably in children and is often categorized by the percent of the width of the posterior oropharynx (e.g., reduce the opening by <25% of opening, by 50%, etc.).

Streptococcal pharyngitis typically produces white or yellow exudates on the tonsils or posterior pharynx, a beefy-red uvula, and palatal petechiae.

Examine the *teeth* for the timing and sequence of eruption, number, character, condition, and position. There is a predictable pattern of tooth eruption. In general, a child will have 1 tooth for each month of age between 6 and 26 months, up to a maximum of 20 primary teeth.

Abnormalities of the enamel may reflect local or general disease.

Carefully inspect the inside of the upper teeth (Fig. 25-13).

Nursing bottle caries; dental caries; staining of the teeth, which may be intrinsic or extrinsic

Dental caries are the most common health problem of children and are particularly prevalent in children living in poverty.

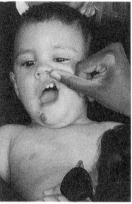

FIGURE 25-13. Lift the lip to check for dental caries.

Look for abnormalities of tooth position.

Malocclusion

Note the size, position, symmetry, and appearance of the *tonsils*.

Peritonsillar abscess

Heart

A challenging aspect to cardiac examination of children is evaluation of *heart murmurs*, particularly distinguishing common benign murmurs from unusual or pathologic ones. Most children have one or more *functional*, or *benign*, heart murmurs at some point in time (Fig. 25-14).

See Table 25-4, Characteristics of Pathologic Heart Murmurs, pp. 493–494.

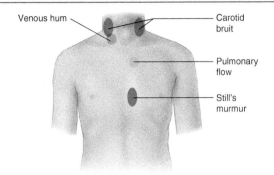

FIGURE 25-14. Location of benign heart murmurs in children.

Abdomen

Most children are ticklish when you first place your hand on their abdomens for palpation. This reaction tends to disappear, particularly if you distract the child.

A pathologically enlarged liver in children usually is palpable more than 2 cm below the costal margin, has a round, firm edge, and often is tender.

A common condition of childhood that can occasionally cause a protuberant abdomen is constipation.

Please check with your institution about a chaperone policy. In many settings, chaperones are recommended during the examination of school-aged children and adolescents (irrespective of the gender of the examiner) when examining the genitalia of either boys or girls and the breasts of girls.

Male Genitalia

Many boys have an active cremasteric reflex causing the testes to retract upward into the inguinal canal and appear undescended. A useful technique is to have the boy sit cross-legged on the examining table.

In precocious puberty, the penis and testes are enlarged, with signs of pubertal changes.

A painful testicle requires rapid treatment and may indicate torsion.

Inguinal hernias in older boys present as they do in adult men.

Female Genitalia

Use a calm, gentle approach, including a developmentally appropriate explanation.

Examine the genitalia in an efficient and systematic manner. The normal hymen can have various configurations (Fig. 25-15).

Vaginal discharge in early childhood can result from perineal irritation (e.g., from bubble baths, soaps), foreign body, vaginitis, or sexually transmitted infections from sexual abuse. Vaginal bleeding, abrasions, or signs of trauma to the external genitalia can result from sexual abuse (see Table 25-5, Physical Signs of Sexual Abuse, p. 495).

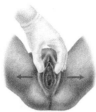

FIGURE 25-15. Separate labia to assess genital structures.

Rectum and Anus

The rectal examination is not routine but should be done whenever intra-abdominal, pelvic, or perirectal disease is suspected.

Tenderness noted on rectal examination of a child usually indicates an infectious or inflammatory cause, such as an abscess or appendicitis.

Musculoskeletal System

Abnormalities of the upper extremities are rare in the absence of injury. To assess the lower extremities, observe the child standing and walking barefoot, and ask the child to touch the toes, rise from sitting, run a short distance, and pick up objects. You will detect most abnormalities by watching carefully.

A screening musculoskeletal examination for children participating in sports can detect injuries or abnormalities that may result in problems during athletics.

Extreme bowing or unilateral bowing may be from pathologic causes such as rickets or tibia vara (*Blount disease*).

A *knock-knee pattern* is common, usually maximal by age 3 years, and gradually corrects by age 7 years.

Nervous System

Beyond infancy, the neurologic examination includes the components evaluated in adults. Again, combine the neurologic and developmental assessments. You can turn this into a game with the child to assess optimal development and neurologic performance (Box 25-15).

Delayed language or cognitive skills can be due to neurologic disease as well as developmental disorders.

Soft neurologic signs can suggest minor developmental abnormalities.

BOX 25-15. Strategies to Assess Cranial Nerves in Young Children

Cranial Nerve		Strategy
I	Olfactory	Testable in older children.
II	Visual acuity	Use Snellen chart after age 3 years.
		Test visual fields as for an adult. A parent may need to hold the child's head.
III, IV, VI	Extraocular movements	Have the child track a light or an object (a toy is preferable). A parent may need to hold the child's head.
V	Motor	Play a game with a soft cotton ball to test sensation.
		Have the child clench the teeth and chew or swallow some food.
VII	Facial	Have the child "make faces" or imitate you as you make faces (including moving your eyebrows) and observe symmetry and facial movements.
VIII	Acoustic	Perform auditory testing after age 4 years.
		Whisper a word or command behind the child's back and have the child repeat it.
IX, X	Swallow and gag	Have the child stick the "whole tongue out" or "say 'ah.'" Observe movement of the uvula and soft palate.
		Test the gag reflex.
XI	Spinal accessory	Have the child push your hand away with his head. Have the child shrug his shoulders while you push down with your hands to "see how strong you are."
XII	Hypoglossal	Ask the child to "stick out your tongue all the way."

ADOLESCENTS, HEALTH HISTORY: GENERAL APPROACH

The key to successfully examining teens is a comfortable, confidential environment that makes the examination relaxed and informative. Adolescents are more likely to open up when the interview focuses on them rather than on their problems.

Consider the patient's cognitive and social development when deciding issues of privacy, parental involvement, and confidentiality. Explain to both teens and parents that the purpose of confidentiality is to improve health care, not keep secrets. Your goal is to help adolescents bring their concerns or questions to their parents. Never make confidentiality unlimited, however. Always state to teens explicitly that you may need to act on information that makes you concerned about safety.

HEEADSSS Assessment

Obtaining an adequate psychosocial history from an adolescent, offers you the ability to contextualize their lives. The HEEADSSS assessment is a good guide (Box 25-16). It is analogous to the "review of systems" and is a valuable tool for assessing the physical, emotional, and social well-being of adolescents.

BOX 25-16. HEEADSSS Assessment

Category	Sample Question Topics
Home environment	Who lives with you? How long have you lived there? Own room? What are relationships like at home? Recent moves or running away?
Education and employment	School/grade performance—any recent changes? Suspension, termination, dropping out? Favorite/least favorite class? Safety at school?
Eating	Likes and dislikes about one's body? Any recent changes in your weight or appetite? Any worries about weight? Worries about having food to eat?
Activities	With peers and family? Church, clubs, sports activities? Video games? History of arrests, acting out, crime?
Drugs and alcohol	Use of tobacco, alcohol, or drugs by peers, by teen, by family members?
Sexuality	Orientation? Dated anyone? Kissed anyone? Degree and types of sexual experience and acts? Number of partners? Sexually transmitted infections, contraception, pregnancy/abortion?
Suicide, depression, and self-harm	Have you thought about hurting yourself or someone else? Have you lost interest in things that you used to really enjoy?
Safety from injury and violence	History of accidents, physical or sexual abuse, or bullying? Violence in home, school, or neighborhood? Access to firearms? Seatbelt use? Ridden with someone who was drunk or high? Any violence in school? Where you live? Ever been picked on or bullied? Ever felt the need to protect yourself?

Sources: American Academy of Pediatrics. *Bright Futures tool and resource kit.* Author; 2010; Smith GL, McGuinness TM. Adolescent Psychosocial Assessment: The HEEADSSS. *J Psychosoc Nurs Ment Health Serv.* 2017;55(5):24–27.

Surveillance of Development: 11 to 20 Years

Adolescence can be divided into three stages: early, middle, and late (Box 25-17).

BOX 25-17. Developmental Tasks of Adolescence

Task	Characteristic	Health Care Approaches
Early Adolescence (10- to 14-year-olds)		
Physical	Puberty (F: 10–14 y; M: 11–16 y)	Confidentiality; privacy
Cognitive	Concrete operational	Emphasis on short-term
Social identity	Am I normal? Peers increasingly important	Reassurance and positive attitude
Independence	Ambivalence (family, self, peers)	Support for growing autonomy
Middle Adolescence (15- to 16-year-olds)		
Physical	Females more comfortable, males awkward	Support if patient varies from normal
Cognitive	Transition; many ideas, often highly emotional thinker	Problem solving; decision making, increased responsibility
Social identity	Who am I? Much introspection; global issues, sexuality	Nonjudgmental acceptance
Independence	Limit testing; experimental behaviors; dating	Consistency; limit setting
Late Adolescence (17- to 20-year-olds)		
Physical	Adult appearance	Minimal unless chronic illness
Cognitive	Formal operational (for many but not all)	Approach as an adult
Social identity	Role with respect to others; sexuality; future	Encouragement of identity to allow growth; safety and healthy decision-making
Independence	Separation from family; toward real independence	Support, anticipatory guidance

Gender and Sexual Identity Formation Among Adolescents

In 2017, the Centers for Disease Control and Prevention (CDC)'s National Youth Risk Behavior Survey found that of 118,803 high school students, 2.4% of youth identified as gay/lesbian, 8% as bisexual, and 4.2% were not sure of their sexual orientation. It also found that 1.8% of youth identified as transgender. It is important to understand that being lesbian, gay, bisexual, transgender, and queer (LGBTQ) is not abnormal and is not inherently a risk factor for high-risk behaviors or adverse health outcomes.

Discussing sexuality and gender may be difficult for adolescents and young adults, and many struggle with their sexual attractions and identity formation. Research shows LGBTQ youth value the opportunity to discuss their gender and sexuality with their clinician, but they often delay disclosing their sexuality until the clinician has built a trusting relationship with them.

When initiating this conversation, the clinician should emphasize and practice confidentiality to allow for a more open discussion. It is not the role of the clinician to inform parents or guardians about a teenager's sexual or gender identity, as doing so could expose the youth to harm. Ostracism, bullying, and parental rejection remain common and can lead to physical and emotional abuse and the possibility of homelessness.

TECHNIQUES OF EXAMINATION

The physical examination of the adolescent is similar to that of the adult. Keep in mind issues particularly relevant to teens, such as puberty, growth, development, family and peer relationships, sexuality, decision making, and risk behaviors. For more details on specific techniques of examination, the reader should refer to the corresponding chapter for the regional examination of interest or concern. Following are special areas to highlight when examining adolescents. Please check with your institution about a chaperone policy. In many settings, chaperones are recommended during the examination of school-aged children and adolescents (irrespective of the gender of the examiner) when examining the genitalia of either boys or girls and the breasts of girls.

Breasts

Assess normal maturational development.

See Table 25-6, Sex Maturity Ratings in Girls: Breasts, p. 496.

Male and Female Genitalia

An important goal when examining adolescent males and females is to assign a sexual maturity rating, regardless of chronologic age.

See Table 25-7, Sex Maturity Ratings in Boys, p. 497, and Table 25-8, Sex Maturity Ratings in Girls: Pubic Hair, p. 498.

Musculoskeletal System

Assessing for Scoliosis. Inspect any child who can stand for *scoliosis*. Make sure the child bends forward with the knees straight (*Adams bend test*). Evaluate any asymmetry in positioning or gait. If you detect scoliosis, use a *scoliometer* to test for the degree of scoliosis (Fig. 25-16).

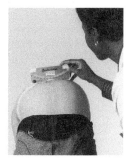

FIGURE 25-16. Measure and record scoliosis with a scoliometer.

Sports Preparticipation Physical Evaluation. Millions of children and adolescents participate in organized sports and often require "medical clearance." Start the evaluation with a thorough medical history focusing on cardiovascular risk factors, prior surgeries, prior injuries, other medical problems, and a family history. A 2-minute preparticipation screening musculoskeletal examination shown in Table 25-9, Screening Musculoskeletal Examination for Sports, p. 499, has been recommended by some experts.

RECORDING YOUR FINDINGS

The format of the pediatric medical record is the same as that of the adult. Thus, although the sequence of the physical examination may vary, convert your written findings back to the traditional format.

Recording the Pediatric Encounter

4/19/2020

Eli is an active, 26-month-old boy accompanied by his father, Matthew Nolan, who is concerned about his development and behavior.

Source and Reliability. Father (Dad), reliable.

Chief Complaint: Slow development and difficult behavior.

History of Present Illness: Eli appears to be developing more slowly than his older sister did. He uses only single words and simple phrases,

continued

rarely combines words, and appears frustrated with not being able to communicate. People understand less than one quarter of his speech. Physical development seems normal to the mother: he can throw a ball, kick, scribble, and dress himself well. He has had no head trauma, chronic illnesses, seizures, or regression in his milestones.

Eli's dad is also concerned about his behavior. Eli is extremely stubborn, frequently has tantrums, gets angry easily (especially with his older sister), throws objects, bites, and physically strikes others when he doesn't get his way. His behavior seems worse around his father who reports that he is "fine" at his childcare center. He moves from one activity to another with an inability to sit still to read or play a game. Of note, he is sometimes affectionate and cuddly. He does make eye contact and plays normally with toys. He has no unusual movements.

Eli is an extremely picky eater who eats a large quantity of junk food and little else. He will not eat fruits or vegetables and drinks enormous quantities of juice and soda. His father has tried everything to get him to eat healthy food, to no avail.

The family has been under substantial stress during the past year because Eli's father has been unemployed. Although Eli now has Medicaid insurance, the parents are uninsured.

Eli sleeps through the night.

Medications. One multivitamin daily.

Past History
Pregnancy. Uneventful. Dad reduced tobacco intake to a half-pack a day and drank alcohol at times. He denies use of other drugs or any infections.

Newborn Period. Born vaginally at 40 weeks; left the hospital in 2 days. Birth weight 2.5 kg (5 lb, 8 oz). Dad does not know why Eli was small at birth.

Illnesses. Only minor illnesses; no hospitalizations.

Accidents. Required sutures last year for a facial laceration secondary to a fall on the road. He did not lose consciousness and had no sequelae.

Preventive Care. Eli has had regular preventive check-ups. At the last appointment 6 months ago, his regular physician said that Eli was a bit behind on some developmental milestones and suggested a childcare center that she knew was excellent, as well as increased parental attention to reading, speaking, playing, and stimulation. Immunizations are up to date. His lead level was elevated mildly last year and Dad reports that he had "low blood." His physician recommended iron supplements and foods high in iron, but Eli really won't eat these foods.

Family History

Strong family history of diabetes (two grandparents, none with diabetes as children) and hypertension. No family history of childhood developmental, psychiatric, or chronic illnesses.

Developmental History: Sat up at 6 months, crawled at 9 months, and walked at 13 months. First words ("mama" and "car") said at approximately 1 year.

Personal and Social History: Parents are married and live with the two children in a rented apartment. Dad has not had a steady job for 1 year but has worked intermittently in a gym. Mom, Wesley Nolan, works as a waitress part-time while Eli is in childcare.

Mom had depression during Eli's first year and attended some counseling sessions but stopped because she could not pay for them or medications. She gets support from her mother who lives 30 minutes away, and many friends, some of whom babysit occasionally.

Despite substantial family stress, Dad describes a loving and intact family. They try to eat dinner together daily, limit television, read to both children (although Eli won't sit still), and go to the nearby park regularly to play.

Environmental Exposures. Both parents smoke, although generally outside the house.

Safety. Dad reports this as a major concern: he can barely leave Eli out of his sight without him getting into something. He fears he will run under a car; the family is thinking of fencing in their small yard. Eli sits in his car seat most of the time; smoke detectors work in the home. Dad's guns are locked; medications are in a cabinet in the parents' bedroom.

Review of Systems

General. No major illnesses.

Skin. Dry and itchy. Last year he was prescribed hydrocortisone for it.

Head, Eyes, Ears, Nose, and Throat (HEENT). Head: No trauma. *Eyes:* Vision fine. *Ears:* Multiple infections in the past year. Frequently ignores parents' requests; they can't tell if this is purposeful or if he can't hear well. *Nose:* Often runny; Dad wonders about allergies. *Mouth:* No dentist visit yet. Brushes teeth sometimes (a frequent source of dispute).

continued

Neck. No lumps. Glands in neck seem large.

Respiratory. Frequent cough and whistle in chest. Dad cannot identify trigger; it tends to go away. He can run around all day without seeming to get tired.

Cardiovascular. No known heart disease. He had a murmur when younger, but it went away.

Gastrointestinal. Appetite and eating habits described above. Regular bowel movements. He is in the process of toilet training and wears pull-ups at night, but not at childcare.

Urinary. Good stream. No prior urinary tract infections.

Genital. Normal.

Musculoskeletal. He is "all boy" and never gets tired. Minor bumps and bruises occasionally.

Neurologic. Walks and runs well; seems coordinated for age. No stiffness, seizures, or fainting. Dad says his memory seems great, but his attention span is poor.

Psychiatric. Generally, seems happy. Cries easily; bounces back and forth from trying to be independent to needing cuddling and comforting.

Physical Examination

General Appearance: Eli is an active and energetic toddler. He plays with the reflex hammer, pretending it is a truck. He appears closely bonded with his father, looking at him occasionally for comfort. He seems concerned that Eli will break something. His clothes are clean.

Vital Signs. Ht 90 cm (90th percentile). Wt 16 kg (>95th percentile). BMI 19.8 (>95th percentile). Head circumference 50 cm (75th percentile). BP 108/58. Heart rate 90 beats per minute and regular. Respiratory rate 30/min; varies with activity. Temperature (ear) 37.5°C. Obviously no pain.

Skin. Normal except for bruises on the anterior aspects of his legs, and patchy, dry skin over external surface of elbows.

HEENT. Head: Normocephalic; no lesions. *Eyes:* Difficult to examine because he won't sit still. Symmetric with normal extraocular movements. Pupils 4 to 5 mm, and symmetrically reactive to light. Discs difficult to visualize; no hemorrhages noted. *Ears:* Normal pinna; no external abnormalities. Normal external canals and tympanic membranes (TMs). *Nose:* Normal nares; septum midline. *Mouth:* Several darkened teeth (inside surface of upper incisors). One clear cavity on upper right incisor. Tongue normal. Cobblestoning of posterior pharynx; no exudates. Tonsils large but adequate gap (1.5 cm) between them. No allergic shiners.

Neck. Supple, midline trachea, no thyroid palpable.

Lymph Nodes. Easily palpable (1.5 to 2 cm), firm, mobile anterior cervical lymph nodes bilaterally. Small (0.5 cm) nodes in inguinal canal bilaterally. All lymph nodes mobile and nontender.

Lungs. Good expansion. No tachypnea or dyspnea. Congestion audible but seems to be upper airway (louder near mouth, symmetric). No rhonchi, rales, or wheezes. Clear to auscultation.

Cardiovascular. PMI in 4th or 5th interspace and midsternal line. Normal S_1 and S_2. No murmurs or abnormal heart sounds. Normal femoral pulses; dorsalis pedis pulses palpable bilaterally. Capillary refill brisk.

Breasts. Normal, with some fat under both.

Abdomen. Protuberant but soft; no masses or tenderness. Liver span 2 cm below right costal margin (RCM) and not tender. Spleen and kidneys not palpable. Bowel sounds present.

Genitalia. Tanner I circumcised penis; no pubic hair, lesions, or discharge. Testes descended, difficult to palpate because of active cremasteric reflex. Normal scrotum both sides.

Musculoskeletal. Normal range of motion of upper and lower extremities and all joints. Spine straight. Gait normal.

Neurologic. Mental Status: Happy, cooperative, active child. *Developmental:* Gross motor—Jumps and throws objects. Fine motor—Imitates vertical line. Language—Does not combine words; single words only, three to four noted during examination. Personal–social—Washes face, brushes teeth, and puts on shirt. Overall—Normal, except for language, which appears delayed. *Cranial Nerves:* Intact, although several difficult to elicit. *Cerebellar:* Normal gait; good balance. *Deep tendon reflexes (DTRs):* Normal and symmetric throughout with downgoing toes. *Sensory:* Deferred.

HEALTH PROMOTION AND COUNSELING: EVIDENCE AND RECOMMENDATIONS

Key Principles of Health Promotion

Current concepts of health promotion include the detection and prevention of disease as well as active promotion of the well-being of children and their families spanning physical, cognitive, emotional, and social health (Box 25-18).

- Every interaction with a child and family is an opportunity for health promotion.
- Parents are the major agents of health promotion for children and your advice is implemented through them.
- Integrate explanations of your physical findings with health promotion.
- Childhood immunizations are a mainstay for health promotion and have been heralded as the most significant clinical achievement in public health worldwide.
- Age-specific screening procedures are performed at specific ages.
- Anticipatory guidance is a major component of the pediatric visit.

BOX 25-18. Key Components of Pediatric Health Promotion

1. Age-appropriate developmental achievement of the child
   - Physical (maturation, growth, puberty)
   - Motor (gross and fine motor skills)
   - Cognitive (developmental milestones, language, school performance)
   - Emotional (self-regulation, mood, self-efficacy, self-esteem, independence)
   - Social (social competence, self-responsibility, integration with family and community, peer interactions)
2. Health supervision visits
   - Periodic assessment of physical, developmental, socio-emotional, and oral health
   - More frequent visits for children with special health care needs
3. Integration of physical examination findings with health promotion
4. Immunizations
5. Screening procedures
6. Oral health

7. Anticipatory guidance
   - Healthy habits
   - Nutrition and healthy eating
   - Safety and prevention of injury
   - Physical activity
   - Sexual development and sexuality
   - Self-responsibility, efficacy, and healthy self-esteem
   - Family relationships (interactions, strengths, supports)
   - Positive parenting strategies
   - Reading aloud with the child
   - Emotional and mental health
   - Oral health
   - Recognition of illness
   - Sleep
   - Screen time
   - Prevention of risky behaviors
   - School and vocation
   - Peer relationships
   - Community interactions
8. Partnership among health care provider, child/adolescent, and family

For the most up-to-date Bright Futures recommendations for preventive health care, see https://www.aap.org/en-us/documents/periodicity_schedule.pdf. Each child and family is unique; therefore, such recommendations are designed for the care of children who are receiving competent parenting, have no manifestation of any important health problems, and are growing and developing in satisfactory fashion.

INTERPRETATION AIDS

TABLE 25-1. Newborn Classification

Weight Small for Gestational Age (SGA) = Birth weight <10th percentile on the intrauterine growth curve

Weight Appropriate for Gestational Age (AGA) = Birth weight within the 10th and 90th percentiles on the intrauterine growth curve

Weight Large for Gestational Age (LGA) = Birth weight >90th percentile on the intrauterine growth curve

Adapted from Sweet YA. Classification of the low-birth-weight infant. In: Klaus MH, et al., ed. *Care of the High-Risk Neonate*. 3rd ed. WB Saunders; 1986. Copyright © 1986 Elsevier. With permission.

TABLE 25-2. Causes of Sustained Hypertension in Children

Newborn	Middle Childhood
Renal artery disease (stenosis, thrombosis)	Primary hypertension
Congenital renal malformations	Renal parenchymal or arterial disease
Coarctation of the aorta	Coarctation of the aorta

Infancy and Early Childhood	Adolescence
Renal parenchymal or artery disease	Primary hypertension
Coarctation of the aorta	Renal parenchymal disease
	Drug induced

TABLE 25-3. Primitive Reflexes

Primitive Reflex		Maneuver	Ages
Palmar Grasp Reflex		Place your fingers into the infant's hands and press against the palmar surfaces. The infant will flex all fingers to grasp your fingers.	Birth to 3–4 mo
Plantar Grasp Reflex	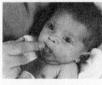	Touch the sole at the base of the toes. The toes will curl.	Birth to 6–8 mo
Rooting Reflex		Stroke the perioral skin at the corners of the mouth. The mouth will open and the infant will turn the head toward the stimulated side and suck.	Birth to 3–4 mo

continued

	TABLE 25-3. Primitive Reflexes *(continued)*		
Primitive Reflex		**Maneuver**	**Ages**
Moro Reflex (Startle Reflex)		Hold the infant supine, supporting the head, back, and legs. Abruptly lower the entire body about 1 foot. The arms will abduct and extend, hands will open, and legs will flex. The infant may cry.	Birth to 4 mo
Asymmetric Tonic Neck Reflex		With the infant supine, turn head to one side, holding jaw over shoulder. The arms/legs on side to which head is turned will extend while the opposite arm/leg will flex. Repeat on other side.	Birth to 2–3 mo

TABLE 25-3. Primitive Reflexes *(continued)*

Primitive Reflex		Maneuver	Ages
Trunk Incurvation (Galant) Reflex		Support the infant prone with one hand and stroke one side of the back 1 cm from midline, from shoulder to buttocks. The spine will curve toward the stimulated side.	Birth to 3–4 mo
Landau Reflex		Suspend the infant prone with one hand. The head will lift up, and the spine will straighten.	Birth to 6 mo
Parachute Reflex		Suspend the infant prone and slowly lower the head toward a surface. The arms and legs will extend in a protective fashion.	8 mo and does not disappear

continued

	TABLE 25-3. **Primitive Reflexes** (continued)	

Primitive Reflex		Maneuver	Ages
Positive Support Reflex		Hold the infant around the trunk and lower until the feet touch a flat surface. The hips, knees, and ankles will extend, the infant will stand up, partially bearing weight, sagging after 20–30 sec.	Birth or 2 mo until 6 mo
Placing and Stepping Reflexes		Hold the infant upright as in positive support reflex. Have one sole touch the tabletop. The hip and knee of that foot will flex and the other foot will step forward. Alternate stepping will occur.	Birth (best after 4 days; variable age to disappear)

TABLE 25-4. Characteristics of Pathologic Heart Murmurs

Congenital Defect	Characteristics of Murmur
Pulmonary Valve Stenosis *Mild* 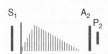 *Severe* 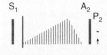	*Location.* Upper left sternal border *Radiation.* In mild degrees of stenosis, the murmur may be heard over the course of the pulmonary arteries in the lung fields. *Intensity.* Increases in intensity and duration as the degree of obstruction increases *Quality.* Ejection, peaking later in systole as the obstruction increases
Aortic Valve Stenosis 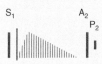	*Location.* Midsternum, upper right sternal border *Radiation.* To the carotid arteries and suprasternal notch; may also be a thrill *Intensity.* Varies, louder with increasingly severe obstruction *Quality.* An ejection, often harsh, systolic murmur

continued

TABLE 25-4. Characteristics of Pathologic Heart Murmurs *(continued)*

Congenital Defect	Characteristics of Murmur
Tetralogy of Fallot *With Pulmonic Stenosis* 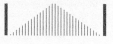 *With Pulmonic Atresia* 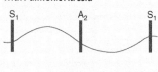	*General.* Variable cyanosis, increasing with activity *Location.* Mid to upper left sternal border. If pulmonary atresia, there is no systolic murmur but the continuous murmur of ductus arteriosus flow at upper left sternal border or in the back. *Radiation.* Little, to upper left sternal border, occasionally to lung fields *Intensity.* Usually grade III–IV *Quality.* Midpeaking, systolic ejection murmur
Transposition of the Great Arteries	*General.* Intense generalized cyanosis *Location.* No characteristic murmur. If present, it may reflect an associated defect such as VSD. *Radiation and quality.* Depends on associated abnormalities
Ventricular Septal Defect *Small to Moderate* 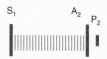	*Location.* Lower left sternal border *Radiation.* Little *Intensity.* Variable, only partially determined by the size of the shunt. Small shunts with a high-pressure gradient may have very loud murmurs. Large defects with elevated pulmonary vascular resistance may have no murmur. Grade II–IV/VI, with a thrill if grade IV/VI or higher.

TABLE 25-5. Physical Signs of Sexual Abuse

Physical Signs That May Indicate Sexual Abuse in Children[a]

- Marked and immediate dilatation of the anus in knee–chest position, with no constipation, stool in the vault, or neurologic disorders
- Hymenal notch or cleft that extends >50% of the inferior hymenal rim (confirmed in knee–chest position)
- Condyloma acuminata in a child older than 3 years
- Bruising, abrasions, lacerations, or bite marks of labia or perihymenal tissue
- Herpes of the anogenital area beyond the neonatal period
- Purulent or malodorous vaginal discharge in a young girl (all discharges should be cultured and viewed under a microscope for evidence of a sexually transmitted infection)

Physical Signs That Strongly Suggest Sexual Abuse in Children[a]

- Lacerations, ecchymoses, and newly healed scars of the hymen or the posterior fourchette
- No hymenal tissue from 3 to 9 o'clock (confirmed in various positions)
- Healed hymenal transections, especially between 3 and 9 o'clock (complete cleft)
- Perianal lacerations extending to external sphincter

A sexual abuse expert must evaluate a child with concerning physical signs for a complete history and sexual abuse examination.

---

[a]Any physical sign must be evaluated in light of the entire history, other parts of the physical examination, and laboratory data.

TABLE 25-6. Sexual Maturity Ratings in Girls: Breasts (Tanner Stages)

Stage 1
Preadolescent—elevation of nipple only

Stage 2

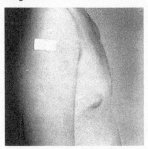

Breast bud stage. Elevation of breast and nipple as a small mound; enlargement of areolar diameter

Stage 3

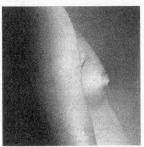

Further enlargement and elevation of breast and areola, with no separation of the contours

Stage 4

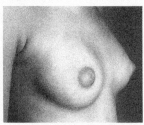

Projection of areola and nipple to form a secondary mound above the level of the breast

Stage 5

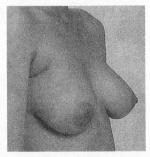

Mature stage; projection of nipple only. Areola has receded to general contour of the breast (although may continue to form a secondary mound).

TABLE 25-7. Sexual Maturity Ratings in Boys (Tanner Stages)

Stage 1: Pubic Hair: Preadolescent—no pubic hair except for the fine body hair (vellus hair) similar to that on the abdomen. **Genitalia: Penis, Testes, and Scrotum:** Preadolescent—same size and proportions as in childhood

Stage 2 	**Pubic Hair:** Sparse growth of long, slightly pigmented, downy hair, straight or only slightly curled, chiefly at the base of the penis **Genitalia** ■ **Penis:** Slight to no enlargement ■ **Testes and Scrotum:** Testes larger; scrotum larger, somewhat reddened, and altered in texture
Stage 3 	**Pubic Hair:** Darker, coarser, curlier hair spreading sparsely over the pubic symphysis **Genitalia** ■ **Penis:** Larger, especially in length ■ **Testes and Scrotum:** Further enlarged
Stage 4 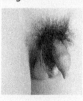	**Pubic Hair:** Coarse and curly hair, as in the adult; area covered greater than in stage 3 but less than adult and not yet on thighs **Genitalia** ■ **Penis:** Further enlarged in length and breadth, with development of the glans ■ **Testes and Scrotum:** Further enlarged; scrotal skin darkened
Stage 5 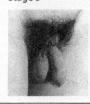	**Pubic Hair:** Hair adult quantity and quality, spread to the medial surfaces of the thighs but not up over the abdomen **Genitalia** ■ **Penis:** Adult in size and shape ■ **Testes and Scrotum:** Adult in size and shape

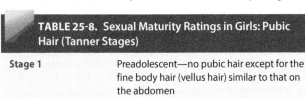

TABLE 25-8. Sexual Maturity Ratings in Girls: Pubic Hair (Tanner Stages)

Stage 1	Preadolescent—no pubic hair except for the fine body hair (vellus hair) similar to that on the abdomen

Stage 2 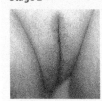	Sparse growth of long, slightly pigmented, downy hair, straight or only slightly curled, chiefly along the labia

Stage 3 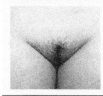	Darker, coarser, curlier hair, spreading sparsely over the pubic symphysis

Stage 4 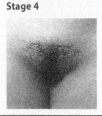	Coarse and curly hair as in adults; area covered greater than in stage 3 but not as great as in the adult and not yet including the thighs

Stage 5 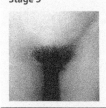	Hair adult in quantity and quality, spread on the medial surfaces of the thighs but not up over the abdomen

TABLE 25-9. Screening Musculoskeletal Examination for Sports

Position and Instruction to Patient

Step 1: Stand straight, facing forward. Note for any asymmetry or swelling of joints.

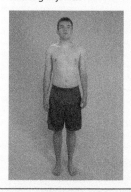

Step 2: Move neck in all directions. Note for any loss of range of motion

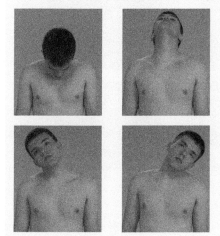

continued

TABLE 25-9. Screening Musculoskeletal Examination for Sports (continued)

Step 3: Shrug shoulders against resistance. Note for any weakness of shoulder, neck, or trapezius muscles.

Step 4: Hold arms out to the side against resistance, and actively raise arms over the head. Note for any loss of strength of deltoid muscle

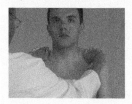

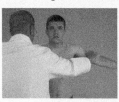

Step 5: Hold arms out to side with elbows bent 90 degrees; raise and lower arms. Note for any loss of external rotation and injury of glenohumeral joint.

Step 6: Hold arms out, completely bend, and straighten elbows (should be able to easily touch the shoulder). Note for any reduced range of motion of elbow.

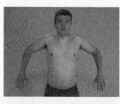

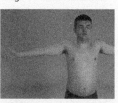

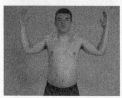

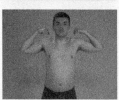

TABLE 25-9. Screening Musculoskeletal Examination for Sports *(continued)*

Step 7: Hold arms down, bend elbows 90 degrees, and pronate and supinate forearms. Note for any reduced range of motion from prior injury to forearm, elbow, or wrist

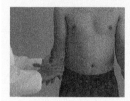

Step 8: Make a fist, clench, and then spread fingers. Note for protruding knuckle, reduced range of motion of fingers from prior sprain or fracture.

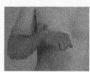

Step 9: Squat and duck-walk for four steps forward. Note for inability to fully flex knees and difficulty standing up from prior knee or ankle injury

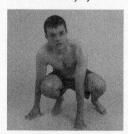

Step 10: Stand straight with arms at sides, facing back. Check whether shoulders, scapula and hips are even. Note for asymmetry from scoliosis, leg-length discrepancy, or weakness from prior injury

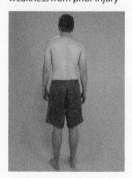

continued

TABLE 25-9. Screening Musculoskeletal Examination for Sports *(continued)*

Step 11: Bend forward with knees straight and touch toes. Note any asymmetry from scoliosis and twisting of back from low back pain

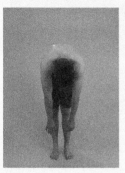

Step 12: Stand on heels and rise to the toes. Note any wasting of calf muscles from prior ankle or Achilles tendon injury

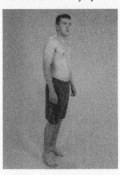

Pregnant Woman

CHANGES DURING PREGNANCY

Multiple physiologic changes occur in the setting of normal pregnancy, many mediated by endocrinologic and hormonal changes (Figs. 26-1 to 26-3). These complex, albeit normal, hormonal variations of pregnancy result in visible changes in anatomy.

See Table 26-1, Physiologic Changes in Normal Pregnancy, pp. 529–532.

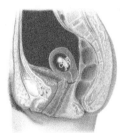

FIGURE 26-1. Sagittal depiction of the gravid abdomen during first trimester (1–12 weeks).

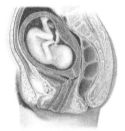

FIGURE 26-2. Sagittal depiction of the gravid abdomen during second trimester (13–26 weeks).

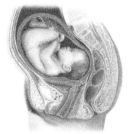

FIGURE 26-3. Sagittal depiction of the gravid abdomen during third trimester (27–40 weeks).

HEALTH HISTORY

Approach to the Initial Prenatal Visit

- Confirmation of pregnancy
- Determining gestational age and expected date of delivery
- Symptoms of pregnancy
- Concerns and attitudes toward the pregnancy
- Current health and past clinical history
- Past obstetric history
- Risk factors for maternal and fetal health
- Family history of patient and father of the newborn
- Plans for genetic screening and aneuploidy testing
- Plans for breastfeeding
- Plans for postpartum contraception

Focus the *initial prenatal visit* on the health status of the mother and fetus. Confirm the pregnancy and estimate gestational age, develop a plan for continuing care, and counsel the mother about her expectations and concerns. At the end of the visit, reaffirm your commitment to the patient's health and any ongoing concerns, review your findings, and discuss any questions or tests or screenings that are needed.

Confirmation of Pregnancy

Has the patient had a confirmatory urine pregnancy test, and when? When was her last menstrual period (LMP)? Has an ultrasound been done to establish dates? Explain that serum pregnancy tests are rarely required to confirm pregnancy.

Gestational Age and Expected Date of Delivery

Accurate dating is best done early and contributes to appropriate management of the pregnancy (Box 26-1). Dating establishes the timeframe for reassuring the patient about normal progress, establishing paternity, timing screening tests, tracking fetal growth, and effectively triaging preterm and postdated labor.

BOX 26-1. Determining Gestational Age and the Expected Date of Delivery

- ■ *Gestational age.* To establish gestational age, count the number of weeks and days from the first day of the LMP. If the actual date of conception is known (as with in vitro fertilization), a conception age which is 2 weeks less than the menstrual age can be used to calculate *menstrual age* (i.e., a corrected or adjusted LMP dating) to establish dating. *Counting this menstrual age from the LMP, although biologically distinct from date of conception, is the standard means of calculating fetal age, yielding an average pregnancy length of 40 weeks.*
- ■ *Expected date of delivery (EDD).* The EDD is 40 weeks from the first date of the LMP. Using the *Naegele rule*, the EDD can be estimated by taking the LMP, adding 7 days, subtracting 3 months, and adding 1 year. For example:
  - ■ LMP = November 26, 2020
  - ■ +7 days = November 2, 2020
  - ■ −3 months = September 2, 2020
  - ■ +1 year = September 2, 2021 = EDD
- ■ *Tools for calculations.* Pregnancy wheels and online calculators are commonly used to calculate the EDD, but they should be checked for accuracy.
- ■ *Limitations on pregnancy dating.* Patient recall of the LMP is highly variable. The LMP can also be biased by hormonal contraceptives, menstrual irregularities, or variations in ovulation that result in atypical cycle lengths. Check LMP dating against physical examination markers such as fundal height, clarifying discrepancies against ultrasound evaluation.

Symptoms of Pregnancy

Has the patient had absence of menses, breast fullness or tenderness, nausea or vomiting, fatigue, or urinary frequency? See Box 26-2.

BOX 26-2. Common Concerns During Pregnancy and Their Explanations

Common Concerns	Trimester	Explanation	
Abdominal pain (lower)	Second	Rapid growth in the second trimester causes tension and stretching of round ligaments that support uterus, causing sharp or cramping pain with movement or position change	See Algorithm 26-1, Approach to the pregnant patient with abdominal pain, p. 526.
Abdominal striae	Second or third	Stretching of skin and tearing of collagen in dermis contribute to thin, usually pink, bands, or *striae gravidarum* (stretch marks). These may persist or fade over time after delivery.	
Amenorrhea (missed periods)	All	High levels of estrogen, progesterone, and hCG build up endometrium and prevent menses, causing a missed period, which is often the first noticeable sign of pregnancy.	
Backache	All	Hormonally induced relaxation of the pelvic ligaments contributes to musculoskeletal aches. Lordosis required to balance the gravid uterus contributes to lower back strain. Breast enlargement may contribute to upper backaches.	
Breast tenderness/ tingling	First	Pregnancy hormones stimulate growth of breast tissue, which causes swelling and possible aching, tenderness, and tingling. Increased blood flow can make delicate veins more visible beneath the skin.	
Constipation	All	Constipation results from slowed gastrointestinal transit due to hormonal changes, dehydration from nausea and vomiting, and supplemental iron in prenatal vitamins.	
Contractions	Third	Irregular and unpredictable uterine contractions (*Braxton Hicks* contractions) are rarely associated with labor. Contractions that become regular or painful should be evaluated for onset of labor.	

Common Concerns	Trimester	Explanation
Edema	Third	Decreased venous return, obstruction of lymphatic flow, and reduced plasma colloid oncotic pressure commonly cause lower extremity edema. However, sudden severe edema and hypertension may signal preeclampsia.
Fatigue	First/Third	Fatigue is related to the rapid change in energy requirements, sedative effects of progesterone, changes in body mechanics due to the gravid uterus, and sleep disturbance.
Heartburn	All	Progesterone relaxes lower esophageal sphincter, allowing gastric contents to reflux into the esophagus. The gravid uterus also exerts physical pressure against the stomach with increasing gestational age.
Hemorrhoids	All	Hemorrhoids may be caused by constipation, decreased venous return from increasing pressure in the pelvis, compression by fetal parts, and changes in activity level during pregnancy.
Loss of mucus plug	Third	Passage of mucus plug is common during labor but may occur prior to the onset of contractions. As long as there are no regular contractions, bleeding, or loss of fluid, loss of the mucus plug is unlikely to trigger the onset of labor.
Nausea and/or vomiting	First	Appears to reflect hormonal changes, slowed gastrointestinal peristalsis, alterations in smell and taste, and sociocultural factors. Up to 75% of women experience nausea in pregnancy. *Hyperemesis gravidarum* is vomiting with weight loss of >5% of prepregnancy weight.
Urinary frequency	All	Increases in blood volume and filtration rate through the kidneys result in increased urine production, while pressure from the gravid uterus reduces potential space for the bladder.
Vaginal discharge	All	Asymptomatic milky white discharge, *leukorrhea*, results from increased secretions from vaginal and cervical epithelium due to vasocongestion and hormonal changes.

Maternal Concerns and Attitudes

Review the mother's feelings about the pregnancy and whether she plans to continue to term. Ask about any fears and about support from the father. Respect diverse family structures, such as extended family support, single motherhood, or pregnancy conceived by sperm donation with or without a partner of either gender.

Current Health and Past Clinical History

Does the patient have any acute or chronic medical concerns, past or present? Pay particular attention to issues that affect pregnancy, such as abdominal surgeries, hypertension, diabetes, cardiac conditions including any that were surgically corrected in childhood, asthma, hypercoagulability states involving lupus or anticardiolipin antibodies, mental health disorders including postpartum depression, HIV, sexually transmitted infections, abnormal Pap smears.

Past Obstetric History

Ask about prior pregnancies and outcomes (Box 26-3). Has she had any complications during past pregnancies? Were there any complications during labor and delivery such as large babies (*fetal macrosomia*), fetal distress, or emergency interventions? Were deliveries by vaginal delivery, assisted delivery (vacuum or forceps), or cesarean section?

BOX 26-3. Nomenclature for Pregnancy Outcomes

This is often part of any oral or written communication related to a woman's reproductive history.

- *Gravidity* refers to the number of times that a woman has been pregnant.
- *Parity* is the number of times that she has given birth to a fetus to a viable age (≥24 gestational weeks), regardless of whether the child was born alive or was stillborn.
- For example:
  - A woman who is described as "gravida 2, para 2" (G2P2) has had two pregnancies and two deliveries after 24 weeks.
  - A woman who is described as "gravida 2, para 0" (G2P0) has had two pregnancies, neither of which survived to a gestational age of 24 weeks.
- Parity is further broken down into *term deliveries, preterm deliveries, abortions* (spontaneous abortions and terminated

pregnancies), and *living children,* which yields the mnemonic "TPAL" when listed in that order.

- ■ A woman with two spontaneous losses prior to 20 weeks' gestation, three living children who were delivered at term, and a current pregnancy, would be referred to as "G6P3023."
- ■ In practice, each pregnancy receives only one count in any of the categories regardless of the number of fetuses, except for *living children,* when all are counted.
- ■ One common error is to assign a multiple pregnancy, for example, twins, as a count of two for either gravity or parity. So, for a first pregnancy with twins delivered at term, the correct designation is G1P1002.

Risk Factors for Maternal and Fetal Health

Does the patient use tobacco, alcohol, or illicit drugs? Does she take any medications, over-the-counter drugs, or herbal prescriptions? Does she have any toxic exposures at work, home, or otherwise? Is her nutritional intake adequate, or is she at risk from obesity? Does she have an adequate social support network and income? Is there unusual stress at home or work? Is there any history of physical abuse or domestic violence?

Family History

Any chronic illnesses or genetically transmitted diseases: sickle cell anemia, cystic fibrosis, muscular dystrophy, and others.

Plans for Genetic Testing and Aneuploidy Screening

All pregnant patients should be offered both aneuploidy screening and diagnostic genetic testing to rule out trisomies 21, 18, and 13 and sex-chromosome abnormalities. Also, carrier screening for certain autosomal-recessive disorders Tay–Sachs disease, spinal muscular atrophy (SMA), cystic fibrosis (CF) and fragile X syndrome is recommended for targeted screening along with hemoglobin electrophoresis to test for hemoglobinopathies.

Plans for Breastfeeding

Education and encouragement during pregnancy increase adoption and duration of breastfeeding.

Plans for Postpartum Contraception

Initiate this discussion early, as postpartum contraception reduces the risk of unintended pregnancy and shortened interpregnancy intervals, which are linked to adverse pregnancy outcomes.

Subsequent Prenatal Visits

During subsequent visits, assess interim changes in the health status of the mother and fetus, review specific physical examination findings related to the pregnancy, and provide counseling and timely preventive screenings. Obstetric visits traditionally follow a set schedule:

- Monthly until 28 gestational weeks, then
- Biweekly until 36 weeks, then
- Weekly until delivery.

Update and document the history at every visit, especially fetal movement, contractions, leakage of fluids and vaginal bleeding. At every visit, assess vital signs (especially blood pressure and weight), fundal height, verification of fetal heart rate (FHR), and fetal position and activity. At each visit, test the urine for infection and protein.

See Algorithm 26-2, Approach to the Pregnant Woman with Vaginal Bleeding, p. 527.

TECHNIQUES OF EXAMINATION

Key Components of the Examination of the Pregnant Woman

- Assess general health, emotional state, nutritional status, and neuromuscular coordination
- Measure height and weight; calculate BMI
- Measure the blood pressure at every visit
- Inspect the head and neck
- Inspect, percuss, and auscultate the thorax and lungs
- Palpate location of the apical impulse
- Auscultate the heart
- Inspect the abdomen
- Palpate the abdomen (masses, fetal movement, uterine contractility and fundal height)
- Auscultate fetal heart tones
- Inspect the external genitalia
- Inspect the internal genitalia by performing speculum and bimanual examinations
    - Speculum examination: Inspect the cervix and vaginal walls; perform a Pap smear if indicated

- ■ Bimanual examination: Palpate the cervix, uterus, adnexa, pelvic floor strength
- ■ Inspect the anus
- ■ Examine the extremities and elicit reflexes
- ■ Perform Leopold maneuvers (if indicated)

Box 26-4 outlines how to prepare for the examination of the pregnant woman.

BOX 26-4. Preparing for the Examination

Be responsive to the patient's comfort and privacy, as well as her individual and cultural sensitivities. During the initial visit, take the history while she is clothed. Ask her to wear her gown with the opening in front to ease the examination of both breasts and the pregnant abdomen.

Positioning

- ■ The semi-sitting position with the knees bent (Fig. 26-4) affords the most comfort and protects abdominal organs and vessels from the weight of the gravid uterus.
- ■ Avoid prolonged periods of lying on the back. Make your abdominal palpation efficient and accurate.
- ■ The pelvic examination also should be relatively quick.

FIGURE 26-4. Semi-sitting position of the pregnant person for examination.

Equipment

- ■ *Gynecologic speculum and lubrication:* Because of vaginal wall relaxation during pregnancy, a larger-than-usual speculum may be needed.
- ■ *Sampling materials:* The cervical brush may cause bleeding, so the "broom" sampling device is preferred during pregnancy. Use additional swabs if needed to screen for sexually transmitted infections, group B strep, and wet mount preparations.
- ■ *Tape measure:* Use a plastic or paper tape measure to assess the size of the uterus after 20 gestational weeks.
- ■ *Doppler fetal heart rate monitor and gel:* Apply a Doppler externally to the gravid abdomen to assess fetal heart rate after 10 weeks of gestation.

General Inspection

Observe the general health, emotional state, nutritional status, and coordination as the pregnant woman comes into the room.

Height, Weight, and Vital Signs

Measure height and weight. Calculate the BMI with standard tables, using 19 to 25 as normal for the prepregnant state.

Weight loss of more than 5% in excessive vomiting, or *hyperemesis*

Measure blood pressure at every visit. In mid-pregnancy, it may be lower than in the nonpregnant state (Box 26-5).

BOX 26-5. Hypertension in Pregnancy

- *Gestational hypertension:* Systolic blood pressure (SBP) >140 mm Hg or diastolic blood pressure (DBP) >90 mm Hg first documented after 20 weeks, without proteinuria or other evidence of preeclampsia, that resolves by 12 weeks postpartum.
- *Chronic hypertension:* SBP >140 mm Hg or DBP >90 mm Hg that predates pregnancy or is diagnosed in the first 20 weeks of gestation.
- *Preeclampsia:*
  - SBP ≥140 mm Hg or DBP ≥90 mm Hg after 20 weeks on two occasions at least 4 hours apart in a woman with previously normal BP or BP ≥160/110 mm Hg confirmed within minutes *and* proteinuria ≥300 mg/24 hrs, protein:creatinine ≥0.3, or dipstick 1+;

    OR
  - New onset hypertension without proteinuria and any of the following: thrombocytopenia (platelets <100,000/μL), impaired liver function (liver transaminase levels more than twice normal), new renal insufficiency (creatinine >1.1 mg/dL or doubles in the absence of renal disease), pulmonary edema, or new onset cerebral or visual symptoms.

Head and Neck

- *Face.* Inspect for the mask of pregnancy, *melasma*, or irregular brownish patches around the forehead and cheeks, across the bridge of the nose, or along the jaw.

Facial edema after 20 weeks in possible preeclampsia

- *Hair.* Hair may become dry, oily, or sparse during pregnancy

Hair loss should not be attributed to pregnancy.

- *Eyes.* Note the conjunctival color.

Anemia of pregnancy may cause conjunctival pallor.

- *Nose,* including nasal congestion

Nosebleeds are more common during pregnancy. Erosion of nasal septum if use of intranasal cocaine.

- *Mouth.* Examine teeth and gums.

Gingival enlargement common

- *Thyroid gland.* Inspect and palpate. Modest symmetric enlargement is common.

Thyroid enlargement, goiters, and nodules are abnormal and should be investigated.

Thorax and Lungs

Inspect the thorax for contours. Observe the pattern of breathing. Auscultate the lungs.

Respiratory alkalosis in later trimesters. Increased respiratory rate, cough, rales, or respiratory distress in infection, asthma, pulmonary embolus, peripartum cardiomyopathy.

Heart

Palpate the apical impulse.

Impulse may be rotated upward and to the left toward the fourth intercostal space by the enlarging uterus.

Auscultate the heart. A venous hum and systolic or continuous *mammary souffle* ("a puff of air," pronounced SOO-*fuhl*) are common.

Murmurs may signal anemia; new diastolic murmurs should be investigated. If signs of heart failure, consider peripartum cardiomyopathy.

Breasts

Inspect the breasts and nipples for symmetry and color. Venous pattern, darkened nipples and areolae, and prominent Montgomery glands are normal.

Inverted nipples at the time of birth may hamper breastfeeding.

Palpate for masses. Tender nodular breasts are normal.

Focal tenderness in mastitis. Investigate any new discrete masses.

Compress each nipple between your index finger and thumb.

This may express colostrum from the nipples; investigate if abnormal bloody or purulent discharge.

Abdomen

Place the pregnant woman in a semi-sitting position with her knees flexed.

- Inspect any scars or striae, the shape and contour of the abdomen, and the fundal height.

Purplish striae and linea nigra are normal.

- Assess the shape and contour to estimate pregnancy size

Growth patterns of the gravid uterus, demonstrating the correlation between gestational age and measurable fundal height (Fig. 26-5).

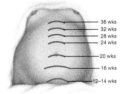

FIGURE 26-5. Uterine fundal height by weeks of pregnancy.

- Palpate for:

  - Organs and masses

  - Fetal movements, usually detected after 24 weeks. The mother can usually feel these movements by 18 to 24 weeks and known as *quickening.*

  Ultrasound confirmation of fetal health and movement may be needed.

  - Uterine contractility

  - Irregular contractions after 12 weeks or after palpation during the third trimester

  Prior to 37 weeks, regular uterine contractions or bleeding are abnormal, suggesting *preterm labor.*

  - If the woman is >20 weeks pregnant, measure *fundal height* with a tape measure from the top of the symphysis pubis to the top of the uterine fundus. After 20 weeks, measurement in centimeters should roughly equal the weeks of gestation.

  If fundal height is more than 4 cm higher than expected, consider multiple gestation, a large fetus, extra amniotic fluid, or uterine leiomyoma. If more than 4 cm lower, consider low level of amniotic fluid, missed abortion, transverse lie, growth retardation, or fetal anomaly.

- Auscultate fetal heart tones, noting FHR, location, and rhythm. A Doppler detects the FHR after 10 weeks. The FHR is audible with a fetoscope after 18 weeks.

  Lack of an audible FHR may indicate pregnancy of fewer weeks than expected, fetal demise, or false pregnancy. If unable to locate the FHR, investigate with formal ultrasound.

  - *Location.* From 10 to 18 weeks, the FHR is in the midline of the lower abdomen; later depends on fetal position. Use modified Leopold's maneuvers to palpate the fetal head and back and identify where to listen.

  - *Rate.* The rate usually is 120 to 160 beats per minute. After 32 to 34 weeks, the FHR should increase with fetal movement.

    Sustained dips in FHR, or "*decelerations*," always warrant investigation, at least by formal FHR monitoring.

  - *Rhythm.* In the third trimester, expect a variance of 10 to 15 beats per minute (BPM) over 1 to 2 minutes.

    Lack of beat-to-beat variability late in pregnancy warrants investigation with an FHR monitor.

Genitalia, Anus, and Rectum

Inspect the external genitalia.

Parous relaxation of the introitus, labial varicosities, enlargement of the labia and clitoris, scars from an episiotomy or perineal lacerations

Palpate Bartholin and Skene glands. Check for a cystocele or rectocele.

Bartholin cyst

Examine the internal genitalia.

Speculum Examination

- Inspect the cervix for color, shape, and healed lacerations.

  Purplish color of pregnancy; lacerations from prior deliveries, cervical erosion, erythema, discharge, or irritation in cervicitis and STIs

- Perform a Pap smear, if indicated.

  Specimens may be needed for diagnosis of vaginal or cervical infection

■ Inspect the vaginal walls.

Bluish or violet color, deep rugae, leukorrhea in normal pregnancy; vaginal discharge in candidiasis and bacterial vaginosis (can affect pregnancy outcome); see Algorithm 26-3, Approach to the pregnant woman with vaginal discharge, p. 528.

Bimanual Examination. Insert two lubricated fingers into introitus, palmar side down, with slight pressure downward on the perineum. Slide the fingers into the posterior vaginal vault. Maintaining downward pressure, gently turn the fingers palmar side up.

■ Assess the cervical os and degree of shortening (*effacement*). Place your finger gently in the os, and then sweep it around the surface of the cervix.

Closed external os if nulliparous; os open to size of fingertip if multiparous

■ Estimate the length of the cervix. Palpate the lateral surface from the cervical tip to the lateral fornix.

Prior to 34 to 36 weeks, cervix should retain normal length of ≥3 cm. Effacement prior to 37 weeks in preterm labor.

■ Palpate the uterus for size, shape, consistency, and position.

Hegar sign, or early softening of the isthmus; pear-shaped uterus up to 8 weeks, then globular

■ Estimate uterine size. With your internal fingers placed at either side of cervix, palmar surfaces upward, gently lift the uterus toward the abdominal hand. Capture the fundal portion of the uterus between your two hands and gently estimate size.

An irregularly shaped uterus suggests uterine myomata or a bicornuate uterus, two distinct uterine cavities separated by a septum.

■ Palpate the left and right adnexa.

Early in pregnancy, it is important to rule out tubal (*ectopic*) pregnancy.

■ Evaluate pelvic floor strength as you withdraw the examining fingers.

■ Inspect the *anus*. Rectal and rectovaginal examinations are usually not indicated.

Hemorrhoids may engorge later in pregnancy.

Extremities

Inspect the legs for varicose veins.

Varicose veins may worsen during pregnancy.

Palpate the hands and legs for edema.

Watch for swelling of preeclampsia or deep venous thrombosis.

Check knee and ankle deep tendon reflexes.

Hyperreflexia may signal preeclampsia.

Special Techniques

Leopold Maneuvers. Identify:

- Upper and lower fetal poles, namely, the proximal and distal fetal parts

- Maternal side where the fetal back is located

- Descent of the presenting part into the maternal pelvis

- Extent of flexion of the fetal head

- Estimated fetal weight and size

Common deviations include *breech presentation* (fetal buttocks present at the outlet of the maternal pelvis) and absence of the presenting part well down into the maternal pelvis at term.

First Maneuver (Upper Fetal Pole). Stand at the woman's side, facing her head. Keep the fingers of both examining hands together. Palpate gently with the fingertips to determine what part of the fetus is in the upper pole of the uterine fundus (Fig. 26-6).

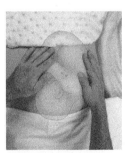

FIGURE 26-6. First Leopold maneuver: determination of what is in the fundus.

Second Maneuver (Sides of the Maternal Abdomen). Place one hand on each side of the woman's abdomen, capturing the fetal body between them (Fig. 26-7). Steady the uterus with one hand and palpate the fetus with the other, looking for the back on one side and extremities on the other.

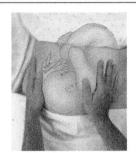

FIGURE 26-7. Second Leopold maneuver: evaluation of the fetal back and extremities.

Third Maneuver (Lower Fetal Pole and Descent into Pelvis). Face the woman's feet. Palpate the area just above the symphysis pubis (Fig. 26-8). Note whether the hands diverge with downward pressure or stay together to learn if the presenting part of the fetus, head or buttocks, is descending into the pelvic inlet.

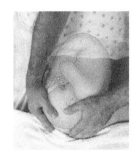

FIGURE 26-8. Third Leopold maneuver: palpation of the presenting part above the symphysis.

Fourth Maneuver (Flexion of the Fetal Head). This maneuver assesses the flexion or extension of the fetal head, presuming that the fetal head is the presenting part in the pelvis. Still facing the woman's feet, with your hands positioned on either side of the gravid uterus as in the third maneuver, identify the fetal front and back sides (Fig. 26-9). Using one hand at a time, slide your fingers down each side of the fetal body until you reach the *cephalic prominence*, that is, where the fetal brow or occiput juts out.

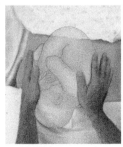

FIGURE 26-9. Fourth Leopold maneuver: determination of the direction and degree of flexion of the head.

RECORDING YOUR FINDINGS

Typically, the write-up follows a standard order: age, Gs and Ps (p. 511), weeks of gestation, means of determining gestational age (ultrasound vs. LMP), followed by chief complaint, chief pregnancy complications, then important history and examination findings.

Recording the Pregnant Woman Physical Examination

"32-year-old G3P1102 at 18 weeks' gestation as determined by LMP presents to establish prenatal care. Patient endorses fetal movement; denies contractions, vaginal bleeding, and leakage of fluids. On external examination, low transverse cesarean scar is evident; fundus is palpable just below umbilicus. On internal examination, cervix is open to fingertip at the external os but closed at the internal os; cervix is 3 cm long; uterus enlarged to size consistent with 18-week gestation. Speculum examination shows leukorrhea with positive Chadwick sign. FHT by Doppler are between 140 and 145 BPM."

This describes a healthy woman at 18 weeks' gestation.

HEALTH PROMOTION AND COUNSELING: EVIDENCE AND RECOMMENDATIONS

Important Topics for Health Promotion and Counseling

- Nutrition and weight gain
- Exercise and physical activity
- Substance use including tobacco, alcohol, and illicit drugs
- Intimate partner violence screening
- Screening for perinatal depression
- Immunizations
- Prenatal laboratory screening
- Prenatal supplementation
- Unintended pregnancy

Nutrition and Weight Gain

Evaluate nutritional status, especially inadequate nutrition and obesity.

- Assess diet history; measurement of height, weight, and body mass index (BMI); and a hematocrit. Prescribe needed vitamin and mineral supplements.
- To help prevent listeriosis, encourage pregnant patients to avoid: unpasteurized milk and foods made with unpasteurized milk; raw and undercooked seafood, eggs, and meat; refrigerated paté, meat spreads, and smoked salmon; and hot dogs, luncheon meats, and cold cuts unless served steaming hot.
- Recommend two servings a week of selected fish low in mercury and shellfish.
- Make a nutritional plan tailored to the patient's BMI. Use the Pregnancy Weight Gain Calculator and Super Tracker at the user-friendly ChooseMyPlate.gov website (http://www.choosemyplate.gov/pregnancy-weight-gain-calculator). This calculator displays the daily recommended intake of each of the five food groups for each trimester, based on height, prepregnancy weight, due date, and levels of weekly exercise.

Monitor weight gain at each visit, with the results plotted on a graph (Box 26-6).

BOX 26-6. Recommendations for Total and Rate of Weight Gain During Pregnancy, by Prepregnancy BMI

Prepregnancy BMI[a]	Total Weight Gain (Range in lbs)	Rates of Weight Gain[b] 2nd and 3rd Trimesters (lbs/wk)	Mean Range
Underweight, or <18.5	28–40	1	1.0–1.3
Normal weight, or 18.5–24.9	25–35	1	0.8–1.0
Overweight, or 25.0–29.9	15–25	0.6	0.5–0.7
Obese, or ≥30.0	11–20	0.5	0.4–0.6

[a]To calculate BMI, go to Calculate Your Body Mass Index, National Heart, Lung, and Blood Institute at http://www.nhlbi.nih.gov/health/educational/lose_wt/BMI/bmicalc.htm.

[b]Calculations assume a 1.1–4.4 lbs-weight gain in the first trimester.

Source: Rasmussen KM, Yaktine AL, eds; Institute of Medicine and National Research Council Committee to Re-examine IOM Pregnancy Weight Guidelines. *Weight Gain During Pregnancy: Re-examining the Guidelines*. National Academies Press; 2009. Available at http://www.ncbi.nlm.nih.gov/books/NBK32799/table/summary.t1/?report=objectonly. Accessed December 29, 2019.

Exercise and Physical Activity

The American Congress of Obstetricians and Gynecologists (ACOG) recommends that pregnant women should engage in ≥30 minutes of moderate exercise on most days of the week unless there are contraindications. Women initiating exercise during pregnancy should be cautious and consider programs developed specifically for pregnant women. Water-based exercises can temporarily help alleviate musculoskeletal aches, but immersion in hot water should be avoided.

After the first trimester, women should avoid exercise in the supine position, which compresses the inferior vena cava and can cause dizziness and decreased placental blood flow. Because the center of gravity shifts in the third trimester, advise against exercises that cause loss of balance. Contact sports or activities that risk abdominal trauma are contraindicated throughout pregnancy. Pregnant women also should avoid overheating, dehydration, and any exertion that causes notable fatigue or discomfort.

Substance Use Including Tobacco, Alcohol, and Illicit Drugs

Promote abstinence as the immediate goal during pregnancy. Pursue universal screening in a neutral manner for:

- *Tobacco.* Tobacco use accounts for up to 20% of all low–birth-weight babies. It doubles the risk of placenta previa, placental abruption, and preterm labor and increases risk of spontaneous abortion, fetal death, and fetal digit anomalies. Cessation is the goal, but any decrease in use is favorable.
- *Alcohol.* Fetal alcohol syndrome is the leading cause of preventable mental retardation in the United States. ACOG strongly recommends that women abstain throughout pregnancy.
- *Illicit drugs including narcotics.* Women with addictions should be referred for treatment immediately and counseled and screened for hepatitis C and HIV.
- *Abuse of prescription drugs.* Ask about commonly abused prescription drugs, including narcotics, stimulants, benzodiazepines.
- *Herbal and unregulated supplements.* Herbal supplements during pregnancy may harm the developing fetus.

Intimate Partner Violence Screening

Pregnancy is a time of increased risk from intimate partner violence ranging from verbal to physical abuse or from mild to severe physical abuse. Up to one in five women experiences some form of abuse during pregnancy, contributing to delayed prenatal care, low infant birth weight, or even murder of the mother and fetus. ACOG recommends universal screening of all women for domestic violence at the first prenatal visit and at least once each trimester. For a direct nonjudgmental approach, ACOG recommends an initial statement and simple questions (Box 26-7).

BOX 26-7. ACOG Screening Approach for Intimate Partner Violence

Initial Statement:

- "Because violence is so common in many women's lives and because there is help available for women being abused, I now ask every patient about domestic violence."

Screening Questions:

- "Within the past year—or since you have been pregnant—have you been hit, slapped, kicked or otherwise physically hurt by someone?"
- "Are you in a relationship with a person who threatens or physically hurts you?"
- "Has anyone forced you to have sexual activities that made you feel uncomfortable?"

Source: Intimate partner violence. Committee Opinion No. 518. American College of Obstetricians and Gynecologists. *Obstet Gynecol.* 2012;119:412–417.

Watch for nonverbal clues of abuse such as frequent last-minute appointment changes, unusual behavior during visits, partners who refuse to leave the patient alone during the visit, and bruises or other injuries. Once the patient acknowledges abuse, ask about the best way for you to help her. Respect limits she places on sharing information, with the caveat that if children are involved, you may be required to report harmful behaviors to the authorities. Plan future appointments at more frequent intervals. Perform as thorough a physical examination as the patient permits and document all injuries on a body diagram.

Maintain an updated list of shelters, counseling centers, hotline numbers, and other trusted local referrals (Box 26-8).

BOX 26-8. National Domestic Violence Hotline

- Website: www.thehotline.org
- 1–800–799-SAFE (7233)
- TTY for hearing impaired: 1–800–787–3224

Screening for Perinatal Depression

A 2018 study reported a 12% incidence of postpartum depression and a 17% overall prevalence of depression among healthy mothers without a prior history of depression. ACOG recommends that clinicians screen women at least once during the perinatal period for depression and anxiety symptoms using a standardized, validated tool. Additionally, the USPSTF recommends that clinicians provide or refer pregnant and postpartum persons who are at increased risk of perinatal depression to counseling interventions (B recommendation). Commonly used depression screening tools for the pregnant or peripartum adult include the Edinburgh Postnatal Depression Scale (EPDS) or the Patient Health Questionnaire-9 (PHQ-9). The EPDS consists of 10 self-reported items, takes <5 minutes to complete, has been translated into 50 different languages, has a low required reading level, and is easy to score. The PHQ-9 is a brief nine-item questionnaire focused on the nine diagnostic criteria for DSM-IV depressive disorders. It is one of the most validated tools in mental health and can be a powerful tool to assist clinicians with diagnosing depression and monitoring treatment response.

Immunizations

Administer Tdap during each pregnancy, ideally at 27 to 36 weeks' gestation, regardless of the prior immunization history, and to caretakers in direct contact with the infant. Give inactivated influenza vaccination in any trimester during the influenza season (Box 26-9).

BOX 26-9. Safe and Unsafe Vaccines During Pregnancy	
Safe During Pregnancy	**Not Safe During Pregnancy**
▪ Pneumococcal polysaccharide ▪ Meningococcal polysaccharide and conjugate ▪ Hepatitis A ▪ Hepatitis B	▪ Measles/mumps/rubella ▪ Polio ▪ Varicella

All women should have rubella titers drawn during pregnancy and be immunized after birth if found to be nonimmune. Check Rh(D) and antibody typing at the first prenatal visit, at 28 weeks, and at delivery. Anti-D immunoglobulin should be given to all Rh-negative women at 28 weeks' gestation and again within 3 days of delivery to prevent sensitization if the infant is Rh-D positive.

Prenatal Laboratory Screenings

Initially include blood type and Rh, antibody screen, complete blood count—especially hematocrit and platelet count, rubella titer, syphilis test, hepatitis B surface antigen, HIV, STI screen for gonorrhea and chlamydia, and urinalysis with culture. Scheduled screenings include an oral glucose tolerance test for gestational diabetes around 24 weeks; a vaginal swab for group B streptococcus between 35 to 37 weeks' gestation; and for obese pregnant patients, a glucose tolerance in the first trimester. Pursue additional testing related to the mother's risk factors, such as screening for aneuploidy, Tay–Sachs, or other genetic diseases, or amniocentesis.

ACOG recommends screening all pregnant women for anemia during pregnancy, though the United States Preventive Services Task Force (USPSTF) states that the evidence is insufficient (I statement) to screen pregnant women who do not have symptoms of iron deficiency anemia.

Prenatal Supplementation

Multivitamin and Mineral Supplementation. Daily prenatal vitamin and mineral supplements should include 600 IU of vitamin D and at least 1,000 mg of calcium. Women should be advised that excess amounts of fat-soluble vitamins like vitamins A, D, E, and K can cause toxicity.

Folic Acid Supplementation. Folate deficiency in pregnancy has a well-documented association with neural tube defects (NTDs). ACOG recommends that all women contemplating pregnancy take 400 µg of folic acid supplementation in addition to a folate-rich diet, which is also supported by the USPSTF (grade A recommendation). Supplementation should be initiated 3 months prior to conception and continued through the first trimester.

Iron Supplementation. Iron requirements increase dramatically during pregnancy, with increasing amounts of iron needed with advancing gestation to support maternal erythrocyte mass, fetal RBC production, and fetoplacental growth. The CDC recommends 30 mg/day of oral iron supplementation be started at the first prenatal visit, which is the dose typically available in iron-containing prenatal vitamins. Additionally, women should be encouraged to ingest iron-rich foods.

Unintended Pregnancy

Almost half of US pregnancies are unintended (2.8 million of the 6.1 million pregnancies).

- If a woman did not want to become pregnant at the time the pregnancy occurred but did want to become pregnant at some point in the future, the pregnancy is considered *mistimed* (27% of pregnancies).

▪ If a woman did not want to become pregnant then or at any time in the future, the pregnancy is considered *unwanted* (18% of pregnancies).

Among pregnancies in adolescents ages 15 to 19 years and younger than age 15 years, the percentage of unintended pregnancy climbs to over 80% and 98%, respectively.

It is important to counsel girls and women about the timing of ovulation in the menstrual cycle and how to plan or prevent pregnancy. Be familiar with the numerous options for contraception and their effectiveness (Box 26-10).

BOX 26-10. Types of Contraception Methods	
Methods	**Types of Contraception**
Natural	Fertility awareness/periodic abstinence, withdrawal, lactation
Barrier	Male condom, female condom, diaphragm, cervical cap, sponge
Implantable	Intrauterine devices (IUD), subdermal implant of levonorgestrel
Pharmacologic/ hormonal	Spermicide, oral contraceptives (estrogen and progesterone; progestin only), estrogen/progesterone injectables and patch, hormonal vaginal contraceptive ring, emergency contraception
Surgery (permanent)	Tubal ligation; transcervical sterilization; vasectomy

▪ Failure rates are lowest for the subdermal implant, IUD, female sterilization, and vasectomy at less than 0.8% per year (<1 pregnancy/ 100 women/yr) and highest for male and female condoms, withdrawal, sponge in parous women, fertility awareness methods, and spermicides at more than 18% per year (or ≥18 pregnancies/100 women/yr).
▪ Failure rates for injectables, oral contraceptives, the patch, vaginal ring, and diaphragm range from 6% to 12% per year (or 6 to 12 pregnancies/ 100 women/yr).

Take the time to understand the patient or couple's concerns and preferences and respect these preferences whenever possible. Continued use of a preferred method is superior to a more effective method that is abandoned. For adolescents, a confidential setting eases discussion of topics that may seem private and difficult to explore.

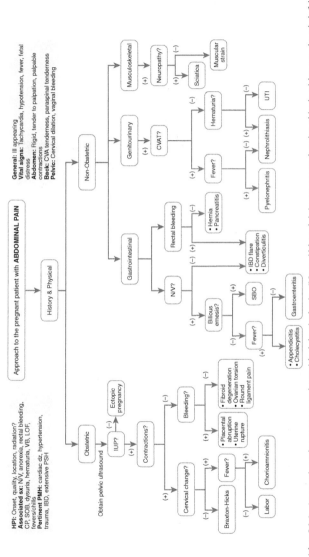

Algorithm 26-1. Approach to the pregnant patient with abdominal pain. (Note: Although it is not comprehensive, this algorithm may be a helpful starting approach for synthesizing information gathered from the history and physical. CP, chest pain; CVAT, costovertebral angle tenderness; HPI, history of present illness; IBD, inflammatory bowel disease; IUP, intrauterine pregnancy; LOF, leakage of fluid; sx, symptoms; N/V, nausea/ vomiting; PMH, past medical history; PSH, past surgical history; SOB, shortness of breath; UTI, urinary tract infection; VB, vaginal bleeding.

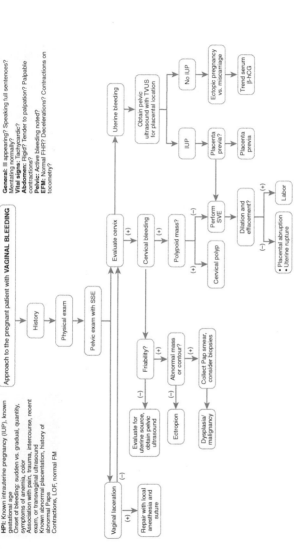

Algorithm 26-2. Approach to the pregnant woman with vaginal bleeding. (Note: Although it is not comprehensive, this algorithm may be a helpful starting approach for synthesizing information gathered from the history and physical.) EFM, external fetal monitoring; FHR, fetal heart rate; FM, fetal movement; hCG, human chorionic gonadotropin; HPI, history of present illness; IUP, intrauterine pregnancy; LOF, leakage of fluid; SSE, sterile speculum exam; SVE, sterile vaginal examination; TVUS, transvaginal ultrasound.

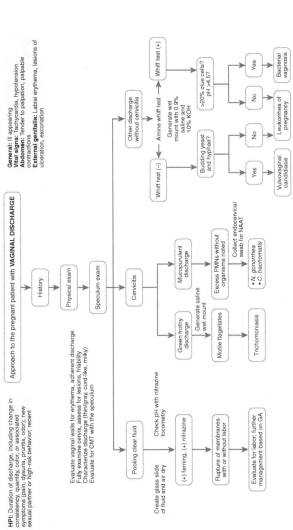

Approach to the pregnant patient with VAGINAL DISCHARGE

HPI: Duration of discharge, including change in consistency, quantity, color, or associated symptoms (pain, dysuria, pruritis, odor); new sexual partner or high-risk behavior; recent

General: Ill appearing
Vital signs: Tachycardia, hypotension
Abdomen: Tender to palpation, palpable contractions
External genitalia: Labial erythema, lesions of ulceration, excoriation

History

Physical exam

Speculum exam

Evaluate vaginal walls for erythema, adherent discharge
Fully examine cervix, assess for lesions, friability
Characterize discharge (thin/gray, curd-like, milky)
Evaluate for CMT with the speculum

Pooling clear fluid

Check pH with nitrazine tocometry

Create glass slide of fluid and air dry

(+) ferning, (+) nitrazine

Rupture of membranes with or without labor

Evaluate for labor; further management based on GA

Cervicitis

Green frothy discharge

Generate saline wet mount

Motile flagellates

Trichomoniasis

Mucopurulent discharge

Excess PMNs without organisms noted

Collect endocervical swab for NAAT

• *N. gonorrhea*
• *C. trachomatis*

Other discharge without cervicitis

Whiff test (−) — Amine whiff test — Whiff test (+)

Budding yeast and hyphae?

Generate wet mount with 0.9% saline and 10% KOH

>20% clue cells? pH >4.5?

Yes — Vulvovaginal candidiasis

No — Leukorrhea of pregnancy

No — Leukorrhea of pregnancy

Yes — Bacterial vaginosis

Algorithm 26-3. Approach to the pregnant woman with vaginal discharge. (Note: Although it is not comprehensive, this algorithm may be a helpful starting approach for synthesizing information gathered from the history and physical.) CMT, cervical motion tenderness; GA, gestational age; HPI, history of present illness; KOH, potassium hydroxide; NAAT, nucleic acid amplification test; PMNs, polymorphonuclear cells (leukocytes).

INTERPRETATION AIDS

TABLE 26-1. Anatomic and Physiologic Changes in Normal Pregnancy

Organ System	Organ of Interest	Change in Normal Pregnancy	Clinical Relevance
Vital signs	Heart rate	↑ (Progresses throughout)	
	Blood pressure	↓ (Nadir in second trimester)	
	Respiratory rate	←→	
	Oxygen saturation	←→	
Skin	Skin	Increased cutaneous blood flow	Dissipation of excess heat due to increased metabolism
		Hyperpigmentation	
		Spider angiomata and palmar erythema	Unclear clinical significance, likely related to hyperestrogenemia
	Hair	Scalp hair thickening	
		Hirsutism	Unclear clinical significance; severe hirsutism with signs of virilization should be investigated
Respiratory	Lungs	↑ Oxygen consumption 20%	Shifts CO_2 waste from fetus to maternal circulation
		↓ Arterial pCO_2	
		↑ Ventilation	ABG will demonstrate *respiratory alkalosis*
		↓ TLV, RV, FRC	
		↑ TV, minute ventilation	Aids in CO_2 removal
		↑ Pulmonary vascular resistance	
		←→ Lung compliance	

continued

TABLE 26-1. Anatomic and Physiologic Changes in Normal Pregnancy (continued)

Organ System	Organ of Interest	Change in Normal Pregnancy	Clinical Relevance
	Diaphragm	Diaphragm elevated 4 cm	Diaphragmatic elevation and increased minute ventilation contribute to sensation of *dyspnea in pregnancy*
Cardio-vascular	Heart	↑ Cardiac output up to 50%	Related to both increased pulse and stroke volume
			Further augmented by almost 20% in *multifetal gestation*
		Heart displaced left and upward	Appearance of cardiomegaly on imaging
		Exaggerated split S1	*Systolic murmurs* are common, in up to 90% of pregnant patients
		Hyperdynamic LV function	
	Peripheral vasculature	↓ Systemic vascular resistance	↑ Venous pooling and *postural hypotension*
		↓ BP (diastolic > systolic)	
		↓ Venous flow in the lower extremities due to compression by the gravid uterus	↑ Dependent edema and varicose veins
			Predisposes to thrombosis
Gastro-intestinal	Stomach	↓ Gastric emptying	Contributes to nausea, acid reflux
		↓ Esophageal sphincter tone	
	Intestinal tracts, large and small	Displaced superiorly and laterally	*Appendicitis may present atypically*
		↓ Motility	Contributes to hemorrhoids, constipation

TABLE 26-1. Anatomic and Physiologic Changes in Normal Pregnancy *(continued)*

Organ System	Organ of Interest	Change in Normal Pregnancy	Clinical Relevance
	Hepatobiliary tree	←—→ Liver size	
		↑ Hepatic blood flow	
		↓ Serum albumin concentration	
		↓ Gallbladder motility	↑ Biliary stasis and incidence of cholesterol gallstones, cholecystitis
			↑ Risk of cholestasis
Hematologic	Plasma	↑ Circulating volume 40%–45%	Provision of nutrients to the fetus/placenta, protection against impaired venous return
	Blood	↑ Erythrocyte production and volume	Protection against blood loss during parturition
		↑ Reticulocyte count	Unclear clinical significance—related to hemodilution and ↑ consumption
		↑ Iron turnover	Leads to iron deficiency anemia, *pica*
		↓ Hemoglobin and hematocrit	
		↑ Leukocytosis	
		↓ Platelets	↑ Risk of epistaxis, nasal congestion
		↑ Inflammatory markers (CRP, ESR)	Unreliable markers of inflammation
	Coagulation	↑ Clotting factors (except factors XI and XIII)	
		↑ Fibrinogen	Maintains balance of coagulation and fibrinolysis—overall *hypercoagulable state*
		↓ Protein C and total protein S	
		↑ Fibrinolysis and D-dimer	D-dimer is an unreliable marker of thrombotic risk

continued

TABLE 26-1. Anatomic and Physiologic Changes in Normal Pregnancy *(continued)*

Organ System	Organ of Interest	Change in Normal Pregnancy	Clinical Relevance
Urinary	Bladder	Hyperplasia of bladder muscle and connective tissue	↑ Urinary frequency and incontinence
		Elevation of trigone	
		↑ Bladder pressure	
	Ureters	Laterally displaced and compressed	Contributes to *hydronephrosis*, more commonly right-sided
		↑ Dilation and relaxation	
	Kidneys	↑ Renin–angiotensin–aldosterone system	Maintains BP in the first trimester
			Hypertension does not result in normal pregnancy due to angiotensin II refractoriness as pregnancy progresses
			Contributes to *urinary frequency*
		↑ Kidney size	
		↑ GFR and plasma flow	
		↓ Serum creatinine	Cr >0.9 mg/dL should be evaluated
		↑ Creatinine clearance 30%	
Musculos-keletal	Spine	Lumbar lordosis	Shifts center of gravity to accommodate the gravid uterus. May contribute to low back pain.
		Pelvic joint relaxation—symphysis pubis, sacroiliac and sacrococcygeal joints	*Pubic symphysis separation* >1 cm may cause significant pain and gait disturbance

CRP, c-reactive protein; BP, blood pressure; CO_2, carbon dioxide; ESR, erythrocyte sedimentation rate; FRC, functional residual capacity; GFR, glomerular filtration rate; LV, left ventricle; RV, residual volume; TLV, total lung volume; TV, tidal volume; VTE, venous thromboembolism.

Older Adult

DEMOGRAPHIC IMPERATIVE

It has been estimated that by the year 2050, the number of people older than 60 years worldwide will exceed 2 billion. Older Americans now number more than 46 million people and are expected to reach 98 million by 2060, nearly 24% of the total population. In fact, the fastest growing age group in the United States is the oldest-old (>85 years), a group projected to reach 20 million in 2060.

Hence, the demographic imperative to societies worldwide is to maximize not only life span but also "health span," so that older adults maintain full function as long as possible, enjoying rich and active lives in their homes and communities. This entails promoting healthy or "successful" aging leading to interactive goals in clinical care—an informed activated patient interacting with a prepared proactive team, resulting in high-quality satisfying encounters and improved outcomes and a distinct set of clinical attitudes and skills (Box 27-1).

Primary aging reflects changes in physiologic reserves over time that are independent of changes from disease. However, these changes can lead to the development of multiple impairments, decline in overall functional capacity, and associated morbidity and mortality. These significant alterations in physiology tend to have the most impact during periods of stress, such as exposure to fluctuating temperatures, dehydration, or even shock.

See Table 27-1. Selected Normal Anatomic and Physiologic Changes with Aging and Related Disease Outcomes, pp. 555–562.

BOX 27-1. Key Points in the Care of the Older Adult in the Primary Care Setting

- It is crucial to recognize geriatric syndromes, multifactorial conditions occurring primarily in older adults, in the primary care setting.
- The most important geriatric syndromes to recognize in primary care are falls, urinary incontinence, frailty, and cognitive impairment.
- Elements of ideal geriatric primary care include assessment of functional status, frequent medication review, careful evaluation of the benefits and burdens of any new test or treatment, and frequent assessment of goals of care and prognosis.
- Innovative delivery systems—either comprehensive care, consulting assessment or hospital-level care for acute conditions at home—can improve geriatric primary care. High-value features of geriatric care systems include ensuring round-the-clock access to care, providing a team-based approach to care, performing medication reconciliation and comprehensive geriatric assessments, and integrating palliative care into treatment planning.

This chapter uses the term *older adult* for persons 65 years and older rather than terms such as "senior," "aged," or "elderly." Take the time to find out which term your older adult patients prefer.

COMMUNICATING EFFECTIVELY WITH OLDER ADULTS

As you talk with older adults, convey respect, patience, and cultural awareness (Box 27-2). Be sure to address patients by their last name.

BOX 27-2. Tips for Communicating Effectively with Older Adults

- Provide a well-lit, moderately warm setting with minimal background noise, chairs with arms, and access to the examining table.
- Face the patient and speak in low tones; make sure the patient is using glasses, hearing devices, and dentures, if needed.
- Adjust the pace and content of the interview to the stamina of the patient; consider two visits for initial evaluations.
- Allow time for open-ended questions and reminiscing; include family and caregivers when indicated, especially if the patient has cognitive impairment.

- Make use of screening instruments, the clinical record, and reports from allied disciplines.
- Provide written instructions and make sure they are in large print and easy to read.
- Always give the patient an updated medication that includes the name of the medication, dosage instructions, and why the medication is being prescribed.

Adjusting the Office Environment

Make sure the office is neither too cool nor too warm. Face the patient directly, sitting at eye level. A well-lit room allows the older adult to see your facial expressions and gestures.

More than 50% of older adults have hearing deficits. Free the room of distractions or noise.

Consider using a "pocket talker," a microphone that amplifies your voice and connects to an earpiece inserted by the patient. Chairs with higher seating and a wide stool with a handrail leading up to the examining table help patients with quadriceps weakness.

Shaping the Content and Pace of the Visit

Older people often reminisce. Listen to this process of life review to gain important insights and help patients as they work through painful feelings or recapture joys and accomplishments.

Balance the need to assess complex problems with the patient's endurance and possible fatigue. Consider dividing the initial assessment into two visits.

Eliciting Symptoms from the Older Adult

Underreporting. Older patients may overestimate their health even when increasing disease and disability are apparent. To reduce the risk of late recognition and delayed intervention, adopt more directed questions or *health screening tools.* Consult with family members and caretakers.

Atypical Presentations of Illness. Acute illnesses present differently in older adults. Be sensitive to unusual presentations of myocardial infarction and thyroid disease. Older patients with infections are less likely to have fever.

Geriatric Syndromes. Recognize the symptom clusters of different *geriatric syndromes,* characterized by interacting clusters of symptoms that lead to functional decline, for example, falls, dizziness, depression, urinary incontinence, and functional impairment. Searching for the usual "unifying diagnosis" may pertain to fewer than 50% of older adults.

Cognitive Impairment. Although cognitive impairment may alter the patient's history, most older adults even with mild cognitive impairment can provide sufficient history to reveal current disorders. Use simple sentences with prompts to trigger necessary information. If impairments are more severe, confirm symptoms with family members or caregivers.

ADDRESSING CULTURAL DIMENSIONS OF AGING

Cultural differences affect the epidemiology of illness and mental health, acculturation, the specific concerns of the elderly, the potential for misdiagnosis, and disparities in health outcomes (Box 27-3). Ask about spiritual advisors and native healers. Cultural values particularly affect decisions about the end of life. Elders, family, and even an extended community group may make these decisions with or for the older patient. Eliciting the stresses of migration and acculturation, using medical interpreters effectively, enlisting *patient navigators* from the family and community, and accessing culturally validated assessment tools will help you provide empathic care of older adults.

BOX 27-3. Geriatric Diversity—Now and in 2060

- In 2014, non-Hispanic single-race Whites, Blacks, and Asians accounted for 78%, 9%, and 4% of the U.S. older population, respectively. Hispanics (of any race) were 8% of the older population.
- Projections indicate that by 2060 the composition of the older population will be 55% non-Hispanic White alone, 12% non-Hispanic Black alone, and 9% non-Hispanic Asian alone. Hispanics will be 22% of the older population in 2060.
- While the older population will increase among all racial and ethnic groups, the older Hispanic population is projected to grow the fastest, from 3.6 million in 2014 to 21.5 million in 2060. They are expected to be larger than the older non-Hispanic Black alone population in 2060.
- The older non-Hispanic Asian alone population is also projected to experience rapid growth. In 2014, nearly 2 million older single-race non-Hispanic Asians lived in the United States; by 2060, this population is projected to be about 8.5 million.

Source: Older Americans 2016: Key Indicators of Well-Being. Available at https://agingstats.gov/docs/LatestReport/Older-Americans-2016-Key-Indicators-of-WellBeing.pdf. Accessed December 29, 2019.

HEALTH HISTORY

Common Concerns

- Functional impairments in activities of daily living and instrumental activities of daily living
- Medication management
- Smoking
- Alcohol
- Nutrition

Other areas of concern among older adults are addressed in more detail in the following sections:

- Acute and persistent pain (see Chapter 8, General Survey, Vital Signs, and Pain, p. 113)
- Cognitive impairment (see Chapter 9, Cognition, Behavior, and Mental Status, p. 130)
- Urinary incontinence (see Chapter 19, Abdomen, p. 303)
- Falls (see Chapter 23, Musculoskeletal System, p. 397)

Place symptoms in the context of your overall *functional assessment*, always focusing on helping the older adult to maintain optimal well-being and level of function.

Activities of Daily Living

Daily activities provide an important baseline for future evaluations (Box 27-4). Ask, "Tell me about your typical day" or "Tell me about your day yesterday." Then move to a greater level of detail: "You got up at 8 AM? How is it getting out of bed?"

BOX 27-4. Activities of Daily Living and Instrumental Activities of Daily Living

Basic Activities of Daily Living (ADLs)	Instrumental Activities of Daily Living (IADLs)
■ Bathing	■ Using the telephone
■ Dressing	■ Shopping
■ Toileting	■ Preparing food
■ Transferring	■ Housekeeping
■ Continence	■ Laundry
■ Feeding	■ Transportation
	■ Taking medicine
	■ Managing money

Medication Management

Adults older than 65 take approximately 30% of all prescriptions. Almost 40% take five or more prescription drugs daily. Older adults have more than 50% of all reported adverse drug reactions. Take a thorough medication history, including name, dose, frequency, and indication for each drug (Box 27-5). Explore all components of polypharmacy, including concurrent use of multiple drugs, underuse, inappropriate use, and nonadherence. Ask about use of over-the-counter medications, vitamin and nutrition supplements, and mood-altering drugs. Medications are the most common modifiable risk factor associated with falls. "Start low, go slow" when prescribing doses. Learn about drug–drug interactions and consult the *2019 American Geriatrics Society (AGS) Updated Beers Criteria® for Potentially Inappropriate Medication Use in Older Adults*, widely used by health care providers, educators, and policymakers.

BOX 27-5. Improving Medication Safety among Older Adults

- Perform a thorough *medication history* including the name, dose, frequency and the *patient's view* of the reason for taking each drug. Ask the patient to bring in all medication bottles and over-the-counter products to develop an accurate medication list.
- Complete a *medication reconciliation* at every visit especially after care transitions.
- Explore all components of *polypharmacy*—a major cause of morbidity—including suboptimal prescribing, concurrent use of multiple drugs, underuse, inappropriate use, and nonadherence.
- Ask specifically about over-the-counter products; vitamin and nutritional supplements; and mood-altering drugs such as opioids, benzodiazepines, and recreational substances.
- Assess medications for drug interactions.

Smoking and Alcohol

Smoking is harmful at all ages. At each visit, advise older adult smokers to quit. From 10% to 15% of older patients in primary care practices have problem drinking. Rates of detection and treatment are low.

Screen all older adults for excess alcohol use, which contributes to drug interactions and worsens comorbid illnesses. Use the Alcohol Use Disorders Identification Test–Consumption (AUDIT-C) to assess unhealthy alcohol use among

See Chapter 3, Health History to review the approach to eliciting information regarding smoking and alcohol habits, pp. 39–40.

older adults (see p. 538). It has three questions about frequency of alcohol use, typical amount of alcohol use, and occasions of heavy use, and takes 1 to 2 minutes to administer. The Cut down, Annoyed, Guilty, Eye-opener (CAGE) tool is well known but only detects alcohol dependence rather than the full spectrum of unhealthy alcohol use.

Nutrition

Taking a diet history and using rapid screening tools (p. 539) are especially important in older adults.

SPECIAL TOPICS IN OLDER ADULT CARE

Frailty

Frailty is a multifactorial geriatric syndrome characterized by an age-related lack of adaptive physiologic capacity occurring even in the absence of identifiable illness. Its prevalence is 4% to 59%. Screen for three key features and pursue related interventions: weight loss of more than 5% over 3 years, inability to do five chair stands, and self-reported exhaustion.

Advance Directives and Palliative Care

Many older patients are interested in discussing end-of-life decisions and would like providers to initiate these discussions before the onset of serious illness. *Advance care planning* involves providing information, invoking the patient's preferences, identifying surrogate decision makers, and conveying empathy and support. Use clear, simple language. Clarify directives which may range from general statements of values to such specific orders as *do not resuscitate (DNR)*, *do not intubate (DNI)*, do not hospitalize, do not provide artificial hydration or nutrition, or do not administer antibiotics. Seek a written *health care proxy* or *durable power of attorney for health care*, "someone who can make decisions reflecting your wishes in case of confusion or emergency." Discuss these decisions in the office rather than in the pressured environments of the emergency room or hospital.

When needed, provide *palliative care* "to relieve suffering and improve the quality of life for patients with advanced illnesses and their families through specific knowledge and skills, including communication with patients and family members; management of pain and other symptoms; psychosocial, spiritual, and bereavement support; and coordination of an array of clinical and social services" (Fig. 27-1).

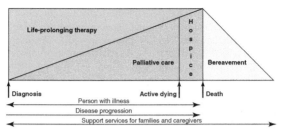

FIGURE 27-1. The place of palliative care within the course of illness. (From Burggraf V, et al. *Healthy Aging: Principles and Clinical Practice for Clinicians.* Wolters Kluwer Health; 2015. Figure 29-1.)

TECHNIQUES OF EXAMINATION

Assessment of the older adult departs from the traditional history and physical examination. Enhanced interviewing, emphasis on daily function and the key topics described above, and functional assessment are especially important.

Assessing Functional Status

Functional status is the ability to perform tasks and fulfill social roles associated with daily living across a wide range of complexity.

The 10-Minute Geriatric Screener (Box 27-6) is brief, has high interrater agreement, and can be used easily by office staff. It covers the three important domains: physical, cognitive, and psychosocial function and addresses key sensory modalities and urinary incontinence, an often-unreported problem.

BOX 27-6. 10-Minute Geriatric Screener

Problem and Screening Measure	Positive Screen
Vision: Two Parts: Ask: "Do you have difficulty driving, or watching television, or reading, or doing any of your daily activities because of your eyesight?" If yes, then: Test each eye with Snellen chart while patient wears corrective lenses (if applicable).	Yes to question and inability to read >20/40 on Snellen chart
Hearing: Use audioscope set at 40 dB. Test hearing using 1,000 and 2,000 Hz.	Inability to hear 1,000 or 2,000 Hz in both ears or either of these frequencies in one ear

Leg mobility: Time the patient after instructing: "Rise from the chair. Walk 20 ft briskly, turn, walk back to the chair, and sit down."	Unable to complete task in 15 sec	
Urinary incontinence: Two Parts: Ask: "In the last year, have you ever lost your urine and gotten wet?" If yes, then ask: "Have you lost urine on at least 6 separate dates?"	Yes to both questions	For identifying causes of transient incontinence, this mnemonic may be helpful: DIAPPERS: **D**elirium, **I**nfection (e.g., urinary tract infection), **A**trophic urethritis or vaginitis, **P**harmaceuticals (e.g., diuretics, anticholinergics, calcium channel blockers, opioids, sedatives, alcohol), **P**sychological disorders (e.g., depression), **E**xcessive urine output (e.g., heart failure, uncontrolled diabetes), **R**estricted mobility (e.g., hip fracture, environmental barriers, restraints), **S**tool impaction.
Nutrition/weight loss: Two parts: Ask: "Have you lost 10 lb over the past 6 mo without trying to do so?" Weigh the patient.	Yes to the question or weight <100 lb	
Memory: Three-item recall	Unable to remember all three items after 1 min	
Depression: Ask: "Do you often feel sad or depressed?"	Yes to the question	
Physical disability: Six questions: "Are you able to …: <ul><li>"Do strenuous activities like fast walking or bicycling?"</li><li>"Do heavy work around the house like washing windows, walls, or floors?"</li><li>"Go shopping for groceries or clothes?"</li><li>"Get to places out of walking distance?"</li><li>"Bathe, either a sponge bath, tub bath, or shower?"</li><li>"Dress, like putting on a shirt, buttoning and zipping, or putting on shoes?"</li></ul>	No to any of the questions	

Source: Reprinted from Moore AA, et al. Screening for common problems in ambulatory elderly: clinical confirmation of a screening instrument. *Am J Med*. 1996;100(4):438–443. Copyright © 1996 Elsevier. With permission.

General Survey

Observe as the patient enters the examining room. Note the patient's hygiene and dress. Assess the patient's apparent state of health, degree of vitality, and mood and affect.

Vital Signs

Measure blood pressure, checking for increased systolic blood pressure (SBP) and widened pulse pressure (PP), defined as SBP minus diastolic blood pressure (DBP).

Isolated systolic hypertension (SBP ≥140) after age 50 years and PP ≥60 increase risk of stroke, renal failure, and heart disease.

For adults ages ≥60 years, JNC8 recommends blood pressure targets of ≤150/90 but notes that if treatment results in SBP <140 and is well tolerated and without adverse effects to health or quality of life, treatment does not need to be adjusted.

Assess the patient for *orthostatic hypotension,* defined as a drop in SBP of ≥20 mm Hg or DBP of ≥10 mm Hg, within 3 minutes of standing. Measure in two positions: supine after the patient rests for up to 10 minutes, then within 2 to 3 minutes after standing up.

Orthostatic hypotension occurs in 10% to 20% of older adults and in up to 30% of frail nursing home residents, especially when they first arise in the morning. Watch for lightheadedness, weakness, unsteadiness, visual blurring, and, in 20% to 30% of patients, syncope.

Assess medications and causes such as autonomic disorders, diabetes, prolonged bed rest, volume depletion, amyloidosis, postprandial state, and cardiovascular disorders.

Measure heart rate, respiratory rate, and temperature. Check the apical heart rate to help detect arrhythmias in older adults. Use thermometers accurate for lower temperatures.

Respiratory rate ≥25 breaths per minute indicates lower respiratory infection or possible CHF or COPD.

Hypothermia is more common in elderly patients.

Weight and height are especially important and needed for calculation of the BMI (p. 547). Weight should be measured at every visit. Obtain oxygen saturation using a pulse oximeter.

Low weight is a key indicator of poor nutrition.

Undernutrition in depression, alcoholism, cognitive impairment, malignancy, chronic organ failure (cardiac, renal, pulmonary), medication use, poor dentition, social isolation, and poverty

Skin

Note physiologic changes of aging, such as thinning, loss of elastic tissue and turgor, and wrinkling.

Dry, flaky, rough, and often itchy

Benign comedones, or blackheads, on the cheeks or around the eyes; cherry angiomas (p. 170); and seborrheic keratoses (p. 169)

Inspect the extensor surface of the hands and forearms.

White depigmented patches (*pseudoscars*); well-demarcated, vividly purple macules or patches that may fade after several weeks (actinic purpura)

Look for changes from sun exposure: *actinic lentigines*, or "liver spots," and actinic keratoses, superficial flattened papules covered by a dry scale (p. 165).

Distinguish such lesions from a basal cell carcinoma and squamous cell carcinoma (p. 165). Dark, raised, asymmetric lesions with irregular borders are suspicious for melanoma

Inspect for painful vesicular lesions in a dermatomal distribution.

Herpes zoster from reactivation of latent varicella-zoster virus in the dorsal root ganglia

In older bedbound patients, especially when emaciated or neurologically impaired, inspect for damage or ulceration.

Pressure sores if obliteration of arteriolar and capillary blood flow to the skin or shear forces with movement across sheets or lifting upright incorrectly

HEENT

Inspect the eyelids, the bony orbit, and the eye.

Senile ptosis arising from weakening of the levator palpebrae, relaxation of the skin, and increased weight of the upper eyelid

Ectropion or entropion of lower lids (p. 196)

Yellowing of the sclera and *arcus senilis*, a benign whitish ring around the limbus

Test visual acuity, using a pocket Snellen chart or wall-mounted chart.

More than 40 million Americans have refractive errors—presbyopia.

Examine the lenses and fundi.

Cataracts, glaucoma, and macular degeneration all increase with aging.

Inspect each lens for opacities.

Cataracts are the world's leading cause of blindness.

Assess the cup-to-disc ratio, usually ≤1:2.

Increased cup-to-disc ratio suggests open-angle glaucoma and possible loss of peripheral and central vision, and blindness.

Inspect the fundi for colloid bodies causing alterations in pigmentation called *drusen*. These may be hard and sharply defined, or soft and confluent with altered pigmentation.

Macular degeneration causes poor central vision and blindness: types include dry atrophic (more common but less severe) and wet exudative (or neovascular).

Test hearing by the whispered voice test (see p. 203) or audioscope. Inspect ear canals for cerumen.

Removing cerumen often quickly improves hearing.

Examine the oral cavity for odor, appearance of the gingival mucosa, any caries, mobility of the teeth, and quantity of saliva.

Malodor in poor oral hygiene, periodontitis, or caries

Gingivitis if periodontal disease

Inspect for lesions on mucosal surfaces. Ask patient to remove dentures so you can check gums for denture sores.

Dental plaque and cavitation if caries. Increased tooth mobility; risk of tooth aspiration

Decreased salivation from medications, radiation, Sjögren syndrome, or dehydration

Oral tumors, usually on lateral borders of tongue and floor of mouth

Thorax and Lungs

Percuss and auscultate the lungs. Note subtle signs of changes in pulmonary function.

Increased anteroposterior diameter, purse-lipped breathing, and dyspnea with talking or minimal exertion in chronic obstructive pulmonary disease

Cardiovascular System

Review blood pressure and heart rate.

Isolated systolic hypertension and a widened pulse pressure are cardiac risk factors. Search for left ventricular hypertrophy (LVH).

Inspect the jugular venous pulsation (JVP), palpate the carotid upstrokes, and listen for any overlying carotid bruits.

A tortuous atherosclerotic aorta can raise pressure in the left jugular veins by impairing drainage into right atrium.

Carotid bruits in possible carotid stenosis.

Assess the point of maximal impulse (PMI), and then heart sounds.

Sustained PMI is found in LVH, hypertension, and aortic stenosis; diffuse PMI in heart failure (see p. 467).

In older adults, S_3 in dilatation of the left ventricle from heart failure or cardiomyopathy; S_4 in hypertension

Listen for cardiac murmurs in all six listening areas (see p. 249). Describe timing, shape, location of maximal intensity, radiation, intensity, pitch, and quality of each murmur.

A systolic crescendo–decrescendo murmur in the second right interspace in aortic sclerosis or aortic stenosis. Both carry increased risk of cardiovascular disease and death.

A harsh holosystolic murmur at the apex suggests mitral regurgitation, common in older adults.

Peripheral Vascular System

Auscultate the abdomen for aortic, renal, femoral artery bruits.

Bruits over these vessels in atherosclerotic disease.

Palpate pulses.

Diminished or absent pulses in arterial occlusion. Confirm with an office ankle–brachial index (see pp. 275–276).

Breasts and Axillae

Palpate the breasts carefully for lumps or masses.

Possible breast cancer

Abdomen

Listen for bruits over the aorta, renal arteries, and femoral arteries.

Bruits in atherosclerotic vascular disease

Inspect the upper abdomen; palpate to the left of the midline for aortic pulsations.

Widened aorta of ≥3 cm and pulsatile mass in abdominal aortic aneurysm.

Female Genitalia and Pelvic Examination

Take special care to explain the steps of examination and allow time for careful positioning. For the woman with arthritis or spinal deformities who cannot flex her hips or knees, an assistant can gently raise and support the legs, or help the woman into the left lateral position.

Inspect the vulva for changes related to menopause; identify any labial masses. Bluish swellings may be varicosities.

Benign masses include condylomata, fibromas, leiomyomas, and sebaceous cysts. Bulging of the anterior vaginal wall below the urethra in urethrocele

Erythema with satellite lesions in *Candida* infection; erythema with ulceration or a necrotic center in vulvar carcinoma.

Chapter 27 ■ Older Adult **545**

Inspect the urethra for caruncles or prolapse of fleshy erythematous mucosal tissue at the urethral meatus.

Clitoral enlargement in androgen-producing tumors or use of androgen creams

Speculum Examination. Inspect vaginal walls, which may be atrophic, and cervix.

Estrogen-stimulated cervical mucus with ferning in use of hormone replacement therapy, endometrial hyperplasia, and estrogen-producing tumors; lichen sclerosus

If indicated, obtain endocervical cells for the Pap smear. Use a blind swab if the atrophic vagina is too small.

See Box 27-10, Screening Recommendations for Older Adults, p. 552.

Removing speculum, ask patient to bear down.

Uterine prolapse, cystocele, urethrocele, or rectocele.

Perform the bimanual examination.

Note any uterine retroversion, retroflexion, porolapse, or myomas (fibroids)

Mobility of cervix restricted if inflammation, malignancy, or surgical adhesion

Palpable ovaries in ovarian cancer.

Perform the rectovaginal examination if indicated.

Enlarged, fixed, or irregular uterus if adhesions or malignancy; rectal masses in colon cancer

Male Genitalia and Prostate

Examine the penis; retract foreskin if present. Examine the scrotum, testes, and epididymis.

Smegma, penile cancer, and scrotal hydroceles

Do a rectal examination.

Rectal masses in colon cancer. Prostate hyperplasia if enlargement; prostate cancer if nodules or masses.

Musculoskeletal System

Screen general range of motion and gait. Conduct timed "get up and go" test.

See Table 27-2, Timed Get Up and Go Test, p. 562.

If joint deformity, deficits in mobility, or pain with movement, conduct a more thorough examination.

Degenerative joint changes in osteoarthritis; joint inflammation in rheumatoid or gouty arthritis.

Nervous System

Review results of 10-Minute Geriatric Screener, p. 541. Pursue further examination if any deficits. Focus especially on memory and affect.	Distinguish delirium from depression and dementia. See Neurocognitive Disorders: Delirium and Dementia, pp. 146–147, Patient Health Questionnaire (PHQ-9), p. 138, Mini-Cog, p. 139, and Montreal Cognitive Assessment (MoCA), p. 141.
Assess gait and balance, particularly standing balance; timed 8-ft walk; stride characteristics like width, pace, and length of stride; and careful turning.	Abnormalities of gait and balance, especially widening of base, slowing and lengthening of stride, and difficulty turning, are correlated with risk of falls.
Although neurologic abnormalities are common in older adults, their prevalence without identifiable disease increases with age, ranging from 30% to 50%.	Physiologic changes of aging: unequal pupil size, decreased arm swing and spontaneous movements, increased leg rigidity and abnormal gait, presence of the snout and grasp reflexes, and decreased toe vibratory sense.
Assess any tremor, rigidity, bradykinesia, micrographia, shuffling gait, and difficulty turning in bed, opening jars, and rising from a chair.	In Parkinson disease, tremor is slow frequency and at rest, with a "pill-rolling" quality, aggravated by stress and inhibited during sleep or movement.
	Essential tremor is often bilateral, symmetric, with positive family history, and diminished by alcohol use.

RECORDING YOUR FINDINGS

As you read through this physical examination, you will notice some atypical findings. Test yourself to see if you can interpret these findings in the context of all you have learned about the examination of the older adult.

Recording the Older Adult Physical Examination

AJ is an older adult who appears healthy but underweight, with good muscle bulk. He is alert and interactive, with good recall of his life history. He is accompanied by his son.

Vital Signs: Ht (without shoes) 160 cm (5′). Wt (dressed) 65 kg (143 lb). BMI 28. BP 145/88 right arm, supine; 154/94 left arm, supine. Heart rate (HR) 98 and regular. Respiratory rate (RR) 18. Temperature (oral) 98.6°F.

10-Minute Geriatric Screener: (see p. 540)

continued

Vision: Patient reports difficulty reading. Visual acuity 20/60 on Snellen chart.

Hearing: Cannot hear whispered voice in either ear. Cannot hear 1,000 or 2,000 Hz with audioscope in either ear.

Leg Mobility: Can walk 20 ft briskly, turn, walk back to chair, and sit down in 14 sec.

Urinary Incontinence: Has lost urine and gotten wet on 20 separate days.

Nutrition: Has lost 15 lb over the past 6 mo without trying.

Memory: Can remember three items after 1 min.

Depression: Does not often feel sad or depressed.

Physical Disability: Can walk fast but cannot ride a bicycle. Can do moderate but not heavy work around the house. Can go shopping for groceries or clothes. Can get to places out of walking distance. Can bathe each day without difficulty. Can dress, including buttoning and zipping, and can put on shoes.

For the physical examination section, carefully describe your findings for each relevant segment of the peripheral examination, using terminology found in the "Recording Your Findings" sections of the prior chapters.

Needs further evaluation for glasses and possibly hearing aid. Needs further evaluation for incontinence, including "DIAPPERS" assessment (see p. 541), prostate examination, and *postvoid residual,* which is normally ≤50 mL (requires bladder catheterization). Needs nutritional screen (see p. 520). Consider an exercise regimen with strength training.

HEALTH PROMOTION AND COUNSELING: EVIDENCE AND RECOMMENDATIONS

Important Topics for Health Promotion and Counseling in Older Adults

- When to screen
- Screening for vision and hearing impairments
- Exercise and physical activity
- Household safety and fall prevention
- Immunizations
- Cancer screening
- Detecting the "3 Ds": delirium, dementia, and depression
- Elder mistreatment and abuse

When to Screen

As the life span for older adults extends into the 80s, base screening decisions on the older adult's individual health and functional status, including presence of comorbidity, rather than age alone.

The American Geriatrics Society (AGS) recommends a five-step approach to screening decisions:

1. Assess patient preferences
2. Interpret the available evidence
3. Estimate prognosis
4. Consider treatment feasibility
5. Optimize therapies and care plans.

If life expectancy is short, give priority to treatment that benefits the patient in the time that remains. Consider avoiding screening if it overburdens the older adults who have multiple clinical problems, shortened life expectancy, or advanced dementia. Tests that help with prognosis and planning may still be warranted even if the patient does not want to pursue treatment.

Screening for Vision and Hearing Impairments

Among adults aged 65 to 69 years, 1% have visual impairment, increasing to 17% of those over age 80 years. About a third of adults over age 65 years have hearing loss, increasing to 80% in those over age 80 years. Although the U.S. Preventive Services Task Force (USPSTF) has cited insufficient evidence (I statements) to support screening for either hearing loss or impaired visual acuity in older adults, geriatricians recommend screening for *vision* and *hearing* insofar as they are vital sensory modalities for daily living. They are key items in the 10-Minute Geriatric Screener.

Exercise and Physical Activity

Exercise is one of the most effective ways to promote healthy aging. Recommendations emphasize combining aerobic exercise with graded resistance training in major muscle groups to increase strength (Box 27-7).

BOX 27-7. CDC Exercise Recommendations for Older Adults

Adults need at least:
- 2 hrs and 30 min (150 min) of moderate-intensity aerobic activity (i.e., brisk walking) every week *and*
- muscle-strengthening activities on two or more days a week that work all major muscle groups (legs, hips, back, abdomen, chest, shoulders, and arms).

OR
- 1 hr and 15 min (75 min) of vigorous-intensity aerobic activity (i.e., jogging or running) every week *and*
- muscle-strengthening activities on two or more days a week that work all major muscle groups (legs, hips, back, abdomen, chest, shoulders, and arms).

OR
- An equivalent mix of moderate- and vigorous-intensity aerobic activity *and*
- muscle-strengthening activities on two or more days a week that work all major muscle groups (legs, hips, back, abdomen, chest, shoulders, and arms).

Household Safety and Fall Prevention

Approximately 30% of adults aged 65 and older fall each year with a direct clinical cost of $50 billion. Many have hip fractures and traumatic brain injuries that impact daily function and independence (Box 27-8).

BOX 27-8. Household Safety Tips for Older Adults

- Install bright lighting and lightweight curtains or shades.
- Install handrails and lights on all staircases. Pathways and walkways should be well-lit.
- Remove items that cause tripping like papers, books, clothes, and shoes from stairs and walkways.
- Remove or secure small throw rugs and other rugs with double-sided tape.
- Wear shoes both inside and outside the house. Avoid bare feet and wearing slippers.
- Store medications safely.
- Keep commonly used items in cabinets that are easy to reach without using a step stool.

- Install grab bars and nonslip mats or safety strips in baths and showers.
- Repair faulty plugs and electrical cords.
- Install smoke alarms and have a plan for escaping fire.
- Secure all firearms.
- Have a clinical alert device/system for calling a universal emergency number such as 911 or emergency contacts.

Immunizations

A number of vaccines are routinely recommended for older adults in the United States (Box 27-9).

BOX 27-9. Older Adult Immunizations, 2018

- *Influenza vaccination:* One high-dose vaccine annually
- *Tetanus, diphtheria, and acellular pertussis (Tdap) vaccination:* Administer 1 dose to older adults who previously did not receive a dose of tetanus toxoid, reduced diphtheria toxoid, and acellular pertussis vaccine (Tdap) as an adult or child
- *Tetanus and diphtheria toxoids (Td):* One dose Td booster every 10 yrs
- *Varicella vaccination:* Administer 2 doses to older adults without evidence of immunity to varicella 4–8 wks apart
- *Zoster vaccination:* Administer 2 doses of recombinant zoster vaccine (RZV) 2–6 mo apart to adults ≥50 yrs regardless of past episode of herpes zoster or receipt of zoster vaccine live (ZVL)
- *Pneumococcal vaccination:* Administer to immunocompetent older adults 1 dose of *13-valent pneumococcal conjugate vaccine* (PCV13, Prevnar13®) at age 65 yrs or older then followed by 1 dose of *23-valent pneumococcal polysaccharide vaccine* (PPSV23, Pneumovax®23) at least 1 year after PCV13. Once a dose of PPSV23 is given at age 65 yrs or older, no additional doses of PPSV23 should be administered.

Cancer Screening

Cancer screening can be controversial because of limited evidence about adults older than age 70 to 80 years. The USPSTF guidelines are summarized in Box 27-10.

BOX 27-10. Screening Recommendations for Older Adults: U.S. Preventive Services Task Force

- **Breast cancer (2016):** Recommends mammography every 2 yrs for women aged 50–74 yrs (grade B) and cites insufficient evidence for screening women aged ≥75 yrs (I statement).
- **Cervical cancer (2018):** Recommends *against* routine screening for women over age 65 yrs if they have had adequate recent screening with normal Pap smears and are not otherwise at high risk for cervical cancer, based on fair evidence (grade D).
- **Colorectal cancer (2016):** Recommends screening beginning age 50 yrs through age 75 yrs (grade A). Available strategies and screening intervals include colonoscopy every 10 yrs, CT colonography every 5 yrs, annual fecal immunochemical test, annual high-sensitivity fecal occult blood test (FOBT), fecal DNA test every 1 or 3 yrs, or flexible sigmoidoscopy every 5 yrs. Recommends that routine screening for adults aged 76–85 yrs be an individual one, considering the patient's overall health and prior screening history due to moderate certainty that the net benefit is small (grade C).
- **Prostate cancer (2018):** Recommends that prostate-specific antigen (PSA)-based screening for prostate cancer for men aged 55–69 yrs be an individual one with incorporation of the patient's values and preferences in the decision due to moderate certainty that the net benefit is small (grade C). Before deciding whether to screen, a discussion of the potential benefits and harms of screening with their clinician should occur. Recommends *against* PSA-based screening for prostate cancer in men 70 yrs and older due to evidence that expected harms are greater than expected benefits.
- **Lung cancer (2014):** For adults aged 55–80 yrs with a 30-pack year smoking history, and those who currently smoke or have quit within the past 15 yrs, recommends annual screening with low-dose computed tomography (grade B). Screening should be *discontinued* once a person has not smoked for 15 yrs or develops a health problem that substantially limits life expectancy or the ability or willingness to have curative lung surgery.
- **Skin cancer (2016):** States that evidence is insufficient to balance the benefits and harms of whole-body skin examination by a clinician (I statement).

The American College of Physicians (ACP) has developed high- and low-value screening strategies that factor in health benefits, frequency of screening, and harms and costs (Box 27-11).

BOX 27-11. Low-Value Screening for Five Types of Cancer in Adults >65 Years

Cancer Type	Screening Strategy	Low Value (not recommended)
Breast	Any screening	Older adult women ≥75 yrs or older adult women ≥65 yrs not in good health and with life expectancy <10 yrs
Cervical	Any screening	Older adult women >65 yrs with previous recent negative screening results
Colorectal	Any screening	Older adults >75 yrs or older adults ≥65 yrs not in good health and with life expectancy <10 yrs
	Colonoscopy	Older adults 65–74 yrs with normal colonic examination results (i.e., without adenomatous polyps) within the last 10 yrs or normal flexible sigmoidoscopy results within the last 5 yrs
Prostate	PSA testing	Older adult men 65–69 yrs who have had an informed discussion and have not expressed a clear preference for testing after the discussion
		Older adult men >69 yrs or older adult men 65–69 yrs and not in good health and have a life expectancy <10 yrs

Detecting the "3 Ds": Delirium, Dementia, and Depression

Delirium. *Delirium* is an acute confusional state characterized by sudden onset, fluctuating course, inattention, and at times alteration of consciousness. Upon hospital admission, approximately 11% to 25% of older adult patients will have delirium and an additional 29% to 31% of older adult patients admitted without delirium will develop delirium. The Confusion Assessment Method (CAM) is recommended for screening at-risk patients (p. 142).

Dementia. *Dementia* is an acquired condition that is characterized by a decline in at least two cognitive domains that is severe enough to affect social or occupational functioning. In the DSM-5, delirium and dementia fall under the new category of *neurocognitive disorders.* One of the aims of this reclassification includes reducing stigma associated with dementia. The most common types are Alzheimer disease (affecting 5 million Americans over age 65 years), Lewy body dementia, and frontotemporal dementia. Diagnosing dementia requires exclusion of delirium and depression. Use recommended screening tests for dementia such as the Mini-Cog (p. 139) or the Montreal Cognitive Assessment (MoCA) (p. 141).

Depression. Depression affects 5% to 7% of community-dwelling older adults and approximately 10% of older men and 18% of older women but is often undiagnosed. Use the Patient Health Questionnaire-PHQ (p. 138) and the Geriatric Depression Scale in older adults (p. 113).

Elder Mistreatment and Abuse

Screen older patients for possible *elder mistreatment,* which includes *abuse, neglect, exploitation,* and *abandonment.* Prevalence ranges from 5% to 10% of older adults; however, many cases remain undetected. *Self-neglect,* or "the behavior of an older adult person that threatens his/her own health and safety," is also a growing national concern and represents more the 50% of adult protective service referrals.

In its 2018 review, the USPSTF found no valid, reliable screening tools in the primary care setting to identify abuse of older or vulnerable adults without recognized signs and symptoms of abuse and therefore cited insufficient evidence for recommending screening (I statement). Consequently, a careful history and high index of suspicion are important.

INTERPRETATION AIDS

TABLE 27-1. Selected Normal Anatomic and Physiologic Changes with Aging and Related Disease Outcomes

Normal Changes in Anatomy and Physiology	Clinical Manifestations and Disease Outcomes
Cardiovascular	
■ Increase in thickness of left ventricular wall, involving both myocyte hypertrophy and increase in collagen deposition secondary to decreased turnover of these cells	1. Decrease in early diastolic cardiac filling, increase in cardiac filling pressure and lower threshold for dyspnea
■ Myocardial thickening combined with lipofuscin deposits, fatty infiltration, and fibrosis	2. Left ventricular stiffness and thus a fourth heart sound
■ Dilation of left atrium	3. Lone atrial fibrillation
■ Loss of about 10% of pacemaker cells every decade	4. Sinus arrest or tachy-brady syndrome
■ Increased fibrosis, myocyte hypertrophy, and calcium deposition	5. Prolonged PR and QRS intervals and right bundle-branch block
■ Increase in dilation, elasticity and rigidity of arterial walls, with decrease in sensitivity to receptor-mediated agents	6. Atherosclerosis
■ Increase in peripheral resistance and decrease in central arterial compliance	7. Systolic hypertension
	8. Stroke
Respiratory	
■ Decrease in number and elasticity of parenchymal elastic fibers, the latter in part because of decrease in collagen levels	1. Gradual loss of elastic recoil of lungs
■ Less effective ciliary action	2. Smaller airway size, with airway collapse in lower lung zone
■ Less compliant and stiffer chest wall	3. Increase in susceptibility to respiratory infections

continued

TABLE 27-1. Selected Normal Anatomic and Physiologic Changes with Aging and Related Disease Outcomes (continued)

Normal Changes in Anatomy and Physiology	Clinical Manifestations and Disease Outcomes
■ Weaker respiratory muscles and diaphragm, the latter by about 25% ■ Decrease in forced expiratory volume and forced vital capacity (30% by age 80) ■ Increase in residual volume by about 20 mL/yr	4. Decrease in both quiet breathing (effort-independent) 5. Decrease in forced breathing (effort-dependent) 6. Decrease in PaO_2 due to ventilation–perfusion mismatching. (*Acceptable PaO2 = 100 – [0.32 age]*) 7. Decrease in pulmonary reserve and exercise tolerance
Gastrointestinal ■ Increase in tongue varicosities ■ Decrease in saliva production ■ Increase in nonperistaltic spontaneous contractions of esophagus ■ Decrease in stomach acid production ■ Decreased gastric acid clearance ■ Slowed gastric emptying after fatty meal, prolonging gastric distention ■ Decrease in gut-associated lymphoid tissue ■ Atrophy of large intestine mucosa ■ Decrease in tensile strength of colonic smooth muscle ■ Decrease in effectiveness of colonic contractions and sensitivity of rectal wall ■ Decrease in calcium absorption ■ Atheromata in large intestine vessels ■ Decrease in liver size and blood flow	1. Increase in oral infections and gum disease 2. Dysphagia 3. Atrophic gastritis (in those >70 yrs, the incidence of atrophic gastritis is 16%) 4. Decrease in vitamin B12 and iron absorption 5. Gastroesophageal reflux disease 6. Increasing meal-induced satiety 7. Impaired response to gastric mucosal injury, thus increasing risk of both gastric and duodenal ulcers 8. Increase in diverticulosis 9. Frequent constipation 10. Bone loss 11. Chronic intestinal ischemia 12. Impaired clearance of drugs requiring phase I metabolism

TABLE 27-1. Selected Normal Anatomic and Physiologic Changes with Aging and Related Disease Outcomes *(continued)*

Normal Changes in Anatomy and Physiology	Clinical Manifestations and Disease Outcomes
▪ Decrease in pancreatic mass and enzyme reserves ▪ Hyperplasia of pancreatic duct ▪ Increase in pancreatic cyst formation, fatty deposition and deposition of lipofuscin granules in acinar cells	13. Decrease in insulin secretion and increase in insulin resistance
Urinary ▪ Decrease in number and length of functional renal tubules ▪ Increase in tubular diverticula and basement membrane thickness ▪ Altered vascular pattern, atherosclerotic changes, altered arteriole-glomerular flow and focal ischemic lesions ▪ Decrease in creatinine clearance and glomerular filtration rate, the latter by about 10 mL/decade ▪ Decrease in concentrating and diluting capacity of kidneys ▪ Decrease in serum renin and aldosterone by about 30–50% ▪ Decrease in vitamin D activation	1. Impaired permeability and decreased ability to resorb glucose 2. Decreased renal blood flow with a selective loss of cortical vasculature 3. Decrease in elimination of drugs and toxins 4. Fluid and electrolyte abnormalities causing increased volume depletion and dehydration, hyperkalemia and decrease in sodium and potassium excretion and conservation 5. Vitamin D deficiency
Immunologic/Hematologic ▪ Average decline in function, including more stimulus and time required for activation ▪ Decrease in T cell function ▪ Decrease in naive T cells and increase in memory T cells ▪ Gradual decrease in B-cell function	1. Reduced primary and secondary responses to infection 2. Reduced body's ability to mount immune response to new pathogens 3. Production of abnormal antibodies

continued

TABLE 27-1. Selected Normal Anatomic and Physiologic Changes with Aging and Related Disease Outcomes *(continued)*

Normal Changes in Anatomy and Physiology	Clinical Manifestations and Disease Outcomes
■ Decrease in response of naive B cells to new antigens ■ Atrophy of thymus ■ Loss of ability of hematopoietic stem cells to self-renew ■ Decrease in rate of erythropoiesis and incorporation of iron into red blood cells	4. Decrease in production and functioning of T lymphocytes 5. Decrease in proliferation of natural killer cells 6. Decrease in production of cytokines needed for maturation of B cells 7. Dysfunctional immune system 8. Slight decrease in average values of both hemoglobin and hematocrit
Sensory Organs Vision ■ Loss of periorbital fat ■ Laxity of eyelids ■ Thickening and yellowing of lens combined with lipid infiltrate accumulations (arcus senilus) ■ Increase in fibrosis of iris ■ Increase in lens size and rigidity due to constant formation of central epithelial cells at front of lens ■ Progressive increase in annular layers of lens ■ Compression of central components that become hard and opaque ■ Decrease in lacrimation Hearing ■ Thickening of tympanic membrane and loss in its elasticity as well as in efficiency of its ossicular articulation	1. Sunken eyes 2. Senile entropion and ectropion 3. Increase in vulnerability to conjunctivitis 4. Decrease in transparency of cornea 5. Decreases accommodation and slows dark adaptation 6. Presbyopia 7. Increase in rate of cataract formation 8. Dry eye syndrome 9. Conductive deafness affecting low-frequency sounds 10. Sensorineural hearing loss of high-frequency sounds 11. Difficulty discriminating source of sound 12. Impaired discrimination of target from noise

TABLE 27-1. Selected Normal Anatomic and Physiologic Changes with Aging and Related Disease Outcomes *(continued)*

Normal Changes in Anatomy and Physiology	Clinical Manifestations and Disease Outcomes
■ Decrease in the elasticity and efficiency of ossicular articulation ■ Increasing deficit in central processing Smell and Thirst ■ Decrease in smell detection by about 50% ■ Decrease in thirst drive ■ Impaired control of thirst by endorphins	13. Diminished ability to enjoy food and decrease in appetite 14. Dehydration
Dermatologic ■ Decrease in skin elasticity ■ Decrease in barrier function ■ Slower cell replacement ■ Ineffective DNA repair ■ Altered mechanical protection and decrease in sensory perception ■ Decrease in immunologic and inflammatory responses ■ Decrease in sweating and effectiveness of thermoregulation ■ Decrease in vitamin D production ■ Loss of melanocytes at base of hair follicles ■ Slowing of linear nail growth	1. Lax skin 2. Dry skin 3. Rough skin with delayed healing 4. Increase in rate of photocarcinogenesis 5. Greater susceptibility to injury 6. Chronic low-grade infections and impaired wound healing, with persistent wounds and weak scars 7. Tendency toward hyperthermia and greater vulnerability to both heat and cold 8. Osteomalacia 9. Gray hair 10. Nails thicker, duller and more brittle, opaque and yellow, with development of longitudinal ridges

continued

TABLE 27-1. Selected Normal Anatomic and Physiologic Changes with Aging and Related Disease Outcomes *(continued)*

Normal Changes in Anatomy and Physiology	Clinical Manifestations and Disease Outcomes
Nervous System Central Nervous System ■ Decrease in weight of brain and cerebral blood flow by about 20% ■ Decrease in number and functioning of nerve cells ■ Less fluid and stiffer cell membranes in brain neurons ■ Irregularity in structure of internal membranes ■ Accumulation of lipofuscin and tangled neurofibrils ■ Decrease in ability of neuron to grow branches of both axons and dendrites[4] Peripheral Nervous System ■ Age-related changes in somatic motor function ■ Slower action potentials and spreading of muscle cell contraction ■ Lower peak strength of muscle contractions, with slower relaxation	1. After age 70, gradual decrease in vocabulary, with increase in semantic errors and abnormal prosody 2. Increased forgetfulness in noncritical areas, which does not affect function or impair recall of important memories 3. After age 80, slower central processing, which prolongs time to complete tasks 4. Decrease in fine motor control 5. Decrease in cells that can be stimulated and decrease in maximum strength of muscular contractions 6. Prolonged time required for impulses to arrive, muscle cells to contract and movements to be initiated 7. Decrease in maximal muscle strength when performing quick movements
Musculoskeletal Muscle ■ Decrease in muscle fibers (mainly type II—fast twitch) ■ Replacement of lost muscle tissue with tough fibrous tissue Bone ■ Decrease in vitamin D absorption, which decreases osteoblasts	1. Decrease in muscle mass (sarcopenia), leading to lean body mass 2. Thin, bony appearance to hands 3. Brittle bone 4. Greater susceptibility to fracture, with slower healing 5. Osteoporosis

TABLE 27-1. Selected Normal Anatomic and Physiologic Changes with Aging and Related Disease Outcomes *(continued)*

Normal Changes in Anatomy and Physiology	Clinical Manifestations and Disease Outcomes
■ Decrease in bone formation and modeling by osteoblasts and osteoclasts, impairing bone microarchitecture Joints ■ Decrease in thickness of articular cartilage, though not in nonarticular cartilage ■ Stiffer collagen, resulting in disordered cartilage matrix	6. Dorsal kyphosis 7. Less ability to handle mechanical stresses 8. Joint breakdown, including inflammation, pain, stiffness and deformity 9. Overall decrease and limitation in movement 10. Decrease in arm swing and steadiness of walking
Endocrine Pituitary gland ■ Minimal changes but on average, decrease in pulsatile secretion pattern, including nocturnal pulsatile secretion of prolactin Pineal gland ■ Decrease in diurnal melatonin rhythm Thyroid gland ■ Atrophy, with increased fibrosis and nodule formation ■ Decrease in T4 production in the very old (If aging is normal, blood thyroxine concentration continues unchanged even though T4 production decreases) Parathyroid glands ■ In women over age 40 yrs, increase in parathyroid hormone and decrease in metabolism, with associated decrease in 1,25 (OH) vitamin D levels and changes in bone mineral homeostasis	1. Decrease in size of various structures 2. Decrease in lean body mass to fat ratio 3. Insomnia 4. Deficit in free-radical defenses 5. Increase in rate of hypo- and hyperthyroidism 6. Vitamin D deficiency 7. Orthostatic hypotension 8. Masculinization of postmenopausal women 9. Decrease in immune function increasing the risk of infection and cancer 10. Changes in skin, hair, muscle, and bone and decrease in body fat, despite increase in leptin 11. Skin changes, increase in LDL and decrease in bone minerals 12. Decrease in body fat

continued

TABLE 27-1. Selected Normal Anatomic and Physiologic Changes with Aging and Related Disease Outcomes *(continued)*

Normal Changes in Anatomy and Physiology	Clinical Manifestations and Disease Outcomes
Adrenal gland ■ Moderate decrease in aldosterone secretion ■ In postmenopausal women, increase in androgen secretion Thymus ■ Decrease in immune function Male gonads ■ Large decrease in estrogen and progesterone ■ After age 70, decrease in leptin	

TABLE 27-2. Timed Get Up and Go Test

Performed with patient wearing regular footwear, using usual walking aid if needed, and sitting back in a chair with armrest.

On the word, "Go," the patient is asked to do the following:

1. Stand up from the armless chair
2. Walk 3 m (in a line)
3. Turn
4. Walk back to chair
5. Sit down

Repeat. Time the second effort.

Observe patient for postural stability, steppage, stride length, and sway.

Scoring:

1. *Normal:* completes task in <10 sec
2. *Abnormal:* completes task in >20 sec
   Low scores correlate with good functional independence; high scores correlate with poor functional independence and higher risk of falls.

Sources: Get-up and Go Test. In: Mathias S, et al. "Balance in elderly patient" The "Get Up and Go" Test. *Arch Phys Med Rehabil.* 1986;67:387–389; Podsiadlo D, Richardson S. The Timed "Up and Go": A test of basic functional mobility for frail elderly persons. *J Am Geriatr Soc.* 1991;39:142–148.

Index

Note: Page numbers followed by "*a*," "*b*," "*f*," and "*t*" indicate algorithm, boxed material, figure, and end-of-chapter tables, respectively.

A

ABCDE rule, for melanoma, 158, 159*b*–160*b*
Abdomen, 60
  auscultation, 305
  in children, 475
  examination techniques, 304–310
  health history, 299–303
  health promotion and counseling, 311–318
  in infant, 468
  inspection, 305–306
  in older adults, 545
  pain in (*See* Abdominal pain)
  palpation, 306, 306*f*
  percussion, 306
  in pregnancy, 514–515, 514*f*
  recording findings, 311
Abdominal aortic aneurysm (AAA), 270, 278–279
  in older adults, 545
  risk factors, 278
  screening for, 278–279
Abdominal masses, 306, 306*f*
Abdominal pain
  acute, 301
  approach to patient with, 314*a*
  chronic, 301
  GI symptoms associated with, 302
  left lower quadrant pain, 301, 317*a*
  mechanisms of, 299–300
  in pregnancy, 506*b*, 526*a*
  referred pain, 300*b*
  right lower quadrant pain, 301, 316*a*
  right upper quadrant pain, 301, 315*a*
  somatic/parietal pain, 300*b*
  visceral pain, 299*b*
Abdominal striae, 506*b*
Abdominal tenderness, 305, 322*t*
  from disease in chest and pelvis, 322*t*
  peritoneal, 322*t*
  visceral, 322*t*

Abnormal uterine bleeding, approach to patient with, 345*a*
Absolute risk difference, 111*b*
Acne vulgaris, 164*t*
Acoustic neuroma, 201*b*
Acromioclavicular arthritis, 406*t*
Actinic keratosis, 165*t*
Actinic lentigines, 543
Adams bend test, 481
Addiction, 123*b*
Adolescents
  breasts, 480
  development surveillance, 479, 479*b*
  examination techniques, 480–481
  gender and sexual identity formation, 480
  health history, 477–480
  HEEADSSS assessment, 478, 478*b*
  male and female genitalia, 480
  musculoskeletal system, 481
  sports preparticipation, 481, 499*t*–502*t*
Advance directives, 26, 539
Affect, in mental status examination, 133, 133*b*
Alcoholic hepatitis, 303*b*
Alcohol Use Disorders Identification Test–Consumption (AUDIT-C), 92, 538
Alcohol use, unhealthy, 91
  behavioral counseling for, 92
  Screening, Brief Intervention, and Referral to Treatment (SBIRT) Program, 92–93
  screening for, 91–92, 91*b*
Algorithm
  abdominal pain, 314*a*–318*a*
  abnormal uterine bleeding, 345*a*
  back pain, 401*a*
  breast discomfort/pain, 294*a*
  breast lump/mass, 293*a*
  chest pain, 259*a*
  cough, 232*a*

Algorithm (*continued*)
depression, 143*a*
dizziness, 207*a*
dyspnea, 231*a*
eyelids, swollen, 194*a*
fatigue, 126*a*
headache, 435*a*
hearing loss, 209*a*
hemoptysis, 233*a*
hoarseness, 215*a*
knee pain, 402
leg discoloration, 282
leg pain, 280*a*
leg swelling, 281
memory impairment, 144*a*
murmur, 261*a*
musculoskeletal complaints, 399*a*
neck mass, 181*a*
nipple discharge, 295*a*
numbness, 436*a*
palpitations, 260*a*
pelvic pain, 347*a*
penile mass/lesion, 328*a*
pregnant patient, abdominal pain
in, 526*a*
red eyes, bilateral, 192*a*
red eyes, unilateral, 193*a*
rhinitis, 208*a*
scrotal mass/pain, 329*a*
shoulder pain, 400*a*
skin primary lesion, 161*a*
urinary incontinence, 318*a*
urinary symptoms, 359*a*
vaginal bleeding in pregnant woman,
527*a*
vaginal discharge in pregnant
woman, 528*a*
vulvovaginal symptoms, 337*a*
weakness, 437*a*
Allen test, 276–277, 276*f*–277*f*
Alopecia, 150
areata, 173*t*
Ambiguous genitalia, 468
Amenorrhea, 336
in pregnancy, 336, 506*b*
primary, 336
secondary, 336
Anagen effluvium, 172*t*
Anal fissure, 355, 361*t*
Anal warts, 355
Anatomic snuffbox, 379, 379*f*
Aneurysm, abdominal aortic, 270, 308
in older adults, 545
risk factors, 278
screening for, 278–279

Angina pectoris, 262*t*
Angioedema, 216*t*
Angular cheilitis, 216*t*
Ankle–brachial index (ABI), 275,
275*b*–276*b*, 278
Ankle jerks, 426
Ankles and feet
examination of, 393–394, 394*f*,
394*t*
range of motion, 394*b*
Anorectal fistula, 361*t*
Anorexia nervosa, 302
Anterior drawer sign, 391, 391*f*
Anus
examination techniques, 355, 356*f*,
357
health history, 354–355
recording findings, 357
Anxiety
risk factors, 128–129
screening questions for, 129*b*
Aorta, palpation, 308, 308*f*
Aortic aneurysm, dissecting, 263*t*
Aortic valve stenosis, 493*t*
Apgar scoring system, 457, 457*b*
Aphasia, 444*t*
Broca, 444*t*–445*t*
Wernicke, 444*t*–445*t*
Aphonia, 444*t*
Aphthous ulcer, 219*t*
Appearance, in mental status
examination, 133
Appendicitis, 310–311
McBurney point, 310, 310*f*
obturator sign, 310
psoas sign, 310
Rovsing sign, 310
Arcus senilis, 543
Arms
brachial pulse, 272, 272*f*
pain in, 269
radial pulse, 272, 272*f*
Arterial insufficiency, chronic, 284*t*
Arterial pulses, 272, 272*b*, 272*f*
Arthritis
acromioclavicular, 406*t*
knee, 407*t*
monoarticular, 366
osteoarthritis, 403*t*–404*t*
rheumatoid, 403*t*–404*t*
Ascites, assessment of, 309, 309*f*
Assessment, documentation of, 71,
71*b*–74*b*
Asterixis, 429
Ataxia, 413

Athetosis, 448*t*
Atrial fibrillation, 121
Atrial septal defect, 467
Attention
    in mental status examination, 132*b*, 135
    in neurocognitive disorders, 147*t*
Automated ambulatory blood pressure monitoring, 116

B

Babinski response, 427, 427*f*
Back pain, low, 369, 396, 405*t*
    approach to patient with, 401*a*
    chronic back stiffness, 405*t*
    lumbar spinal stenosis, 405*t*
    mechanical, 405*t*
    nocturnal back pain, 405*t*
    pain referred from abdomen/pelvis, 405*t*
    prevalence of, 396
    radicular, 405*t*
    red flags for, from underlying systemic disease, 369*b*
Bacterial vaginosis, 350*b*
Balloon sign, 392, 392*f*
Barlow test, 469, 469*f*
Basal cell carcinoma (BCC), 166*t*
    nodular, 166*t*
Behavior
    in mental status examination, 133
    in neurocognitive disorders, 146*t*
Behavioral counseling, 84
    guidelines for adults, 86*b*, 90*b*
    for healthful diet, 87–88, 87*b*, 88*b*
    motivational interviewing, 85, 85*b*
    for physical activity, 89–90, 89*b*
    for sexually transmitted infections, 93
    for tobacco use, 92–93, 93*b*
    transtheoretical model for behavioral change, 84, 84*b*–85*b*
    for unhealthy alcohol use, 91–92
    for weight loss, 86, 86*b*
Benign prostatic hyperplasia (BPH), 355, 362*t*
    BPH symptom score index, 360*t*
Bias
    anchoring, 69*b*
    attrition, 110*b*
    in clinical encounters, 11, 11*b*
    confirmation, 69*b*
    detection, 110*b*
    explicit, 11
    implicit, 11
    institutional, 11

performance, 109*b*
    selection, 109*b*
    visceral, 69*b*
Bicipital tendinitis, 406*t*
Blepharitis, 197*t*
Blindness, legal, 191
Bloating, 301
Blood in stool, 355
Blood pressure
    categories, 255*b*
    cuff selection, 117*b*
    diastolic, 120, 120*b*
    and dietary sodium, 125
    inaccuracy in measurement of, 118*b*
    during infancy, 461, 461*f*
    isolated systolic, 120
    measurement of, 116, 119*b*, 245
    of older adults, 542
    orthostatic (postural), 120
    screening for, 254
    steps for measurement of, 118*b*
    systolic, 119, 120*b*
Blount disease, 476
Body dysmorphic disorder, 145*t*
Body mass index (BMI), 82, 82*b*, 116
    calculation of, 116*b*
Bowel sounds, 311
Bradycardia, 461
Brain, 410, 410*f*. *See also* Nervous system
Braxton Hicks contractions, 506*b*
Breast cancer
    peau d'orange sign, 297*t*
    relative risk factors, 298*t*
    retraction signs, 297*t*
    risk assessment, 290–291, 291*b*
    risk factors, 290*b*
    screening, 291, 291*b*–292*b*
    visible signs of, 297*t*–298*t*
Breast discomfort/pain
    approach to patient with, 294*a*
    health history, 285
Breast lump/mass
    approach to patient with, 293*a*
    health history, 285
    palpable masses, 296*t*
Breasts
    axillae, 289
    examination techniques, 286–289
    female breast, 286–288, 286*f*–288*f*
    health history, 285
    health promotion and counseling, 290–292
    male breast, 289
    in pregnancy, 506*b*, 513
    recording findings, 289

Breathing, abnormalities in, 239*t*
Breech presentation, 517
Broca aphasia, 444*t*–445*t*
Brudzinski sign, 428
Bruits, 246, 305, 305*f*
   arterial, 305
   hepatic, 305
Bulge sign, 392, 392*f*
Bulimia nervosa, 127*t*
Bullae, 163*t*
Burrows, 165*t*

C

Cancer
   oral cavity, 214
   prostate, 362*t*
   rectum, 362*t*
   skin, 157–160
   thyroid, 180
Candida vaginitis, 350*t*
Canker sore, 219*t*
Carcinoma
   of cervix, 351*t*
   of lip, 217*t*
   of penis, 332*t*
   of tongue, 219*t*
   of vulva, 349*t*
Cardiac examination
   auscultation, 248–249, 248*f*, 249*f*
   inspection and palpation, 247–248,
      247*f*
   murmurs, 250, 251*b*
   patient positions and sequence for,
      247*b*
   squatting and standing, 251
   Valsalva maneuver, 250
Cardiovascular disease (CVD), 253
   CVD risk calculators, 254, 254*b*
   diabetes and, 255, 255*b*, 257*b*
   dyslipidemias and, 256, 257*f*
   family history and, 256–258
   hypertension and, 254, 255*b*
   lifestyle modifications for risk
      reduction, 258, 258*b*
   metabolic syndrome and, 256
   obesity and, 256–258
   risk factors, screening for,
      253–258
   smoking and, 256–258
Cardiovascular system, 60
   examination techniques, 244–250
   health history, 243–244
   health promotion and counseling,
      252–258
   recording findings, 252

Carotid pulse, 246
Carpal tunnel syndrome, 378
   testing for, 381*f*, 382*f*
Caviar lesions, 219*t*
Cellulitis, 269
Central nervous system (CNS), 409,
      409*f*. *See also* Nervous system
   brain, 410, 410*f*
   spinal cord, 410
Cerebrovascular disease, prevention of,
      433–434, 433*b*–434*b*
Cerumen, 202
Cervical cancer
   prevention of, 343
   risk factor for, 343
   screening, 344, 344*b*
Cervical lymph nodes, palpation of,
      177–178
Cervicitis, mucopurulent, 340, 351*t*
Cervix
   abnormalities of, 351*t*
   carcinoma of, 351*t*
   inspection, 341
Chalazion, 197*t*
Chancroid, 331*t*
Cherry angioma, 170*t*
Chest pain, 243, 262*t*–263*t*
   anterior, 243
   anxiety/panic disorder and, 263*t*
   approach to patient with, 259*a*
   cardiovascular problem and,
      262*t*–263*t*
   gastrointestinal problem and,
      263*t*
   pulmonary disease and, 262*t*
Chest wall pain, 263*t*
Children, 453. *See also* School-aged
      children/early childhood
   body mass index for age, 471
   clinical encounter with, 454,
      454*b*
   cognitive development, 453
   development principles, 453
   health history, 455–456
   health promotion in, 486–487,
      486*b*–487*b*
   heart murmurs in, 474, 475*f*
   hypertension in, 471
   immunizations, 456
   language development, 453
   otoscopic examination in, 474,
      473*b*
   physical development, 453
   physical examination, 456
   recording findings, 481–485

screening, 456
sexual abuse in, 495*t*
social and emotional development, 453
surveillance of development, 453
visual acuity in, 471*b*
Chills, 112
Cholecystitis, acute, 311
Chorea, 448*t*
Clinical breast exam (CBE), 291
Clinical encounter, 1, 1*f*
clinician-centered approach, 1
closing session, 10
documentation of, 15–17
enhanced Calgary-Cambridge Guides, 1*f*
environment for, 2
explaining and planning, 9–10
greeting patient in, 3
information gathering, 8–9
initial rapport, establishing, 3, 3*b*–4*b*, 5, 5*b*–6*b*
initiating encounter, 2–7
oral presentation, 76, 76*b*–78*b*
patient-centered approach, 1
patient's perspective of illness in, 8, 8*b*, 9*b*
physical examination, 9
structure and sequence of, 2–10, 2*b*
Clinical evidence
biases affecting, 109, 109*b*
critical appraisal of, 108–111
differential diagnosis, 102
evaluation of, 102–111
Fagan nomogram, 106, 107*f*
Kappa score, 106–107, 108*b*
likelihood ratios, 105–106, 106*b*
precision, 108
predictive values, 104, 104*t*
prevalence of disease, 104–105, 104*b*
reproducibility of findings, 106–108
sensitivity and specificity, 103–104
statistics use, 110, 110*b*–111*b*
validity of findings, 103–105
Clinical reasoning, process of, 65
basic structure of, 65*b*
clinical hypothesis, 67, 67*b*
clinical information, organizing and interpreting, 68
cognitive errors in, 69, 69*b*
diagnostic and treatment strategy, 69–70
differential diagnosis, memory aids for, 67, 67*b*–68*b*

illness scripts, 68, 68*b*
initial patient information, gathering, 65
problem representation, 66, 66*b*–67*b*
and progress note, 75, 75*b*–76*b*
testing hypotheses, 68
working diagnosis, 69
Clinical record, 2, 14
abbreviations in, 17, 17*b*–18*b*
purpose of, 14
quality, checklist for, 15*b*–16*b*
Clubbing of fingers, 174*t*
Cognitive functions, in mental status examination, 133*b*, 135–136
Cogwheel rigidity, 449*t*
Cold sore, 216*t*
Colorectal cancer, screening for, 313, 313*b*
Coma
Glasgow Coma Scale, 451*t*
metabolic and structural, 450*t*
Comatose patient
assessment of, 429–431
doll's eye movement, 430, 431*f*
level of consciousness, 429, 429*b*
neurologic examination, 430–431
pupils in, 452*t*
Communication
Ask-Tell-Ask framework, 27
broaching sensitive topics, 24, 24*b*
disclosing serious news, SPIKES protocol for, 26, 26*b*–27*b*
informed consent, 24
interpreters, use of, 24–25, 25*b*
interprofessional, 27, 27*b*
nonverbal, 23
skilled interviewing (*See* Interviewing, skilled)
Condylomata acuminata. *See* Genital warts
Confusion Assessment Method (CAM), 142*b*
Congenital hip dysplasia, 469
Consciousness, level of, 429, 430*b*
Constipation, 302
in pregnancy, 506*b*
Constitutional symptoms, 112
Control event rate (CER), 111*b*
Conversion disorder, 145*t*
Coordination, testing, 421, 421*f*
Corneal light reflex test, 471, 471*f*
Cough, 236*t*–238*t*
approach to patient with, 232*a*
Cover–uncover test, 471, 471*f*

Cozen test, 377, 377*f*
Cranial nerves (CNs), 411
  CN I (olfactory), 416
  CN II (optic), 416
  CN II, III (optic and oculomotor), 416
  CN III, IV, VI (oculomotor, trochlear, and abducens), 416
  CN IX, X (glossopharyngeal and vagus), 417
  CN V (trigeminal), 416, 416*f*
  CN VII (facial), 417
  CN VIII (vestibulocochlear), 417
  CN XI (spinal accessory), 417–418, 417*f*
  CN XII (hypoglossal), 418
  function, 411*b*
  in young children, assessment of, 477*b*
Crohn disease, 320*t*
Cryptorchidism, 333*t*
Cultural humility
  defined, 12
  5Rs of, 12*b*
Cyst
  Baker, 408*t*
  epidermoid, 348*t*
  epididymal, 334*t*
  pilar, 164*t*
Cystocele, 353*t*
Cystourethrocele, 353*t*

D

Decisional capacity, 14, 14*b*
Deep venous thrombosis (DVT), 269, 271, 273
Delirium, 130, 146*t*–147*t*
  in older adults, 553
  screening for, 142, 142*b*
Dementia, 130, 146*b*, 146*t*–147*t*
  clinical features, 146*b*
  in older adults, 553–554
  screening for, 137–140, 139*b*–140*b*
Dental caries, in children, 474, 474*f*
Depression, 129
  approach to patient with, 143*a*
  Patient Health Questionnaire (PHQ-9), 138*b*–139*b*
  perinatal, 523
  screening for, 137, 138*b*
  screening questions for, 129*b*–130*b*
Dermatitis, seborrheic, 162*t*
Dermatofibroma, 164*t*
Dermatomes, 423, 423*f*
Developmental delay, causes of, 470

Diabetes
  diagnosis of, 256*b*
  screening for, 255*b*
Diabetic retinopathy
  nonproliferative, moderately severe, 198*t*
  nonproliferative, severe, 198*t*
  proliferative, advanced, 198*t*
  proliferative, with neovascularization, 198*t*
Diagnostic and Statistical Manual of Mental Disorders, Fifth Edition (DSM-5), 128
Diarrhea, 302, 319*t*–320*t*
  acute, 302, 319*t*
  chronic, 302, 319*t*–320*t*
  drug-induced, 319*t*
  osmotic, 320*t*
  secretory, 320*t*
  voluminous, 320*t*
Diastolic blood pressure (DBP), 120, 120*b*
Diphtheria, 220*t*
Diplopia, 184, 413
Discriminative sensation, testing, 424, 424*f*
Dissociative disorder, 145*t*
Dizziness, 412
Dress, in mental status examination, 133
Drop-arm test, 376*b*
Drusen, 544
Dysarthria, 413, 444*t*
Dysesthesias, 423
Dyslipidemias, 256, 257*f*
Dysmenorrhea, 337
  primary, 337
  secondary, 337
Dyspepsia, 301
Dysphagia, 176, 302
Dysphonia, 444*t*
Dysplastic nevus, 168*t*
Dyspnea, 176, 234*t*–235*t*, 243–244
  approach to patient with, 231*a*
  orthopnea, 243
  paroxysmal nocturnal, 243
Dysuria, 303

E

Ears
  dizziness, 199; approach to patient with, 207*a*
  examination techniques, 201–205
  health history, 199–201
  health promotion and counseling, 206–209

hearing loss, 199, 209*a*
presyncope, 201
recording findings, 205–206
tympanic membrane abnormalities, 210*t*
vertigo, 199, 200*b*–201*b*
Eating disorders, 127*t*
Ecchymosis, 171*t*
Ectropion, 196*t*
Edema, 244
in pregnancy, 506*b*
scrotal, 332*t*
Edinburgh Postnatal Depression Scale (EPDS), 523
Elbow
Cozen test, 377, 377*f*
examination of, 376–377, 377*b*, 377*f*
range of motion, 394*b*
Elder abuse, 83
Electronic thermometer, 122*b*
Empty can test, 376*b*
Endocervical polyp, 351*t*
Entropion, 196*t*
Epidermoid cyst, 348*t*
Epididymis, 325
abnormalities of, 334*t*
cyst of, 334*t*
Epididymitis, acute, 334*t*
Epigastric pain, 300
Episcleritis, 197*t*
Epistaxis, 201
Epitrochlear nodes, 272
Esophageal spasm, diffuse, 263*t*
Ethical dilemma, clinical, 14, 14*b*–15*b*
Exercise
for older adults, 549, 550*t*
during pregnancy, 521
Exophthalmos, 196*t*
Experimental event rate (EER), 110*b*
Extraocular muscles, assessment of, 186, 186*f*
Eyelids
physical findings in, 196*t*
swollen, approach to patient with, 194*a*
Eyes
double vision, 184
examination techniques, 184–190
health history, 183–184
health promotion and counseling, 191
pain, redness, or tearing, 184
physical findings in and around, 196*t*–197*t*
recording findings, 204

red, bilateral, approach to patient with, 192*a*
red, unilateral, approach to patient with, 193*a*
vision, change in, 183

F
Facial expressions, in mental status examination, 133
Facial paralysis, 446*t*
Factitious disorder, 145*t*
Failure to thrive, 460
Fainting. *See* Syncope
Falls, in elderly
prevention of, 397–398, 550
risk factors, 397
Fasciculations, 448*t*
Fatigue, 112
approach to patient with, 126*a*
in pregnancy, 506*b*
Female genitalia
examination techniques, 338–342
external, 338–339, 338*f*
health history, 336–337
health promotion and counseling, 343–344
internal examination, 339–342, 339*b*, 340*f*–342*f*
menopause, 337
menstruation, 336–337
pelvic pain, 337
postmenopausal bleeding, 337
recording findings, 343
rectovaginal examination, 342, 342*f*
vulvovaginal symptoms, 337
Fetal alcohol syndrome, 521
Fetal exposure to diethylstilbestrol (DES), 351*t*
Fever, 112–113, 121
blister, 216*t*
causes of, 121
Finkelstein test, 381*f*
Folate deficiency, in pregnancy, 524
Furuncles, 164*t*
Furunculosis, 164*t*

G
Gait
inspection of, 385–386, 385*f*, 421–422
older adults, assessment in, 547
tandem walking, testing, 421, 421*f*
Gastroesophageal reflux disease (GERD), 263*t*
pain in, 300
symptoms, 301

General survey, 58
  apparent state of health, 114
  body and breath odors, 115
  dress, 115
  facial expression, 115
  gait and motor activity, 115
  grooming and personal hygiene, 111
  of infant, 460
  level of consciousness, 114
  of older adults, 542
  posture, 115
  signs of distress, 115
  skin color and lesions, 115
Genital herpes, 330t, 348t
Genitalia
  female, 336–353 (*See also* Female genitalia)
  male, 323–335 (*See also* Male genitalia)
Genital warts, 330t
Gestational hypertension, 512b
Giant cell arteritis, 440t
Glasgow Coma Scale, 451t
Glass thermometer, 122b
Glaucoma, 191
  in older adults, 543
  screening for, 191
Glaucomatous cupping, 188b
Goiter, 176
  multinodular, 182t
Groin hernias, 326, 335t
Guttate psoriasis, 163t

H

Habit tic deformity, 174t
Hair
  examination, 149–152, 154
  health history, 148–149
  loss, 150, 154, 171t–173t
  pull test, 154, 154f, 172t
  tug test, 154, 154f
Halitosis, 212
Hawkins impingement sign, 375b
Head
  components of examination, 176–177
  examination of, 176–178
  recording findings, 178
Headache, 412
  analgesic rebound, 439t
  approach to patient with, 435a
  brain tumor and, 440t
  cluster, 438t
  from eye disorders, 439t
  giant cell arteritis and, 440t
  glaucoma and, 439t
  meningitis, 440t
  migraine, 438t
  postconcussion, 441t
  primary, 438t
  secondary, 439t–441t
  from sinusitis, 439t
  tension, 438t
  thunderclap, 440t
  trigeminal neuralgia and, 441t
Head, eyes, ears, nose, throat (HEENT), 42
  in older adults, 543–544
Health care, disparities in
  cultural humility, 12, 12b
  racism and bias, 11, 11b
  social determinants of health, 10
Health history, 33
  alcohol history, 39
  in ambulatory care clinic, 44b
  chief complaint (CC) in, 34–35, 36b, 45, 46b–47b
  components of, 33, 33b–34b
  documentation of, 45–48, 49b–52b
  in emergency care, 44b
  familial and social relationships, 38–39
  family history, 37
  history of present illness, 35, 45–47, 46b, 48b
  in home, 45b
  illicit drug use history, 40
  in intensive care unit, 44b
  medications in, 37
  mental, 37
  in nursing home, 45b
  past medical history, 36–37, 48
  physical and sexual abuse, clues to, 39b
  review of systems, 42–44
  sexual history, 40, 40b–41b
  sexual orientation and gender identity, 38
  social history, 37–41, 38b
  spiritual history, 41, 41b–42b
  subjective *versus* objective data in, 34, 34b
  symptom, attributes of, 35b
  tobacco use history, 39
Health maintenance and screening
  behavioral counseling, 84–86
  guideline recommendations, 79, 79b–80b
  immunization, 95–101

primary prevention, 79
screening recommendations, 80,
80*b*–81*b*
secondary prevention, 79
Health promotion and counseling
abdominal aortic aneurysm,
278–279
blood pressure and dietary sodium,
125
breast cancer, 290–291, 290*b*,
291*b*–292*b*
cardiovascular disease, 253
carotid artery stenosis,
asymptomatic, 434
cerebrovascular disease, 433–434,
434*b*
cervical cancer, 343, 344*b*
colorectal cancer, 313, 313*b*
dementia, 137
depression, screening for, 137,
138*b*
diabetic peripheral neuropathy, 434
glaucoma screening, 191
hearing loss, 206
hypertension, 125
latent tuberculosis, 230
low back pain, 396
lung cancer, 230
menopause and hormone
replacement therapy, 344
obstructive sleep apnea, 230
for older adults, 548–554
oral and pharyngeal cancer, 214
oral health, 180
osteoporosis, 396–398, 397*b*,
398*b*
peripheral arterial disease, 278,
278*b*
during pregnancy, 519–525
suicide risk assessment, 137
testicular cancer, 327
thyroid cancer, screening for, 180
thyroid dysfunction, screening for,
180
viral hepatitis, 312–313,
312*b*–313*b*
visual impairment, 191
Hearing loss, 202, 206
approach to patient with, 209*a*
conductive loss, 199, 203
health promotion and counseling,
206
patterns of, 204*b*
Rinne test, 203
sensorineural, 417
sensorineural loss, 199, 203
Weber test, 203
whispered voice test, 203, 203*b*
Heart
examination of (*See* Cardiac
examination)
infant, 467–468
in pregnancy, 513
Heartburn, in pregnancy, 507*b*
Heart rate, 121, 121*f*
infant/child, 461, 461*b*
Heart sounds, 248, 264*t*
first, variations in, 265*t*
second, variations in, 266*t*–267*t*
Hegar sign, 516
Height, measurement of, 115
Hematemesis, 302
Hematochezia, 355
Hemoptysis, approach to patient with,
233*a*
Hemorrhoids
external, 361*t*
in pregnancy, 507*b*, 516
Hepatitis, 301, 303*b*, 312
hepatitis A, 312, 312*b*
hepatitis B, 312, 312*b*–313*b*
hepatitis C, 313
Hepatomegaly, 307
Herbal supplements, during pregnancy,
521
Hereditary hemorrhagic telangiectasia,
216*t*
Hernia
femoral, 326, 335*t*, 342
in groin, 326, 335*t*
inguinal, 326, 335*t*, 342, 475
scrotal, 332*t*
Herpes simplex virus vesicles, 163*t*
Hips
examination of, 385–387, 385*f*,
386*f*, 386*b*–387*b*, 387*f*
FABER/Patrick test, 387, 387*f*
gait inspection, 385, 385*f*
palpation, 385, 386*f*
range of motion, 386*b*–387*b*
HIV infection
prevention of, 95
screening for, 94
Hoarseness, 211–212
approach to patient with, 215*a*
Housemaid's knee, 407
Hydrocele, 332*t*
Hyperemesis gravidarum, 507*b*
Hyperopia, 183
Hyperpyrexia, 121

Hypertension, 254, 255*b*
  in childhood, 471, 488*t*
  dietary changes in, 127*t*
  masked, 117*b*
  nocturnal, 117*b*
  in pregnancy, 512*b*
  primary (essential), 125
  screening for, 125
  secondary, 125
  types of, 116, 117*b*
  white-coat, 117*b*
Hypertonia, 449*t*
Hypopyrexia, 121
Hypospadias, 332*t*
Hypothermia
  causes of, 122
  in older adults, 542
Hypotonia, 449*t*

I

Illness anxiety disorder, 145*t*
Immunization, 95
  hepatitis A vaccine, 97
  hepatitis B vaccine, 97
  herpes zoster vaccine, 101
  human papillomavirus vaccine, 98
  influenza vaccine, 98
  pneumococcal vaccine, 99, 99*b*
  recommendations for, 95, 96*b*–97*b*
  tetanus, diphtheria, pertussis vaccine, 100
  varicella vaccine, 100–101
Infant
  abdomen, 468
  blood pressure, 461, 461*f*
  breasts, 468
  ears, 464, 464*b*
  examination techniques, 459*b*
  eyes, 463, 464*b*
  facies, abnormal, 463, 463*b*
  female genitalia, 468
  general survey, 460
  head, 462
  head circumference, 460, 460*f*
  hearing assessment, 464*b*
  heart and peripheral vascular system, 467–468
  heart rate, 461, 461*b*
  height and weight, 460
  liver size, 468*b*
  lymph nodes, 465, 465*f*
  male genitalia, 468
  mental and physical status, 459
  mouth and pharynx, 464
  musculoskeletal system, 469
  neck, 465, 465*f*
  nervous system, 470
  nose, 464
  respiration and breathing, 466*b*
  respiratory rate, 461
  skin, 462
  sutures and fontanelles, 462, 462*f*
  temperature, 461
  thorax and lungs, 465–466, 466*b*
  upper airway and lower airway sounds, 467*b*
  visual milestones, 464*b*
Informed consent, 24
Inguinal nodes, superficial, 273, 273*f*
Insect bites, 163*t*
Insight, in mental status examination, 132*b*, 135
Intermittent claudication, 269–270
Interviewing, skilled, 19
  "Ask Me Three" approach, 21–22
  empowering the patient, 21, 21*b*
  nonstigmatizing language, use of, 22, 23*b*
  nonverbal communication in, 23
  teach-back method, 22, 22*b*
  techniques for, 19*b*–21*b*
Intimate partner violence
  during pregnancy, 521–522, 522*b*
  screening for, 83–84
Involuntary movements, 414–415, 418, 448*t*
  athetosis, 448*t*
  chorea, 448*t*
  fasciculations, 448*t*
  intention tremor, 448*t*
  postural tremor, 448*t*
  resting static tremors, 448*t*
Irritable bowel syndrome, diarrhea in, 319*t*
Ischiogluteal bursa, 386

J

Joint pain
  acute, 367
  articular/nonarticular, 366
  assessment of, tips for, 366*b*
  causes of, by age, 368*b*
  chronic, 366
  inflammation and, 366
  location, 366
  monoarticular, 366
  morning stiffness and, 368
  onset and timing, 367
  patterns of, 403*t*–404*t*
  polyarticular, 366

quality, 367
remitting/exacerbating factors, 367
severity, 367
symmetric/asymmetric, 366
Joints, 363. *See also* Joint pain
anatomy, terminology related to, 363*b*
cartilaginous, 364*b*
examination of, steps for, 370
fibrous, 364*b*
inflammation, signs of, 370*b*
synovial, 364*b*, 365*b*
Jolt accentuation of headache (JAH), 428
Judgment
in mental status examination, 133*b*, 135
in neurocognitive disorders, 146*t*
Jugular venous pressure (JVP), 245, 245*f*
Jugular venous pulsations, 245

K

Keloid, 164*t*
Keratosis
actinic, 165*t*
seborrheic, 169*t*
Kernig sign, 428, 428*f*
Kidneys, 304*b*, 308
costovertebral angle (CVA) tenderness, 308, 308*f*
Klinefelter syndrome, 333*t*
Knees
anterior cruciate ligament test, 391, 391*f*
balloon sign, 392, 392*f*
bulge sign, 392, 392*f*
effusion assessment, 392–393
examination of, 387–392, 388*f*, 390*f*–392*f*, 390*t*
inspection, 389
Lachman test, 391, 391*f*
lateral collateral ligament test, 391, 391*f*
McMurray test, 390, 390*f*
medial collateral ligament test, 390, 390*f*
medial structure, 388, 388*f*
patellofemoral compartment, 389
posterior cruciate ligament test, 391, 391*f*
range of motion, 390*b*
tibiofemoral joint, 389
Knees, painful, 407*t*–408*t*
anterior cruciate tear/sprain, 408*t*
approach to patient with, 402*a*

arthritis, 407*t*
Baker cyst, 408*t*
bursitis, 407*t*
collateral ligament sprain/tear, 408*t*
meniscal tear, 407*t*
patellofemoral instability, 407*t*
Koplik spots, 220*t*
Korotkoff sounds
pulsus alternans, 246
pulsus paradoxus, 246

L

Labyrinthitis, acute, 200*b*
Language, in mental status examination, 133*b*, 134
Lead-pipe rigidity, 449*t*
Leg discoloration, 270
approach to patient with, 282*a*
Leg pain, 269
approach to patient with, 280*a*
Legs
dorsalis pedis pulse, 274, 274*f*
examination of, 273–274
popliteal pulse, 274, 274*f*
Leg swelling, 269
approach to patient with, 281*a*
Leopold maneuvers, 517–518, 517*f*, 518*f*
Lesbian, gay, bisexual, transgender, and queer (LGBTQ) patients, 6–7, 480
establishing initial rapport with, 7*b*
Leukocoria, 463
Level of consciousness, 133, 134*b*
in mental status examination, 132*b*, 133, 134*b*
in neurocognitive disorders, 146*t*
Lid retraction, 196*t*
Lipoma, 164*t*
Lips
abnormalities of, 216*t*–217*t*
angioedema, 216*t*
angular cheilitis, 216*t*
carcinoma of, 217*t*
hereditary hemorrhagic telangiectasia, 216*t*
herpes simplex vesicles, 216*t*
Peutz–Jeghers syndrome, 217*t*
syphilitic chancre, 217*t*
Liver
examination, 306–307
palpation, 307, 307*f*
percussion, 306, 306*f*
Liver damage, toxic, 303*b*
Liver diseases, risk factors for, 303*b*

Low back pain. *See* Back pain, low
Lumbosacral radiculopathy, testing for, 428, 428*f*

M

Macular degeneration, 544
Macules, 162*t*
Major depressive disorder (MDD), 130*b*
Malabsorption syndrome, 320*t*
Male genitalia
  anatomy of, 324*f*
  examination techniques, 324–326
  health history, 323
  health promotion and counseling, 327
  penile discharge/lesions, 323
  recording findings, 327
  scrotal swelling, 324
  sexually transmitted infections of, 324, 330*t*–331*t*
  testicular swelling/pain, 323
Mammography, 291
Mass(es)
  abdominal, 306, 306*f*
  breast mass, 285, 293, 296*t*
  neck, 176, 181
  penile, 328*a*
  scrotal, 329*a*
McBurney sign, 310
Medical ethics, 13
  core values of, 13*b*
Melanoma, 157–158
  amelanotic, 167*t*
  and mimics, 167*t*–169*t*
  screening for, 158, 159*b*–160*b*
  in situ, 168*t*
Melanoma Risk Assessment Tool, 157–158
Melanonychia, 174*t*
Melena, 302, 355
Memory
  in mental status examination, 132*b*, 135
  in neurocognitive disorders, 147*t*
  recent, 135
  remote, 135
Memory problems, 130. *See also* Neurocognitive disorders
  after head injury, 131
  approach to patient with, 144*a*
  sudden-onset, 130
Meniere disease, 199, 200*b*
Meningitis, 440*t*
Menopause, 337

Mental disorders, 142
  examination techniques (*see* Mental status examination)
  health history, 128–131
  health promotion and counseling, 136–140
  medically unexplained symptoms and, 130
  recording findings, 136
  screening for, 131, 131*b*
  and substance use disorders, 142
Mental status examination
  appearance and behavior in, 133
  cognitive function in, 135–136
  components of, 132
  insight and judgment in, 135
  mood in, 134
  speech and language in, 134
  terminology related to, 132*b*–133*b*
  thoughts and perceptions in, 134
Metabolic syndrome, 256
Metacarpophalangeal joints, 379, 379*f*
Migraine, 438*t*
Mini-Cog (screening test for dementia), 139*b*–140*b*
Mini Mental State Examination, 137
Montreal Cognitive Assessment (MoCA), 140, 141*b*
Mood
  depressed (*see* Depression)
  in mental status examination, 133*b*, 134
  in neurocognitive disorders, 146*t*
Morbilliform drug eruption, 162*t*
Motor behavior, in mental status examination, 133
Motor disorders, 447*t*
Movements, involuntary. *See* Involuntary movements
Mucopurulent cervicitis, 351*t*
Murmurs, 249–250, 268*t*
  approach to patient with, 261*a*
  in children, 475, 475*f*, 493*t*–494*t*
  continuous, 268*t*
  crescendo, 50
  crescendo–decrescendo, 250
  decrescendo, 250
  diastolic, 251*b*, 268*t*
  in infants, 468
  midsystolic, 268*t*
  in older adults, 545
  pathologic, 493*t*–494*t*
  plateau, 250
  in pregnancy, 513
  systolic, 250–251, 251*b*, 268*t*

Murphy sign, 311
Muscle
  bulk and tone, 418
  strength, 418–420, 419*b*
Muscle tone, disorders of, 449*t*
Musculoskeletal system, 43
  ankles and feet, 393–394, 394*b*, 394*f*
  children, 476
  complaints, approach to patient
    with, 399*a*
  elbow, 376–377, 377*b*, 377*f*
  health history, 365–369
  health promotion and counseling,
    396–398
  hips, 385–387, 385*f*, 386*f*,
    386*b*–387*b*, 387*f*
  infant, 469
  joint anatomy, 363–365, 364*b*, 365*b*
  joint examination, 370, 370*b*
  knees, 388–393, 388*f*, 390*f*–393*f*,
    390*t*
  leg length, measuring, 395, 395*f*
  in older adults, 546
  range of motion, measuring, 395,
    395*f*
  recording findings, 395
  shoulder, 372–376, 372*f*,
    373*b*–374*b*, 375*b*–376*b*
  spine, 382–384, 383*b*, 383*f*, 384*b*
  temporomandibular joint, 371,
    371*b*, 371*f*
  wrists and hands, 377–382,
    378*f*–382*f*, 380*t*
Myocardial infarction, 262*t*
Myoma of uterus, 352*t*
Myopia, 183

N
Nails
  findings in or near, 174*t*–175*t*
  inspection of, 151, 151*f*
  terry, 175*t*
Neck
  examination techniques, 176–177,
    178*f*
  health history, 176
  health promotion and counseling,
    180
  recording findings, 178
Neck mass, 176
  approach to patient with, 181*a*
Neck pain, 368
  cervical myelopathy and, 404*t*
  cervical radiculopathy and, 404*t*
  mechanical, 404*t*

Neer impingement sign, 375*b*
Negative predictive value (NPV), 104*b*
Nervous system, 60–61, 409
  asterixis, 429
  central, 409, 409*f*, 410
  comatose patient, assessment of,
    429–431
  cranial nerves, 411, 411*b*, 416–418
  cutaneous/superficial stimulation
    reflexes, 427–428
  health history, 412–416
  health promotion and counseling,
    433–434
  infant, 469
  lumbosacral radiculopathy, 428
  meningeal signs, 427–428
  motor system, 418–422
  muscle stretch reflexes, 425–426
  in older adults, 547
  peripheral, 409–412, 409*f*
  recording findings, 431–433
  scapular winging, 429, 429*f*
  sensory system, 422–425
Neural tube defects (NTDs), 524
Neurocognitive disorders, 137. *See also
    specific disorder*
  delirium, 130, 146*t*–147*t*
  dementia, 130, 146*t*–147*t*
  mild, 130
  screening for, 137–140
Neuropathic ulcer, 284*t*
Nevi, intradermal, 167*t*
Newborn
  Apgar score, 457, 457*b*
  appropriate for gestational age
    (AGA), 488*t*
  assessment hours after birth, 458–459
  birth, assessment at, 458–459
  classifications, 458*b*
  gestational age and birth weight,
    458, 458*b*
  health history, 456
  large for gestational age (LGA), 488*t*
  small for gestational age (SGA), 488*t*
  umbilical cord examination, 459
Nicotine replacement therapy (NRT),
    93
Night sweats, 112
Nipple
  discharge, 285; approach to patient
    with, 295*a*
  inspection of, 287
  Paget disease of, 287, 297*t*
  palpation, 288
  retraction and deviation, 297*t*

Nocturia, 304
Nodule, 164*t*
Nose
  epistaxis, 201
  examination techniques, 201–205
  health history, 201
  recording findings, 205
  rhinorrhea, 201
Number identification, 425
Number needed to treat (NNT), 111*b*
Numbness, 413
  approach to patient with, 436*a*
Numeric Rating Scale (NRS), 113*f*
Nutrition
  Choose MyPlate, 88, 89*b*
  counseling, 87–88, 87*b*–88*b*
  for older adults, 538
  during pregnancy, 520, 520*b*

O

Obesity, 116
Obturator sign, 310
Odynophagia, 302
Older adults, 533
  abdomen, 545
  activities of daily living, 537, 537*b*
  advance directives and palliative care,
    539, 540*f*
  breasts and axillae, 545
  cardiovascular system, 544–545
  care of, 534, 535*b*
  changes with aging, 533, 547,
    554*t*–562*t*
  cognitive impairment in, 536
  communication with, 534–536,
    534*b*–535*b*
  cultural diversity and care of, 535,
    536*b*
  delirium in, 553
  dementia in, 553–554
  eliciting symptoms from, 535–536
  exercise and physical activity for,
    549, 550*t*
  female genitalia and pelvic
    examination, 545–546
  frailty and care of, 539
  functional status, assessment of,
    540–541
  general survey, 542
  10-Minute Geriatric Screener,
    540*b*–541*b*
  health history, 537–539
  health promotion and counseling,
    548–554
  hearing loss, screening for, 549

HEENT examination, 543–544
household safety and fall prevention
  for, 550, 550*b*–551*b*
male genitalia and prostate, 546
medication safety and management,
  538, 538*b*
mistreatment and abuse, 554
musculoskeletal system, 546
nervous system, 547
nutrition for, 539
peripheral vascular system, 545
recording findings, 547–548
screening decisions, five-step
  approach to, 549
screening for cancer in, 551–553,
  552*b*
skin, 543
smoking and alcohol use by, 538
thorax and lungs, 544
timed get up and go test, 546, 562*t*
vaccines for, 551, 551*b*
visual impairment, screening for,
  549
vital signs, 542
Onycholysis, 175*t*
Onychomycosis, 175*t*
Ophthalmoscope, use of, 187*b*
Optic disc
  abnormalities of, 188*b*–189*b*
  examination of, 188, 188*f*,
    189*b*–190*b*
  glaucomatous cupping, 188*b*
  normal, 188*b*
  optic atrophy, 189*b*
  papilledema, 188*b*
Oral candidiasis (thrush), 465
Oral cavity
  breath malodor, 212
  cancer, 214
  examination techniques, 212–213
  gum bleeding, 211
  health history, 211
  health promotion and counseling,
    214
  inspection of, 180
  lips, abnormalities of, 216*t*–217*t*
  mouth inspection, 212–213
  pharynx, abnormalities of, 220*t*
  tongue, abnormalities of,
    218*t*–219*t*
Orchitis, acute, 333*t*
Orientation
  in mental status examination, 132*b*,
    135
  in neurocognitive disorders, 146*t*

Orthostatic (postural) hypotension, 245
  in older adults, 542
Ortolani test, 469, 469*f*
Osteoarthritis, 403*t*–404*t*
Osteoporosis, 396–397
  risk factors for, 397*b*
  treatment, 397–398
  WHO bone density criteria, 397*b*
Otitis externa, 199, 202
Otitis media, 199, 202, 210*t*
  acute, 472
  with purulent effusion, 210*t*

P

Paget disease of nipple, 287, 297*t*
Pain, 113–114
  in abdomen (*See* Abdominal pain)
  acute, 113
  assessment, 113*f*, 114*b*
  chronic, 113
  with defecation, 355
  eye, 184
  in knees, 407*t*–408*t*
  low back pain (*See* Back pain, low)
  management, 123–124
  in neck, 404*t*
  osteoarthritis, 403*t*–404*t*
  rheumatoid arthritis, 403*t*–404*t*
  in shoulders, 406*t*
  on urination, 303
Painful arc test, 375*b*
Palliative care, 539, 540*f*
Palpitations, 244
  approach to patient with, 260*a*
Papilledema, 188*b*, 463
Pap smears, 341, 341*f*
Papules, 163*t*
Paradoxical breathing, 466
Paradoxical pulse. *See* Pulsus paradoxus
Paravertebral muscle spasm, 383
Paresthesia, 413
Paronychia, 174*t*
Paroxysmal nocturnal dyspnea (PND), 243
Paroxysmal supraventricular tachycardia, 467
Patches, 162*t*
Patient situations
  alert, 134*b*
  with altered state or cognition, 28
  angry/aggressive, 29
  bedbound, 61
  comatose, 134*b*
  with confusing narrative, 28
  discriminatory/racist, 29
  dying, 31
  with emotional lability, 29
  flirtatious, 29
  with hearing loss, 30
  lethargic, 134*b*
  with limited intelligence, 30
  with limited language proficiency, 31
  with low/impaired vision, 30
  with low literacy, 30
  nonadherent, 29
  obese, 62
  obtunded, 134*b*
  with personal problems, 30
  postprocedure, 62
  silent, 28
  stuporous, 134*b*
  verbose, 28
  wheelchair bound, 62
Patient-centeredness, in computerized clinical settings, 31, 31*b*–32*b*
Patient Health Questionnaire (PHQ-9), 137, 138*b*–139*b*, 523
Patient Problem List, 74–75, 75*b*
Patrick test, 387, 387*f*
Pediatric medical record, 481–485
Pelvic floor, relaxations of, 353*t*
Pelvic pain
  acute, 337
  approach to patient with, 347*a*
  chronic, 337
Penile mass/lesion, approach to patient with, 328*a*
Penis
  abnormalities of, 332*t*
  inspection of, 324
  palpation of, 325
Perceptions
  in mental status examination, 132*b*, 134
  in neurocognitive disorders, 146*t*
Pericarditis, 262*t*
Peripheral arterial disease (PAD), 269, 275, 276*f*–277*f*
  assessing for, 275, 275*b*–276*b*, 278
  prevalence, 278
  risk factors for, 278, 278*b*
  warning signs, 270*b*
Peripheral nervous system (PNS), 409, 409*f*. *See also* Nervous system
  cranial nerves, 411, 411*b*
  peripheral nerves, 410

Peripheral vascular system, 60
abdomen, 273, 327*f*
arms, 271–272, 272*f*
examination techniques, 271–277
health history, 269–270
health promotion and counseling,
278–279
legs, 273–275, 274*f*
in older adults, 545
recording findings, 277
Persistent depressive disorder (PDD),
130*b*
Petechia/Purpura, 170*t*
Peutz–Jeghers syndrome, 217*t*
Peyronie disease, 332*t*
Phalen sign, 382, 382*f*
Pharyngitis, 213
Pharynx
abnormalities of, 220*t*
diphtheria, 220*t*
exudative pharyngitis, 220*t*
inspection, 212
Koplik spots, 220*t*
pharyngitis, 220*t*
Physical activity
counseling for, 89–90
guidelines for Americans, 89*b*
Physical dependence, 123*b*
Physical examination, 53
bedbound patient, 61
documentation of, 62, 63*b*–64*b*
equipment for, 54, 54*b*
head-to-toe examination, 57–61,
57*b*–58*b*
lighting and environment for, 54
obese patient, 62
patient in pain, 62
patient privacy and comfort for, 55
postprocedure patient, 62
preparing for, steps in, 53–54
sequence and positioning for, 57
for specific patient situations,
61–62
standard and MRSA precautions,
55
universal precautions during, 55,
56*b*
wheelchair bound patient, 62
Pilar cysts, 164*t*
Pinguecula, 197*t*
Plaque psoriasis, 163*t*
Plaques, skin, 163*t*
Pleuritic pain, 262*t*
Pneumatic otoscope, 472, 472*f*
Point of maximal impulse (PMI), 544

Polydactyly, 469
Polyps of rectum, 361*t*
Polyuria, 304
Positive predictive value (PPV), 104*b*
Posterior drawer sign, 391, 391*f*
Postmenopausal bleeding, 337
Posture, in mental status examination,
133
Precocious puberty, 475
Preeclampsia, in pregnancy, 512*b*
Pregnancy
abdominal pain in, 506*b*; approach
to patient with, 526*a*
in adolescents, 525
aneuploidy screening and genetic
testing, 509
backache in, 506*b*
breastfeeding, plans for, 509
confirmation of, 504
contraception options and, 525, 525*b*
current health and past clinical
history, 508
exercise and physical activity during,
521
family history, 509
folic acid supplementation in, 524
gestational age and expected date of
delivery, determination of, 504,
505*b*
health promotion and counseling,
519–525
hypertension in, 512*b*
immunizations during, 523, 523*b*
initial prenatal visit, approach to,
504
intimate partner violence, screening
for, 521–522, 522*b*
iron supplementation in, 524
laboratory screenings, prenatal, 524
maternal concerns and attitudes,
508
multivitamin and mineral
supplementation in, 524
nomenclature for outcomes of,
508*b*–509*b*
nutrition and weight gain during,
520, 520*b*
past obstetric history, 508
perinatal depression, screening for,
523
physiologic changes in, 503, 503*f*,
529*t*–532*t*
postpartum contraception, plans for,
509–510
risk factors related to health, 509

subsequent prenatal visit, 510
substance use during, 521
symptoms of, 505, 506b–507b
unintended, 524–525
Pregnant woman. *See also* Pregnancy
abdomen, 514–515, 514f
bimanual examination, 516
blood pressure of, 512, 512b
breasts, 513
examination of, 510–511
extremities examination, 517
fetal heart rate (FHR) monitoring, 515
fetal movements, detection of, 514
fundal height, measurement of, 514
general inspection, 512
head and neck inspection, 512–513
heart, 513
height and weight, 512
Leopold maneuvers, 517–518, 517f, 518f
preparation for examination of, 511b
recording physical examination findings, 519
speculum examination, 515–516
thorax and lungs, 513
Premenstrual syndrome, 337
Presbyopia, 183
Pressure injuries, 155
revised staging system, 155b
skin inspection for, 155
stages, 156f
Preterm labor, 514
Primary open-angle glaucoma (POAG), 191
Primitive reflexes, 470, 489t–492t
asymmetric tonic neck reflex, 490t
Landau reflex, 491t
Moro reflex, 490t
palmar grasp reflex, 489t
parachute reflex, 491t
placing and stepping reflex, 492t
plantar grasp reflex, 489t
positive support reflex, 492t
rooting reflex, 489t
trunk incurvation reflex, 491t
Problem representation, 65, 66
documentation of, 70, 70b
Progress note, 75
sample, 71b–74b
Subjective, Objective, Assessment, and Plan (SOAP) format, 75, 75b–76b

Pronator drift, test for, 422, 422f
Proprioception, test for, 424, 424f
Prostate
examination techniques, 355–357, 356f
health history, 354–355
recording findings, 357
Prostate cancer, 357
risk factors, 357
screening, 358b
Prostatitis, acute, 362t
Psoas sign, 310
Ptosis, 196t
Pulmonary valve stenosis, 493t
Pulsus alternans, 246
Pulsus paradoxus, 246
Pupils in comatose patients, 452t
large, 452t
midposition fixed, 452t
one fixed and dilated pupil, 452t
small/pinpoint, 452t
Pupils, inspection of, 185–186
Pustules, 164t

R
Range of motion
ankles and feet, 394b
cervical spine, 383b
elbow, 377b
hip, 386b–387b
knee, 390b
measurement of, 395
shoulder, 373b–374b
temporomandibular joint, 371b
thoracolumbosacral spine, 384b
wrist, 380b
Raynaud disease, 271
Rectal examination, abnormalities on, 361t
acute prostatitis, 362t
anal fissure, 361t
anorectal fistula, 361t
benign prostatic hyperplasia, 362t
cancer of prostate, 362t
cancer of rectum, 362t
external hemorrhoids, 361t
polyps of rectum, 361t
Rectocele, 353t
Rectum
cancer of, 356f, 362t
examination techniques, 354f, 355–357
health history, 354–355
recording findings, 357

Reflex(es), 425
  abdominal, 427, 427*f*
  Achilles/ankle, 426, 426*f*
  anal, 427
  ankle clonus, 426, 426*f*
  biceps, 426, 426*f*
  brachioradialis, 426, 426*f*
  grading, 425*b*
  oculocephalic, 430, 431*f*
  plantar response, 427, 427*f*
  primitive, 470, 489*t*–492*t* (*See also*
    Primitive reflexes)
  quadriceps/patellar, 426, 426*f*
  red retinal, 463
  triceps, 426, 426*f*
Relative risk, 111*b*
Relative risk difference, 111*b*
Respiratory rate, 116
Retinoblastoma, 463
Rheumatoid arthritis, 403*t*–404*t*
Rhinitis, 201
  approach to patient with, 208*a*
Rhythm
  of breathing, 121
  heart, 121
Ringworm. *See* Tinea capitis
Rinne test, 417
Romberg test, 422
Rotator cuff tendinitis, 406*t*
Rovsing sign, 310

S
Scabies, 165*t*
Scapular winging, 429, 429*f*
School-aged children/early childhood
  abdomen, 475
  blood pressure, 471
  ears, 472, 473*b*
  eyes, 471, 472*b*
  female genitalia, 475–476, 476*f*
  health history, 470
  heart, 474, 475*f*
  male genitalia, 475
  mental and physical status, 470–471
  mouth and pharynx, 473–474
  musculoskeletal system, 476
  nervous system, 476, 477*b*
  rectum and anus, 476
Sciatica, 405*t*
Scoliometer, 481
Scoliosis, 481, 481*f*
Screening
  abdominal aortic aneurysm,
    278–279
  alcohol use, unhealthy, 91–92, 91*b*

breast cancer, 291, 291*b*–292*b*
  cardiovascular risk factors, 253–255
  carotid artery stenosis, 434
  cervical cancer, 343, 344*b*
  colorectal cancer, 313, 313*b*
  delirium, 142, 142*b*
  dementia, 137–138, 139*b*–140*b*
  depression, 137, 138*b*–139*b*
  diabetic peripheral neuropathy,
    434
  elder abuse, 83
  glaucoma, 191
  hypertension, 125
  intimate partner violence, 83–84
  melanoma, 158, 159*b*–160*b*
  mental health, 131, 131*b*
  misuse of prescription and illicit
    drugs, 82–83
  musculoskeletal examination for
    sports, 499*t*–502*t*
  peripheral arterial disease, 275,
    278
  prostate cancer, 357–358, 358*b*
  recommendations, 80, 80*b*–81*b*
  sexually transmitted infections, 94
  skin cancer, 158–160
  substance use disorders, 82
  thyroid cancer, 180
  tobacco use, 92
  unhealthy weight and diabetes
    mellitus, 82, 82*b*
Scrotal edema, 332*t*
Scrotal hernia, 332*t*
Scrotal mass/pain, approach to patient
  with, 329*a*
Scrotal transillumination, 326
Scrotum
  abnormalities of, 332*t*
  examination of, 325–326
Seborrheic dermatitis, 162*t*
Seborrheic keratosis, 169*t*
  inflamed, 169*t*
Seizure, 414
Semantic qualifiers, 70, 70*b*
Sensory system, examination
  techniques, 422–425
Sex maturity ratings, in boys, 497*t*
Sex maturity ratings, in girls
  breasts, 496*t*
  pubic hair, 497*t*–498*t*
Sexual abuse, in children, 495*t*
Sexually transmitted infections,
  94, 94*b*
  behavioral counseling for, 95
  chancroid, 331*t*

genital herpes simplex, 330*t*
genital warts, 330*t*
of male genitalia, 323, 330*t*–331*t*
primary syphilis, 331*t*
screening for, 94
Shortness of breath, 243. *See also*
Dyspnea
Shoulder
examination of, 372, 372*f*,
373*b*–374*b*, 373*f*, 375*b*–376*b*
pain, approach to patient with, 400*a*
palpation, 372–375, 372*f*, 373*f*
range of motion, 373*b*–374*b*
SITS muscle assessment,
375*b*–376*b*
Sinuses, 201
examination techniques, 205
SITS (Supraspinatus, Infraspinatus,
Teres minor, and Subscapularis)
muscle, 375, 375*b*–376*b*
Skin, 58
bedbound patient and pressure
injuries, 155, 155*b*, 156*f*
examination techniques, 149–156
health history, 148–149
health promotion and counseling,
157–160
integrated examination, 152
lesion, 148, 161*a*, 162*t*–164*t*
in older adults, 543
rashes and itching on, 148
recording findings, 156–157
seated and standing position,
examination in, 149–151,
149*f*–151*f*
self-skin examination, 153,
153*b*–154*b*
supine and prone position,
examination in, 152, 152*f*
Skin cancer, 157–158
melanoma, 157–158
prevention of, 157–158
screening, 158–160
sun exposure and, 158
Skin lesions, 148
approach to patient with, 161*a*
brown, 167*t*–169*t*
pink, 166*t*
primary, 165*t*, 165*t*
rough, 165*t*
vascular and purpuric, 170*t*–171*t*
Skin tags, 163*t*, 167*t*
Solar lentigo, 168*t*
Somatic symptom disorder, 145*t*
Somatoform disorders, 145*t*

Speech
disorders of, 444*t*–445*t*
in mental status examination, 134
in neurocognitive disorders, 146*t*
Spermatic cord, 334
abnormalities of, 334*t*
torsion of, 334*t*
varicocele of, 334*t*
Spermatocele, 334*t*
Spider angioma, 170*t*
Spider vein, 170*t*
Spinal cord, 410, 410*f. See also*
Nervous system
Spine
anatomy of back, 383*f*
examination of, 382–384, 383*b*,
383*f*, 384*b*
range of motion, 383*b*, 384*b*
Spirituality, 12
Spleen
palpation, 307, 307*f*
percussion, 307
Squamous cell carcinoma (SCC),
166*t*
Static finger wiggle test, 185, 185*f*
Steatorrhea, 302
Stereognosis, 424
Sternocleidomastoid muscles, 418
Stools
black tarry, 355
bloody, 355
Straight-leg raise test, 428, 428*f*
Streptococcal pharyngitis, 211, 473
Stroke, 433
hemorrhagic, 433
prevention of, 433*b*–434*b*
types of, 442*t*–443*t*
warning signs and symptoms,
433*b*
Sty, 197*t*
Subacromial and subdeltoid bursitis,
406*t*
Subcutaneous mass/cyst, skin, 164*t*
Substance use disorders, mental
disorders and, 142
Suicide, 137
risk assessment, 137
Summary Statement, 66. *See also*
Problem representation
Sunscreen, use of, 158
Syncope, 244, 414
Syndactyly, 469
Syphilis
primary, 331*t*
secondary, 349*t*

Syphilitic chancre, 217*t*, 349*t*
Systolic blood pressure (SBP), 116–120, 120*b*

T

Tachycardia, 461
Tanning beds, 158
Teeth
  children, 474, 474*f*
  natal, 465
Telogen effluvium, 154, 172*t*
Temperature
  oral, 122, 122*b*
  rectal, 121, 122*b*
  temporal artery, 122, 122*b*
  tympanic membrane, 122, 122*b*
Temporomandibular joint (TMJ), 371, 371*b*, 371*f*
Tennis elbow, 376, 377*f*
Testicles, undescended, 468
Testicular cancer, 327
  risk factors for, 327
  screening for, 327–328
Testicular self-examination (TSE), 327
Testis
  abnormalities of, 333*t*
  examination of, 325*f*
  small, 333*t*
  tumor of, 333*t*
Test(s)
  Adams bend test, 481
  anterior cruciate ligament test, 391, 391*f*
  Barlow test, 469, 469*f*
  corneal light reflex test, 471, 471*f*
  cover–uncover test, 471, 471*f*
  Cozen test, 377, 377*f*
  drop-arm test, 376*b*
  empty can test, 376*b*
  hair pull test, 154, 154*f*, 172*t*
  hair tug test, 154, 154*f*
  hand grip strength, 381, 381*f*
  Hawkins impingement sign, 375*b*
  Lachman test, 391, 391*f*
  lateral collateral ligament test, 391, 391*f*
  McMurray test, 390, 390*f*
  medial collateral ligament test, 390, 390*f*
  Neer impingement sign, 375*b*
  Ortolani test, 469, 469*f*
  painful arc test, 375*b*
  Patrick test, 387, 387*f*
  posterior cruciate ligament test, 391, 391*f*

  for pronator drift, 422, 422*f*
  Rinne test, 203
  Romberg test, 422
  for scapular winging, 429, 429*f*
  straight-leg raise test, 428, 428*f*
  thumb tenosynovitis, 381, 381*f*
  timed get up and go test, 546, 562*t*
  Tinel sign, 381, 381*f*
  Weber test, 203
  whispered voice test, 203, 203*b*
Tetralogy of Fallot, 493*t*–494*t*
Thoracoabdominal paradox, 466
Thorax
  chest disorders, physical findings in, 242*t*
  deformities of, 240*t*–241*t*
  examination techniques, 223–229
  health history, 221–222
  health promotion and counseling, 230
  recording findings, 229
Thought content
  in mental status examination, 132*b*, 134
  in neurocognitive disorders, 146*t*
Thought processes
  in mental status examination, 132*b*, 134
  in neurocognitive disorders, 146*t*
Throat
  examination techniques, 212–213
  health history, 211
  health promotion and counseling, 214
  hoarseness, 211–212, 215
  pharynx inspection, 213
  recording findings, 213
  sore, 211
Thyroid cancer, screening for, 180
Thyroid gland
  abnormalities of, 182*t*
  diffuse enlargement, 182*t*
  dysfunction, screening for, 180
  function, assessment of, 176
  inspection of, 178
  multinodular goiter, 182*t*
  palpation of, 178, 178*f*
  single nodule, 176, 182*t*
Tibial torsion in infants, 469
Tinea capitis, 173*t*
Tinnitus, 199
Tobacco use
  behavioral counseling, 92–93, 93*b*
  during pregnancy, 521
  screening for, 92

Tolerance, 123*b*
Tongue
    abnormalities of, 218*t*–219*t*
    aphthous ulcer, 219*t*
    candidiasis, 218*t*
    carcinoma of, 217*t*
    fissured, 218*t*
    geographic, 218*t*
    hairy, 218*t*
    hairy leukoplakia, 218*t*
    inspection, 213
    mucous patch of syphilis, 219*t*
    smooth, 218*t*
    varicose veins, 219*t*
Torsion of spermatic cord, 334*t*
Transient ischemic attack (TIA), 433
Transmission-based precautions, in
        patient care facilities, 55, 56*b*
Transposition of great arteries, 494*t*
Trapezius muscles, 417, 417*f*
Tremors/involuntary movements, 414.
    See also Involuntary movements
Trichomonas vaginitis, 350*t*
Trochanteric bursa, 386, 386*f*
Tug test, 154
Tumor of testis, 333*t*
Tympanic membrane
    examination, 201–202, 202*f*
    otitis media with purulent effusion,
        210*t*
    perforation, 210*t*
    serous effusion, 210*t*
    tympanosclerosis, 210*t*

U

Ulcer
    aphthous, 219*t*
    of feet and ankles, 284*t*
    neuropathic, 284*t*
Ulcerative colitis, 320*t*
Ultraviolet radiation, and skin cancer,
        158
Urethritis, 342, 342*f*
Urinary frequency, 303
Urinary incontinence, 304, 321*t*
    approach to patient with, 319*a*
    functional incontinence, 321*t*
    overflow incontinence, 304, 321*t*
    secondary to medications, 304
    stress incontinence, 304, 321*t*
    urge incontinence, 304, 321*t*
Urinary symptoms, 355, 360*a*
Urinary tract
    health history, 303–304
    infection, 303

Urinary urgency, 303
Urticaria, 165*t*
Uterine myomata, 516
Uterus
    anteverted, 352*t*
    bicornuate, 516
    myoma of, 352*t*
    prolapsed, 353*t*
    retroflexed, 352*t*
    retroverted, 352*t*

V

Vaccination. *See also* Immunization
    hepatitis A, 312, 312*b*
    hepatitis B, 312, 312*b*–313*b*
    human papillomavirus infection,
        343
    older adults, 551, 551*b*
    during pregnancy, 523–524, 523*b*
Vaginal bleeding, in pregnant woman,
        approach to patient with, 527*a*
Vaginal discharge, 337, 350*t*
    in bacterial vaginosis, 350*t*
    in *Candida* vaginitis, 350*t*
    in early childhood, 504
    in pregnancy, 506*b*; approach to
        patient with, 528*a*
    in *Trichomonas* vaginitis, 350*t*
Valsalva maneuver, 250
Varicocele, 334*t*
Varicose veins, during pregnancy,
        517
Venereal wart, 348*t*
Venous insufficiency, chronic, 283*t*
Venous pulsation, waves of, 246
Venous stasis ulcers, 269
Ventricular septal defect, 494*t*
Vertigo, 199, 412
    benign positional, 200*b*
    central, 210*b*
    peripheral, 200*b*
Vesicles, 163*t*
Vibration, test for, 424, 424*f*
Visual acuity, testing, 184
Visual fields
    altitudinal defect, 195*t*
    bitemporal hemianopsia, 195*t*
    defects, 195*t*
    homonymous hemianopsia, 195*t*
    homonymous quadrantic defect,
        195*t*
    testing of, 185, 185*f*
    unilateral blindness, 195*t*
Visual impairment, 191
Visual loss, 184

Vital signs, 58, 116
  blood pressure, 116–124
  heart rate, 121, 121*f*
  infant, 461
  of older adults, 542
  respiratory rate, 121
  temperature, 121–122, 122*b*
Vitiligo, 162*t*
Vulnerable adult, 83
Vulva
  carcinoma of, 349*t*
  epidermoid cyst, 348*t*
  genital herpes, 348*t*
  lesions of, 348*t*–349*t*
  secondary syphilis, 349*t*
  syphilitic chancre, 349*t*
  venereal wart, 348*t*
Vulvovaginal symptoms, 337
  approach to patient with, 346*a*

W

Warts, 165*t*
Weakness, 112, 413
  approach to patient with, 437*a*
  distal, 413
  proximal, 413
Weber test, 417

Weight
  gain, 113
  loss, 113
  measurement of, 116, 116*b*
Weight loss, 113
  behavioral counseling for, 86
  steps to promote optimal weight, 87*b*
Wernicke aphasia, 444*t*–445*t*
Wheals, 165*t*
Whispered voice test, 203, 203*b*
Wong-Baker FACES Pain Rating Scale,
    113*f*
Wrists and hands
  examination of, 377–382, 378*f*–382*f*,
      380*t*
  hand grip strength, testing, 381, 381*f*
  inspection of, 378
  palpation of, 378–379, 378*f*, 379*f*
  Phalen sign, 382, 382*f*
  range of motion, 380–381, 380*b*,
      380*f*, 381*f*
  thumb tenosynovitis, testing, 381,
      381*f*
  Tinel sign, 381, 381*f*

X

Xanthelasma, 197*t*